The Temporal Lobes and the Limbic System

The Temporal Lobes and the Limbic System

Edited by

MICHAEL R. TRIMBLE

Consultant Physician in Psychological Medicine and Raymond Way Reader in Behavioural Neurology, Institute of Neurology, Queen Square, London, UK

and

TOM G. BOLWIG

Professor of Psychiatry, State University Hospital, Rigshospitalet, Copenhagen, Denmark

WRIGHTSON BIOMEDICAL PUBLISHING LTD

Petersfield

Editorial Office:

Wrightson Biomedical Publishing Ltd
Ash Barn House, Winchester Road, Stroud,
Petersfield, Hampshire GU32 3PN, UK
Telephone: 0730 265647
Fax: 0730 260368

British Library Cataloguing in Publication Data
A catalogue record for this book is available from the British Library.

ISBN 1 871816 14 9

Composition by Scribe Design, Gillingham, Kent
Printed in Great Britain by Biddles Ltd, Guildford.

Contents

Contributors vii

Preface xi

1 The Limbic System Concept
Paul D. MacLean 1

2 Excitatory Hippocampal Synapses: Functional Properties and Regulation
Per Andersen 15

3 Organizational Principles of Hippocampal Connections
Menno P. Witter and Henk J. Groenewegen 37

4 Excitotoxins, Limbic Pathology and Excitatory Amino Acid Antagonists
Brian S. Meldrum 61

5 Hippocampal Kindling: Some Structure/Activity Relationships
Tom G. Bolwig, Jørn Kragh and Ole Steen Jørgensen 71

6 Antiepileptics and the Hippocampus
Markus Schmutz, Felix Brugger, Hugo Bürki, Thomas Ferrat, Adelheid Hausdorf, Klaus Klebs, Chantal Portet, Mario Pozza, Martin Steinmann and Hans-Rudolf Olpe 91

7 *In vivo* Imaging of the Temporal Lobe Limbic System
Jerome Engel Jr 101

8 Localization Related Epileptic Syndromes
Mogens Dam 115

9 The Aetiology of Mesial Temporal Sclerosis
Agnete Mouritzen Dam ... 129

10 The Gastaut–Geschwind Syndrome
Michael R. Trimble ... 137

11 Psychosis and Epilepsy: The Link to the Temporal Lobe
Bettina Schmitz ... 149

12 Behavioural Consequences of Temporal Lobe Resections
Heinz Gregor Wieser ... 169

13 Cerebrovascular Disease and Tumours in the Limbic System
Olaf B. Paulson and Tom G. Bolwig ... 189

14 Memory and the Temporal Lobes
Michael Kopelman ... 199

15 Neuropathology of Psychoses: Towards a Common Biology
Gareth Wyn Roberts and Katherine Horton ... 213

16 Quantification of Human Brains from Schizophrenics
Bente Pakkenberg ... 239

17 The Temporal Lobes and Affective Disorders
Robert M. Post, Susan R.B. Weiss, Terence A. Ketter, Mark S. George, Mike Clark and Jeffrey Rosen ... 247

18 Brain and Consciousness
J.R. Smythies ... 267

Index ... 277

Contributors

Per Andersen, *Institute of Neurophysiology, PO Box 1104 Blindern, 0317 Oslo, Norway*

Tom G. Bolwig, *Department of Psychiatry, State University Hospital, Rigshospitalet, DK-2100 Copenhagen, Denmark*

Felix Brugger, *Research and Development Department, Pharmaceuticals Division, Ciba-Geigy Ltd, CH-4002 Basel, Switzerland*

Hugo Bürki, *Research and Development Department, Pharmaceuticals Division, Ciba-Geigy Ltd, CH-4002 Basel, Switzerland*

Mike Clark, *Biological Psychiatry Branch, National Institute of Mental Health, 9000 Rockville Pike, Bethesda, MD 20892, USA*

Mogens Dam, *University Clinic of Neurology, Hvidovre Hospital, DK-2650 Hvidovre, Denmark*

Jerome Engel Jr, *Reed Neurological Research Center, 710 Westwood Plaza, Los Angeles, CA 90024-1769, USA*

Thomas Ferrat, *Research and Development Department, Pharmaceuticals Division, Ciba-Geigy Ltd, CH-4002 Basel, Switzerland*

Mark S. George, *Biological Psychiatry Branch, National Institute of Mental Health, 9000 Rockville Pike, Bethesda, MD 20892, USA*

Henk J. Groenewegen, *Department of Anatomy and Embryology, Vrije University, Van der Boechorststraat 7, 1081 BT Amsterdam, The Netherlands*

Adelheid Hausdorf, *Research and Development Department, Pharmaceuticals Division, Ciba-Geigy Ltd, CH-4002 Basel, Switzerland*

Katherine Horton, *Serious Mental Afflictions Research Team, St Mary's Medical School, Imperial College of Science, Technology and Medicine, London W2 1PG, UK*

Ole Steen Jørgensen, *Institute of Neuropsychiatry, University of Copenhagen, Denmark*

Terence A. Ketter, *Biological Psychiatry Branch, National Institute of Mental Health, 9000 Rockville Pike, Bethesda, MD 20892, USA*

Klaus Klebs, *Research and Development Department, Pharmaceuticals Division, Ciba-Geigy Ltd, CH-4002 Basel, Switzerland*

Michael Kopelman, *Division of Psychiatry, United Medical and Dental Schools of Guy's and St Thomas' Hospitals, St Thomas' Campus, London SE1 7EH, UK*

Jørn Kragh, *Laboratory for Experimental Neuropsychiatry, Department of Psychiatry, State University Hospital, Rigshospitalet, DK-2100 Copenhagen, Denmark*

Paul D. MacLean, *National Institute of Mental Health, PO Box 289, Poolesville, MD 20837, USA*

Brian S. Meldrum, *Department of Neurology, Institute of Psychiatry, De Crespigny Park, London SE5 8AF, UK*

Agnete Mouritzen Dam, *Brovænget 36, DK-2830 Virum, Denmark*

Hans-Rudolf Olpe, *Research and Development Department, Pharmaceuticals Division, Ciba-Geigy Ltd, CH-4002 Basel, Switzerland*

Bente Pakkenberg, *Neurological Research Laboratory, Bartholin Instituttet, Kommunehospitalet, 1399 Copenhagen K, Denmark*

Olaf B. Paulson, *Department of Neurology, State University Hospital, Rigshospitalet, DK-2100 Copenhagen, Denmark*

Chantal Portet, *Research and Development Department, Pharmaceuticals Division, Ciba-Geigy Ltd, CH-4002 Basel, Switzerland*

Robert M. Post, *Biological Psychiatry Branch, National Institute of Mental Health, 9000 Rockville Pike, Bethesda, MD 20892, USA*

Mario Pozza, *Research and Development Department, Pharmaceuticals Division, Ciba-Geigy Ltd, CH-4002 Basel, Switzerland*

Gareth Wyn Roberts, *Serious Mental Afflications Research Team, St Mary's Medical School, Imperial College of Science, Technology and Medicine, London W2 1PG, UK*

Jeffrey Rosen, *Biological Psychiatry Branch, National Institute of Mental Health, 9000 Rockville Pike, Bethesda, MD 20892, USA*

Bettina Schmitz, *Institute of Neurology, The National Hospital, Queen Square, London WC1N 3BG, UK and Department of Neurology, Rudolf Virchow Clinic, Spandauer Damm 130, 1000 Berlin 19, Germany*

Markus Schmutz, *Research and Development Department, Pharmaceuticals Division, Ciba-Geigy Ltd, CH-4002 Basel, Switzerland*

J.R. Smythies, *Department of Neuropsychiatry, Institute of Neurology, The National Hospital, Queen Square, London WC1N 3BG, UK*

Martin Steinmann, *Research and Development Department, Pharmaceuticals Division, Ciba-Geigy Ltd, CH-4002 Basel, Switzerland*

Michael R. Trimble, *Institute of Neurology and The National Hospital, Queen Square, London WC1N 3BG, UK*

Susan R.B. Weiss, *Biological Psychiatry Branch, National Institute of Mental Health, 9000 Rockville Pike, Bethesda, MD 20892, USA*

Heinz Gregor Wieser, *Department of Neurology, University Hospital, Frauenklinikstrasse 26, CH-8091 Zürich, Switzerland*

Menno P. Witter, *Department of Anatomy and Embryology, Vrije University, Van der Boechorststraat 7, 1081 BT Amsterdam, The Netherlands*

Preface

In seeking the neural underpinnings of behaviour, several areas of the brain have received significant attention in recent years. The concept that the temporal lobes could be involved with behaviour was consolidated in the 1930s with the classical experiments of Klüver and Bucy. Their experimental results banished forever the idea that the 'rhinencephalon' was only related to olfactory function, and led to a succession of investigations which ultimately resulted in the development of the concept of the limbic system. Over time arguments about the validity of the concept have arisen and different authors have had varying definitions of what actually should be included in the limbic system. Generally it is conceded that medial temporal structures and their downstream connections form the central features of neuronal circuitry whose functions have become closely allied with the feeling and expression of emotional behaviour. As a corollary, it has become more and more accepted that limbic system dysfunction may be associated with several psychopathological states, and that lesions in the limbic system, due to a variety of neurological insults, may lead to a patient presenting primarily with behavioural problems, as opposed to traditional neurological signs and symptoms.

In the last few years, considerable amounts of experimental data have been gathered on the neuroanatomy, neurochemistry and neuropathology of the limbic system which have had a bearing on both neurological and psychiatric practice. For those interested in behavioural neurology, or neuropsychiatry, much of this work forms a foundation stone bridging psychiatry and neurology, such inter-disciplinary specialities developing *pari passu* with that of basic research.

This book has been produced in order to review and redefine recent research in these areas attempting to integrate information from the basic sciences with clinical practice, and recognizing that, if the brain is taken as the starting point, then separations between neurology and psychiatry which had become so fossilized in clinical practice, are no longer tenable.

The first chapter is written by Paul MacLean, who has given his imagination, energy and enthusiasm to the development of the limbic system idea since he so clearly defined the concept in the 1950s. This is followed by an update on the neuroanatomy, neurochemistry and neurophysiology of the limbic system including discussion of such topics as endogenous neurotoxins and kindling.

The second part of the book has to do with describing some temporal lobe syndromes which cover the gamut from more purely localized neurological problems, for example, tumours and cerebrovascular disease, to conditions which truly belong to neuropsychiatry, for example the psychopathology associated with epilepsy, or the growing evidence for neurological underpinnings of schizophrenia and the involvement of limbic system structures in this condition.

The final chapter of the book is an attempt to readdress the mind–body dilemma from a distinguished neurophilosopher, Professor Smythies. The presence of this chapter should remind us that it is the endeavour of all of us interested in these problems to continue to develop holistic theories of brain function, based on an expanding knowledge, allowing us to understand more fully the relationship of mind and brain.

The Editors gratefully acknowledge the educational grant given by Ciba-Geigy of the Nordic Countries for the support of this work. They are especially grateful to Lars Christian Andersen for his enthusiasm and encouragement of the project.

MICHAEL R. TRIMBLE
TOM G. BOLWIG
May 1992

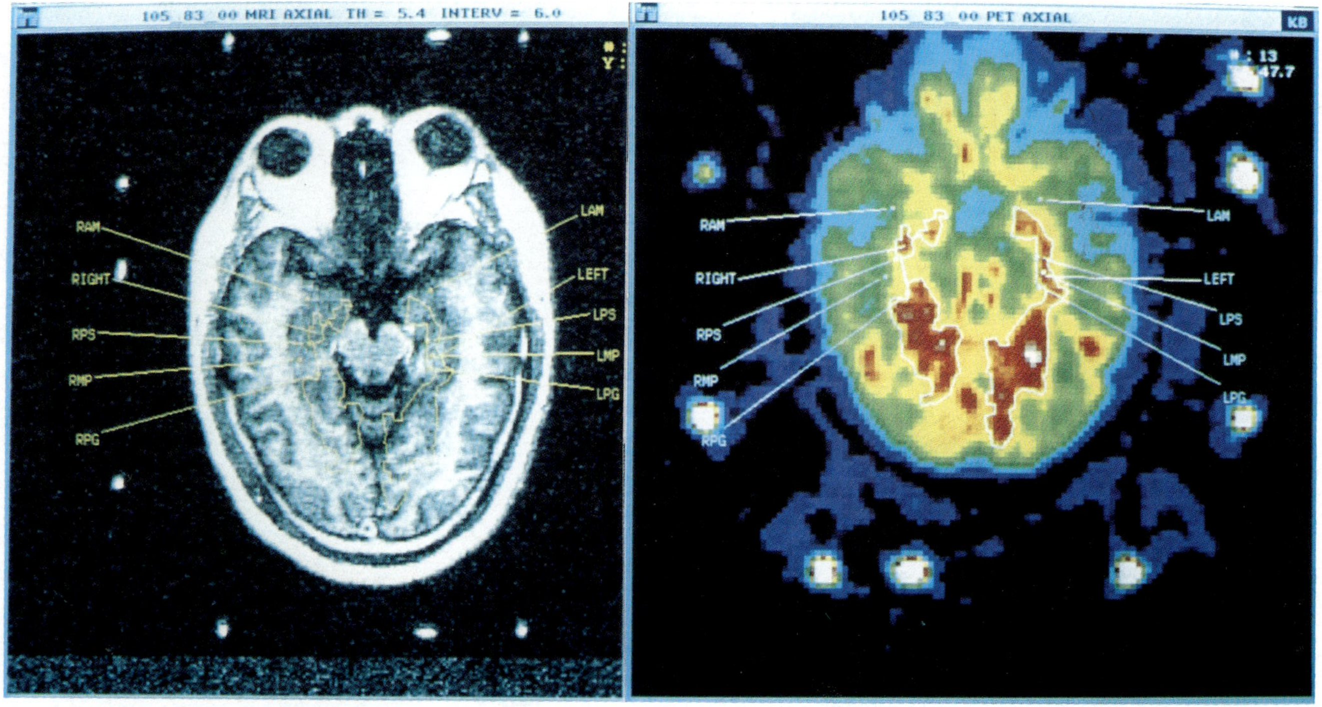

Plate 1. (*See* Chapter 7.) Regions of interest drawn on a PET image (right) can be transferred to an MR image (left) on a similar plane. R=right, L=left, AM=amygdala, PS=presubiculum, MP=midhippocampal pes, PG=posterior hippocampal gyrus. (Reproduced with permission, from Zhang *et al.*, 1990.)

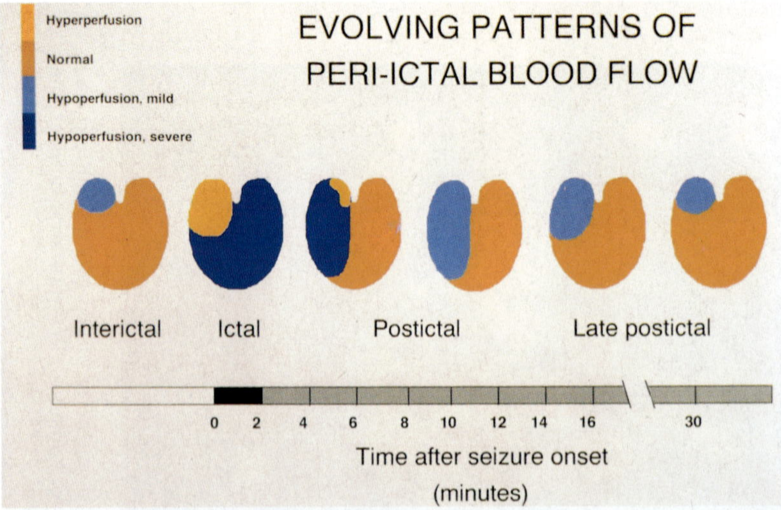

Plate 2. (*See* Chapter 7.) Evolution of the patterns of peri-ictal blood flow. Ictal hyperperfusion is extensive, involving a large portion of the temporal lobe. There is surrounding hypoperfusion. Early in the postictal period, the hyperperfusion is less apparent and predominantly restricted to the anteromesial temporal lobe. Hypoperfusion is widespread and persists longer into the postictal period. Interpretation of postictal studies must therefore take into account the time elapsed since seizure cessation, with a shift in emphasis from hyperfusion to lateral hypoperfusion. (Reproduced with permission, from Rowe *et al.*, 1991.)

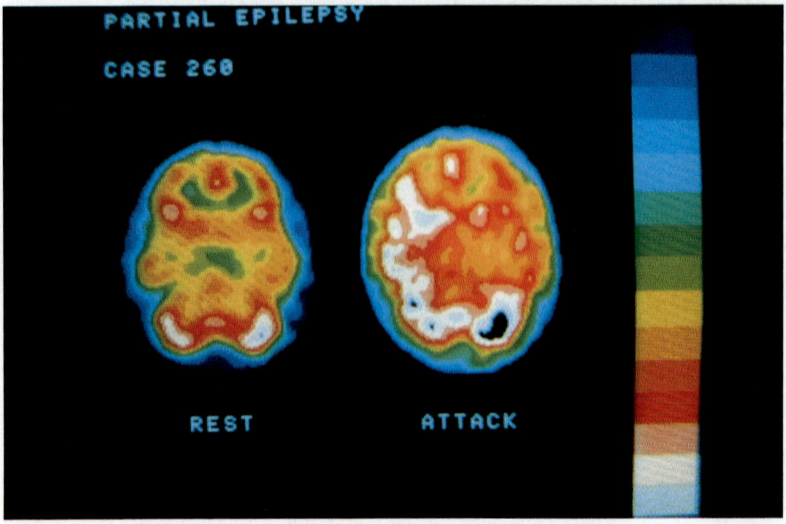

Plate 3. (*See* Chapter 13.) SPECT study of a patient with temporal lobe epilepsy in the interictal state (left, rest) and during a seizure (right, attack). A hypoperfused area in the resting state is highly activated. The tracer used is ^{99m}Tc HMPAO (Ceretec®).

The Temporal Lobes and the Limbic System
Edited by M.R. Trimble and T.G. Bolwig
1992 Wrightson Biomedical Publishing Ltd

1

The Limbic System Concept

PAUL D. MACLEAN
National Institute of Mental Health, Poolesville, Maryland, USA

INTRODUCTION

As background for explaining the limbic system concept it will be helpful to begin with a short statement about the evolution of the mammalian forebrain. Based on the fossil record and comparative findings, it is inferred that the forebrain of human beings and other advanced mammals has evolved as a triune structure (Fig. 1) consisting of three neural assemblies that anatomically and chemically reflect ancestral commonalities with reptiles, early mammals, and late mammals (see MacLean, 1990). The neural assembly identified with early mammals is found as an intermediate development interconnected with the reptilian and neomammalian formations. Anatomically, its cortical representation envelops a large convolution that Paul Broca (1878) called the great limbic lobe because it *surrounds* the brainstem (Fig. 2). The cortex of this lobe, together with its primary connections with structures of the brainstem, corresponds to the so-called limbic system, a designation that I introduced in 1952 as a substitute for the former name *rhinencephalon* that implied primarily olfactory functions (MacLean, 1952).

With this brief statement of the location of the limbic cortex in the forebrain, we proceed to consider the limbic system concept which, in a modular sense, implies that the limbic cortex and its primary brainstem connections constitute an anatomically and functionally integrated system. Perhaps the most compelling evidence of such integration is provided by mapping the propagation of afterdischarges in the limbic system (e.g. Kaada, 1951; Creutzfelt, 1956; MacLean, 1957). Somewhat like stampeding cattle within a corral, the propagating nerve impulses stay within the confines of

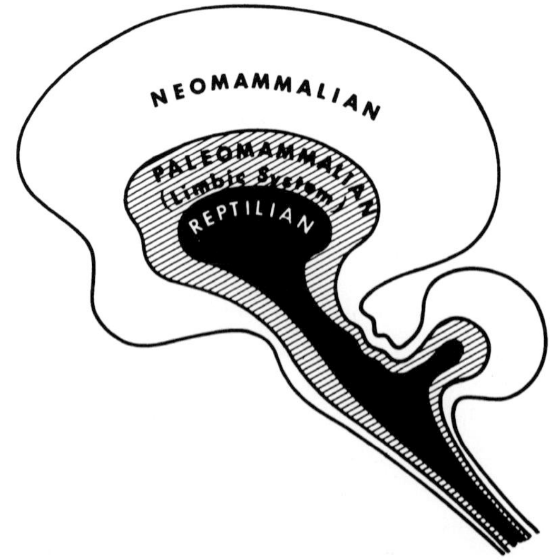

Figure 1. Symbolic representation of triune evolution of three main neural assemblies comprizing the brain of human beings and other advanced mammals. Labelling is placed at the level of the forebrain where each assembly, respectively, reflects anatomical and biochemical commonalities with reptiles, early mammals, and late mammals. (Reproduced from MacLean, 1967.)

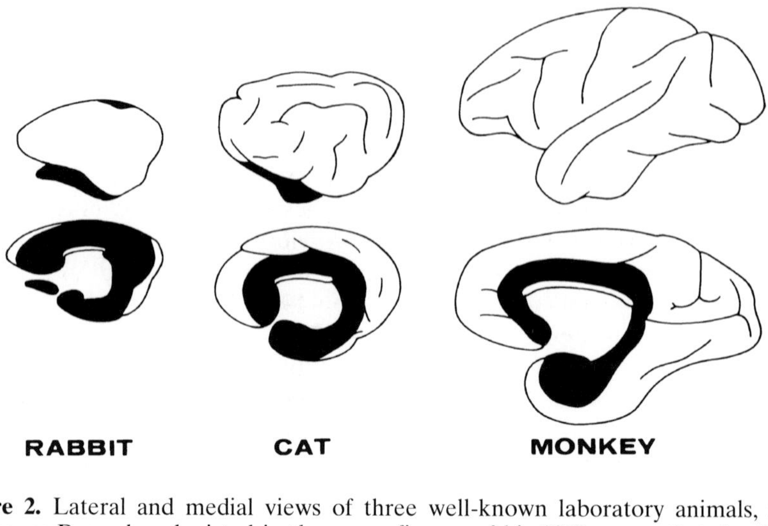

Figure 2. Lateral and medial views of three well-known laboratory animals, illustrating, as Broca has depicted in the many figures of his 1878 paper, that the limbic lobe has evolved as a common denominator of the mammalian brain. The limbic cortex is shown in black and the neocortex in white. (After MacLean, 1954.)

limbic circuitry. Nothing can be more persuasive of limbic integration than to witness this phenomenon time after time in experiment after experiment. If, so to speak, the nerve impulses 'jump the fence' and invade the neocortex, it usually results in a generalized seizure. Parallel observations have been made during therapeutic neurosurgical procedures (e.g. Pagni, 1963).

DEVELOPMENT OF THE LIMBIC SYSTEM CONCEPT

It was Broca's special contribution (1878) to identify the presence of the limbic lobe in a wide variety of mammalian species and on that basis infer that it was a part of the brain common to all mammals (Fig. 2). He mentioned that 40 years earlier Gerdy had referred to the lobe as the 'annular convolution'. As regards function, Broca's comparative findings led him to infer that the limbic lobe operated at an animalistic level, whereas the rest of the cortex subserved intelligence, and in his paper of the subsequent year (1879) actually referred to a 'cerveau brutal' and a 'cerveau intellectuel'. Being impressed by the robust connections of the olfactory bulb with the forward part of the limbic lobe, Broca speculated that the entire convolution was involved in olfactory functions. This notion gained wide appeal, and textbooks appeared in the 1890s referring to the entire limbic lobe as the rhinencephalon (see MacLean, 1990, p. 263). Since olfaction was regarded as an unimportant sense in human beings, the rhinencephalon was treated like an unwanted child in the teaching of brain anatomy. As one neuroanatomist wrote in a book, *The Human Brain: From Primitive to Modern*, published in 1957, the rhinencephalon 'probably has not contributed greatly to the evolution of the human brain and will, therefore, not be considered further' (Lassek, 1957).

Despite such negative attitudes, the temporal olfactory structures were mentioned from time to time in connection with other functions. In 1919, Elliot Smith, in his Croonian Lectures, suggested that unlike other sensory systems, the olfactory structures might provide an 'affective tone' linking together anticipation and consummation into one experience and thereby provide a germ for memory. Years later in 1935, Raymond Dart, a former student of Smith, proposed that the parahippocampal cortex plays a role in governing 'reactions associated with the expression of emotion' (Dart, 1935). Around the same time, C. Judson Herrick (1933) concluded an article on functions of the olfactory cortex by saying that this part of the brain may influence the 'internal apparatus' accounting for general bodily attitude, disposition, and affective tone.

But prior to 1937, there appears to have been no author who considered the entire limbic lobe in regard to non-olfactory functions. In that year the comparative neuroanatomist and neurologist, James Wenceslas Papez,

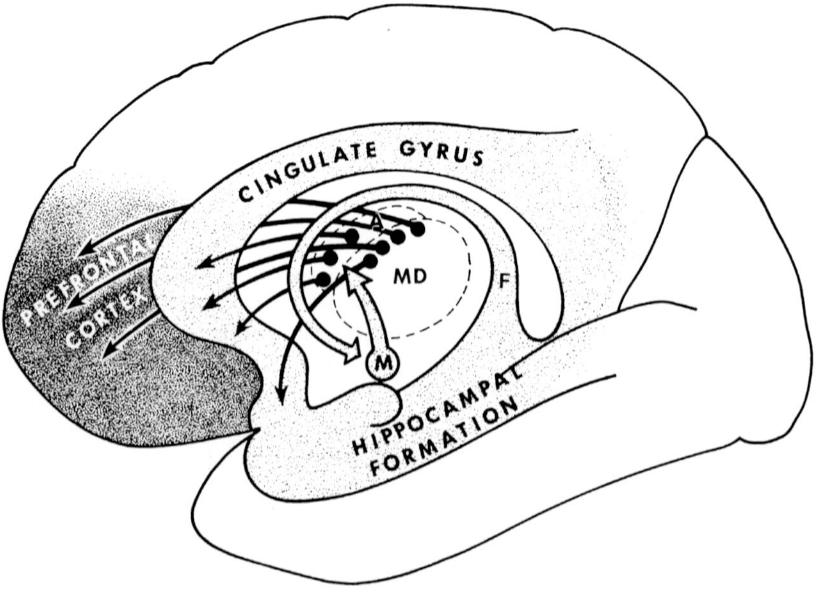

Figure 3. Diagram of 'the Papez circuit' (light shading), in this instance focusing on the part that in evolution becomes related to the 'prefrontal' neocortex (dark shading). Abbreviations: A, anterior thalamic nuclei; F, fornix; M, mammillary bodies; MD, medial dorsal nucleus. (Reproduced from MacLean, 1973.)

published a paper entitled 'A Proposed Mechanism of Emotion' (Papez, 1937). Taking into account what was then known about the role of the hypothalamus in the expression of emotion, Papez pointed out that the limbic lobe was the only part of the hemisphere known to be strongly connected with the hypothalamus. In citing case material to support his argument, he summed up his view of the underlying mechanism as follows (Fig. 3): 'The central emotive process of cortical origin may then be conceived as being built up in the hippocampal formation and as being transferred to the mammillary body and thence through the anterior thalamic nuclei to the cortex of the gyrus cinguli. The cortex of the cingulate gyrus may be looked on as the receptive region for the experiencing of emotion as the result of impulses coming from the hypothalamic region, in the same way as the area striata is considered the receptive cortex for photic excitations coming from retina' (Papez, 1937). The serially connected structures just mentioned have become known as 'the Papez circuit'.

The 'limbic system concept' derives in large part from the clinical study of psychomotor epilepsy ('temporal lobe epilepsy', 'limbic epilepsy', 'complex partial seizures') and at the same time has helped to explain the symptomatology of that condition. In 1948, 11 years after the appearance of the Papez paper, Gibbs *et al.* published a landmark paper entitled 'Psychomotor Epilepsy'. Their work, and particularly the localizing neurosurgical findings of Penfield and Jasper (1954), channelled the way to the best evidence, and indeed the only subjective evidence, that the limbic lobe plays a primary role in the elaboration and expression of emotional feelings. During the aura at the beginning of an epileptic storm, the patient's mind may light up with one or more feelings that in one case or another involve a wide range of emotional feelings. Of great epistemological significance, as will be commented upon later, some patients experience an altered sense of self or exaggerated, free-floating feelings of what is real, true, and important.

In the years 1947 to 1949, I had a US Public Health fellowship in Dr Stanley Cobb's department of the Massachusetts General Hospital. For my research I had devised an improved nasopharyngeal electrode for recording the bioelectrical activity at the base of the brain and became involved in recording the basal electroencephalogram in patients with symptoms of psychomotor epilepsy whose standard EEG had shown either no abnormality or no localizing disturbance. Using the sleep activated method of Gibbs *et al.* (1948), we found in a majority of cases that spiking activity appeared and reached greatest amplitude at the site of the left or right nasopharyngeal electrodes—the electrodes nearest the hippocampal formation, a supposedly rhinencephalic structure (MacLean and Arellano, 1950)

How would such a localization account for the emotional symptomatology of such patients, and more incomprehensible still, the symptoms involving the visual, auditory, or somatic sensory systems? In searching for an answer I stumbled upon Papez's 1937 paper and was immediately struck by its relevance to our findings. By good fortune, I arranged to visit him in Ithaca, NY, asking particularly about the visual, auditory, and somatic connections (see MacLean, 1978). With human material he demonstrated potential pathways to the hippocampal formation from the visual, auditory, and somatic cortical areas.

Subsequently, I wrote a paper published in 1949 in which I focused on 'new developments bearing on the Papez theory of emotion'. I suggested that an overlapping of inputs to the hippocampal gyrus from intero- and exteroceptive systems might permit an integration of neural activity requisite for various affective feelings. In the title of the paper I used the term 'visceral brain' instead of rhinencephalon as a means of reducing the previous accent on olfactory functions. In its original sixteenth century meaning, visceral applies to strong inward feelings and implicitly to accompanying visceral manifestations. In terms of Freudian psychology, I speculated that 'the visceral brain is not at all unconscious (. . .not even in certain stages of sleep) but rather eludes the grasp of the intellect because its animalistic and primitive structure makes it impossible to communicate in verbal terms'. In conclusion, I suggested that whereas our intellectual functions are mediated in the newest and most highly developed part of the brain, 'our affective behaviour continues to be dominated by a relatively crude and primitive system'. 'This situation', I said, 'provides a clue to understanding the difference between what we "feel" and what we "know"'.

In regard to the question of inputs into the hippocampal formation, our neuronographic studies (MacLean and Pribram, 1953; Pribram and MacLean, 1953) and subsequent anatomical studies by other workers (e.g. Jones and Powell, 1970; Van Hoesen and Pandya, 1975) were indicative of step-by-step connections of the somatic, auditory, and visual cortical areas with the hippocampal gyrus. Hodologically more significant, our later microelectrode studies in awake sitting Saimiri monkeys provided evidence of more direct

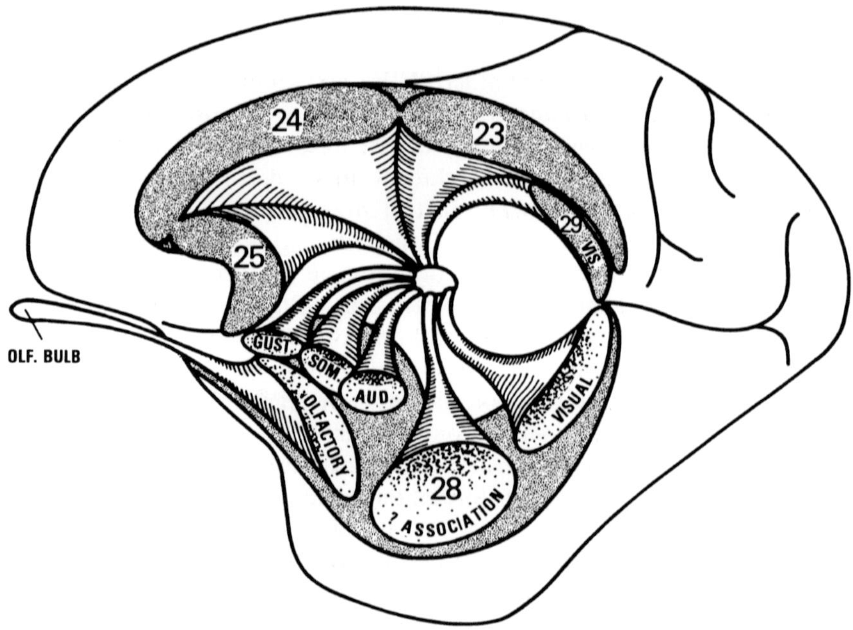

Figure 4. Diagram of inferomedial aspect of squirrel monkey's brain, showing limbic areas of unit responses to excitation of respective extero- and interoceptive systems in chronically prepared, awake, sitting subjects. Areal locations of responses are as follows: visual (VIS.), posterior parahippocampal cortex and retrosplenial cingulate area 29; auditory (AUD.), insular cortex overlying caudal claustrum; somatic (SOM.), insular cortex over mid-claustrum; gustatory (GUST.), insular cortex overlying rostral claustrum; olfactory, anterior hippocampal gyrus and hippocampus (not shown); vagal, cingulate areas 25, 24, 23, rostral insula, and hippocampus (not shown). Vertices for all but the olfactory 'biocones' are pictured as stemming from brainstem. (Reproduced from MacLean, 1990.)

inputs to respective limbic areas (Fig. 4) not only from the five exteroceptive systems, but also from interoceptive systems via the vagus nerve (see MacLean, 1990, pp. 496–498).

I should interject at this point that when I joined the Department of Physiology at Yale in 1949, I became aware that the term visceral brain seemed to give some of my colleagues rather uncomfortable feelings because as physiologists, the term viscera applied only to the glands and hollow organs, including the blood vessels. As a way around this, I found myself referring to the limbic cortex and its brainstem connections as the *limbic system.* Broca originally chose the word limbic because it is purely descriptive and implies no theory about function. At any rate, that is how the term limbic system was introduced into the literature in 1952.

NEUROBEHAVIOURAL ANALYSIS

The emphasis given to the role of the limbic system in emotional experience and expression has tended to obscure what appear to be the basic factors in its evolution. In some writings for instance, the limbic system seems to be regarded as though it functioned globally in generating diffuse emotional feelings. However, as will be mentioned in a moment, it consists of three main subdivisions, each of which is inferred to generate feelings that are germane to its respective functions.

In speaking of limbic evolution it would be more descriptive to say directional evolution because, in the evolution of some 20 orders of extant mammals, the same structures keep cropping up in all of them. In terms of bodily structures, however, there could be no better illustration of directional evolution than the mammal-like reptiles (therapsids) which for very persuasive reasons are believed to be the antecedents of mammals. Dating back to middle Permian times, the successive changes toward the mammalian condition are best seen in the Karroo Beds of South Africa. As Robert Broom (1932) commented, the study of the successive beds 'is like examining the pages of a book of history'. The fossil record shows that several lines of these animals were approaching the mammalian condition so that finally the most reliable distinction is the presence in the therapsid jaw joint of two small bones that in mammals become the malleus and incus of the middle ear.

In our neurobehavioural studies of reptiles we chose to work with lizards because the ear bones and other skeletal features come the closest to resembling those of the mammal-like reptiles. A comparative analysis of reptilian and mammalian behaviour reveals that both share the basic forms of behaviour seen in the daily master routine and in the four main displays used in social communication. In addition, the analysis indicates that the evolutionary transition from reptiles to mammals is characterized by three cardinal forms of behaviour—namely, (i) nursing, conjoined with maternal care; (ii) audiovocal communication for maintaining maternal–offspring contact; and (iii) playful behaviour.

Most lizards lay their eggs and then leave them to hatch on their own. And most lizards do not vocalize, which for the young hatchlings appears life-saving because if they were to make a separation cry typical of mammals, the chances are that their parents or other adult lizards might seek them out and eat them. The young of the giant Komodo lizards must take to the trees for the first year of life so as to avoid being cannibalized.

The three cardinal forms of behaviour typical of mammals appear to have depended on the progressive evolution of the limbic system. Indeed one might say that *the history of the evolution of the limbic system is the history of the evolution of mammals, while the history of the evolution of mammals is the history of the development of a family way of life.*

THREE MAIN SUBDIVISIONS

On the basis of anatomy and function, the limbic system can be divided into three main subdivisions. Before summarizing their anatomy and respective functions, it will be useful to characterize, in general, the features of the limbic cortex. The Australian anatomist Abbie (1942) developed the concept that the cortex evolves from around the brainstem by 'successive waves of circumferential differentiation'. The limbic cortex (Fig. 5) consists of two main types of cortex, an inner ring corresponding to archicortex and its transition into an outer ring of mesocortex, which as shown in the figure occupies most of the cingulate cortex. Elliot Smith (1901) referred to the outer ring of cingulate cortex as 'neopallium' (alias neocortex), but several anatomists have pointed out that it shows features that are transitional with neocortex. Sanides (1969) elaborated on Abbie's scheme, referring to it as the 'growth ring hypothesis', and characterized the outer ring of cingulate cortex by Vogts' term *proisocortex* connoting rudimentary neocortex. But Rose's (1926) original term *mesocortex* continues to be the more typical expression.

Given that background, we consider the three main subdivisions of the limbic system shown schematically in Fig. 5. The limbic and perilimbic cortex (overlain by the small numeral '1') innervated by nuclei of the amygdala constitute the amygdalar division. The second division correspondingly identified by the numeral '2' forms the septal division. Experimental work indicates that the amygdalar division is primarily concerned with self-preservation as it pertains to feeding, the search for food, and the fighting and defence that may be required in obtaining food. The septal division, on the other hand, appears to promote survival of the species as evidenced by

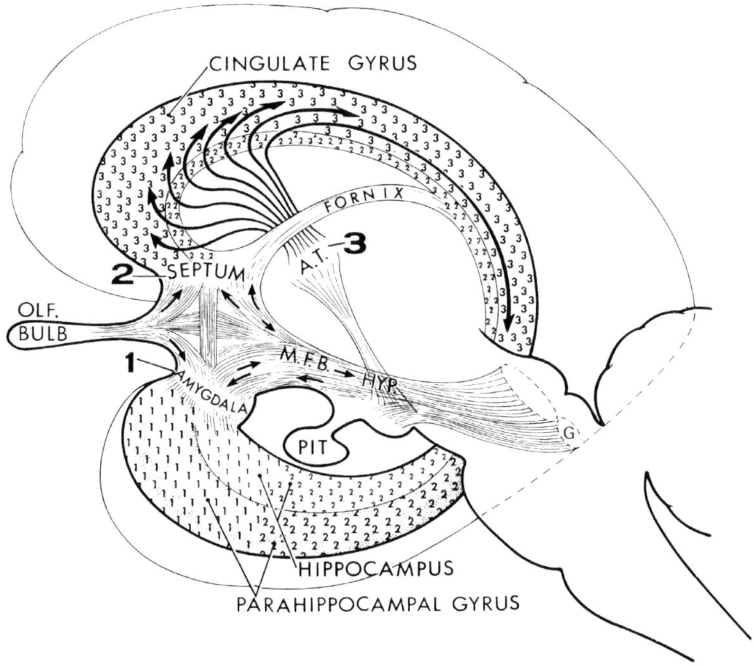

Figure 5. Three main subdivisions of the limbic system. Large numerals 1, 2, and 3 identify nuclear groups that are nodal, respectively, for the amygdalar, septal, and thalamocingulate divisions. Small numerals overlie limbic cortical areas predominantly interconnected with these respective nuclear groups. See text regarding functions. Abbreviations: AT, anterior thalamic nuclei; G, dorsal and ventral tegmental nuclei of Gudden; HYP, hypothalamus; M, mammillary bodies; MFB, medial forebrain bundle; PIT, pituitary; OLF, olfactory. (After MacLean, 1973.)

its involvement in primal sexual functions and manifestations conducive to sociability and reproduction.

It is to be noted that the main pathway to the third subdivision bypasses the olfactory apparatus. It is appropriately referred to as the thalamocingulate division because it is represented by the cingulate mesocortex that is mainly innervated by the anterior thalamic nuclei. It is this division that appears to be chiefly implicated in the above-mentioned triad of behaviours typical of mammals. Significantly, there is no definite foreshadow of its existence in the reptilian brain. Neurobehavioural studies have revealed that ablations in respective parts of the cingulate gyrus eliminate or interfere with acts of maternal behaviour, the utterance of the separation cry, and play (see MacLean, 1990, chapter 21).

Clinical findings on crying and laughter: relevance to emotion and limbic integration

The question as to what cerebral structures account for crying and laughter continues to present one of the most difficult problems in clinical neurology. Our finding that ablation of the rostral cingulate cortex in adult Saimiri monkeys eliminates the spontaneous production of the separation cry made it desirable to review clinical case material in regard to the localization of epileptogenic foci and lesions associated with epileptic crying and laughter, as well as locations where electrical stimulation resulted in these manifestations during neurosurgical intervention. The outcome of the review is too detailed to be described here, but it may be summarized by saying that both with respect to the somatic manifestations and lacrimation, the involved structures were located along the 'Papez circuit'—namely, the rostral hippocampal formation and adjacent amygdala, the mammillary bodies, the anterior thalamus, and the midline frontocingulate cortex (MacLean, 1990, pp. 534–538).

Just as in everyday life, the alternation of crying and laughter that may occur under ictal conditions suggests that these manifestations have an underlying reciprocal innervation. The above clinical review gains in interest in the light of the experimental findings implicating the thalamocingulate division in play that in human beings combines with laughter to promote familial and other forms of affiliation. If it were agreed that a condition that makes being a mammal so painful is separation, then the thalamocingulate division would have the distinction of having a representation of a reciprocal innervation of two manifestations that rank closely to language in expressing what it is to be human.

In an evolutionary sense, the possibility suggests itself that the painful aspects of separation are traceable to the fatal consequences of separation of mother and offspring when nursing became a family way of life. In this respect it is notable that the rostral cingulate cortex implicated in the call is innervated by nuclei involved in the perception of pain (see MacLean, 1990, p. 541; Vogt and Grabiel, 1992).

Such considerations run counter to past and current claims that there is no evidence that the cingulate gyrus is involved in emotional experience or expression. Moreover, the multiplicity of sites along the Papez circuit at which crying and laughter can be triggered is a reminder that these manifestations occur under conditions other than separation or reunion—as, for example, in defeat or triumph. Factors of this kind, together with the acknowledged robust anatomical interlinkage of limbic structures are not consistent with the claim that 'the limbic system. . .is not functioning as a limbic system' (Poletti, 1986), a statement based on the finding that only 17% of cingulate units in four squirrel monkeys showed an alteration of discharge, but granting that only '50% of the electrode tracks sampled cortical layers 1 and 4—shown to receive thalamic afferents' (Dagi and Poletti, 1983).

CONCLUDING COMMENTS

It may be said of psychomotor epilepsy that this cruel affliction provides more windows for viewing the human psyche than any other clinical entity. In conclusion, it is of basic interest to comment on some epistemic implications in regard to a sense of self and reality apropos of the memory of ongoing experience and matters of belief.

Memory of ongoing experience

Following the manifestations of the aura, patients engage in automatisms that range in individual cases from simple to very complex forms of behaviour. Subsequently, there is absolutely no recall of what took place during that period. They behave, so to speak, during the automatism like a disembodied spirit, showing in some cases cognitive capabilities and the ability to carry out highly complicated tasks. In case after case, Penfield and coworkers (e.g. Feindel and Penfield, 1954; Penfield and Jasper, 1954) observed that the reproduction of a patient's symptomatology by electrical stimulation in the amygdala-hippocampal region invariably resulted in amnesia for anything that occurred after the onset of the automatism.

What is the explanation of the amnesia? It may be posed as part of the limbic system concept that a sense of self and a sense of reality depend on an integration of internally and externally derived experience by limbic structures. Whereas the neocortex is primarily oriented toward the external environment, receiving most of its information from the visual, auditory, and somatic systems, the limbic system is closely tuned to the internal environment by interoceptive systems, and, most importantly also, is supplied, as was noted, by inputs from the exteroceptive systems (Fig. 4). I have suggested that a bilateral propagation of limbic seizures may interfere with the integration of internally and externally derived experience and that the situation compares to a temporary functional ablation having an effect like that of bilateral disease or damage to certain critical structures in the Papez circuit. Without a sense of self and reality, there is, so to speak, nothing on which to attach a memory of *ongoing experience.* Accordingly, therefore, the amnesia associated with automatisms would be similar to the anterograde amnesia of a patient, say, with bilateral damage to the hippocampus.

Feelings of belief

Finally, it is of profound epistemic significance in regard to human belief that the symptomatology of psychomotor epilepsy suggests that the limbic cortex generates free-floating, affective feelings conveying a sense of what is real, true and important. The same applies to feelings of discovery. Does this mean that this ancient part of the brain with an incapacity for verbal communication accounts for the feelings of conviction that we attach to our beliefs regardless of whether they are true or false? It is one thing to have this animalistic mind to assure us of the reality of food or mate, but what can we intellectually believe, if it is also requisite to assure the authenticity of our ideas, concepts, and theories? It would seem that this question, along with the impossibility of resolving the logical problems of self-reference attributable to neocortical function, will forever keep us humble about what we can believe regarding scientific and other intellectual matters. At the very least, it will present human beings a challenge that should last a few lifetimes—a challenge that deals with perhaps the most fundamental of all human questions: how is it that we subjectively sense mental emanations for which there are no known quanta in the cosmic universe?

REFERENCES

Abbie, A.A. (1942). Cortical lamination in a polyprotodont marsupial. *Parameles nasuta. J. Comp. Neurol.*, **76**, 509–536.

Broca, P. (1878). Anatomie comparée des circonvolutions cérébrales. Le grand lobe limbique et la scissure limbique dans la série des mammifères. *Rev. Anthropol.*, **1** (Ser. 2), 385–498.

Broca, P. (1879). Localisations cérébrales, Recherches sur les centres olfactifs. *Rev. Anthropol.*, **2**, 385–455.

Broom, R. (1932). *The Mammal-Like Reptiles of South Africa and the Origin of Mammals* , H.F. and G. Witherby, London.

Creutzfelt, O.D. (1956). Die Krampfausbreitung im Temporallappen der Katze. Die Krampfentladungen des Ammonshorns und ihre Beziehungen zum ubrigen Rhinencephalon und Isocortex. *Arch. Suisses Neurol. Psychiatry*, **77**, 163–194.

Dagi, T.F. and Poletti, C.E. (1983). Reformulation of the Papez circuit: absence of hippocampal influence on cingulate cortex unit activity in the primate. *Brain Res.*, **259**, 229–236.

Dart, R.A. (1935). The dual structure of the neopallium: its history and significance. *J. Anat.*, **69**, 3–19.

Feindel, W. and Penfield, W. (1954). Localization of discharge in temporal lobe automatism. *Arch. Neurol. Psychiatry*, **72**, 605–630.

Gibbs, E.L., Gibbs, F.A. and Fuster, B. (1948). Psychomotor epilepsy. *Arch. Neurol. Psychiatry*, **60**, 331–339.

Herrick, C.J. (1933). The functions of the olfactory parts of the cerebral cortex. *Proc. Natl Acad. Sci. USA*, **19**, 7–14.

Jones, E.G. and Powell, T.P.S. (1970). An anatomical study of converging sensory pathways within the cerebral cortex of the monkey. *Brain*, **93**, 793–820.

Kaada, B.R. (1951). Somato-motor, autonomic and electrocorticographic responses to electrical stimulation of 'rhinencephalic' and other structures in primates, cat and dog. A study of responses from the limbic, subcallosal, orbito-insular, piriform and temporal cortex, hippocampus-fornix and amygdala. *Acta Physiol. Scand.*, **23** (Suppl. 83), 1–285.

Lassek, A.M. (1957). *The Human Brain. From Primitive to Modern*, Charles C. Thomas, Springfield, p. 65.

MacLean, P.D. (1949). Psychosomatic disease and the 'visceral brain'. Recent developments bearing on the Papez theory of emotion. *Psychosom. Med.*, **11**, 338–353.

MacLean, P.D. (1952). Some psychiatric implications of physiological studies on frontotemporal portion of limbic system (visceral brain). *Electroencephalogr. Clin. Neurophysiol.*, **4**, 407–418.

MacLean, P.D. (1954). Studies on limbic system ('visceral brain') and their bearing on psychosomatic problems. In: Cleghorn, R.A. and Wittkower, E. (Eds), *Recent Developments in Psychosomatic Medicine*, Pitman, London, pp. 101–125.

MacLean, P.D. (1957). Chemical and electrical stimulation of hippocampus in unrestrained animals. I. Methods and electroencephalographic findings. *Arch. Neurol. Psychiatry*, **78**, 113–127.

MacLean, P.D. (1967). The brain in relation to empathy and medical education, *J. Nerv. Ment. Dis.*, **144**, 374–382.

MacLean, P.D. (1973). *A Triune Concept of the Brain and Behavior*, University of Toronto Press, Toronto.

MacLean, P.D. (1978). Challenges of the Papez heritage. In: Livingston, K. and Hornkiewicz, O. (Eds), *Limbic Mechanisms*, Plenum, New York, pp. 1–15.

MacLean, P.D. (1990). *The Triune Brain in Evolution. Role in Paleocerebral Functions*, Plenum Press, New York.

MacLean, P.D. and Arellano Z, A.P. (1950). Basal lead studies in epileptic automatisms. *Electroencephalogr. Clin. Neurophysiol.*, **2**, 1–16.

MacLean, P.D. and Pribram, K.H. (1953). Neuronographic analysis of medial and basal cerebral cortex. I. Cat. *J. Neurophysiol.*, **16**, 312–323.

Pagni, C.A. (1963). Étude électro-clinique des post-décharges amydalo-hippocampiques chez l'homme par moyen d'électrodes de profondeur placées avec méthode steréotaxique. *Confin. Neurol.*, **23**, 477–499.

Papez, J.W. (1937). A proposed mechanism of emotion. *Arch. Neurol. Psychiatry*, **38**, 725–743.

Penfield, W. and Jasper, H. (1954). *Epilepsy and the Functional Anatomy of the Human Brain*, Little Brown, Boston.

Poletti, C.E. (1986). Is the limbic system a limbic system? Studies of hippocampal efferents: their functional and clinical implications. In: Doane, B.K. and Livingston, K.E. (Eds), *The Limbic System: Functional Organization and Clinical Disorders*, Raven Press, New York, pp. 79–94.

Pribram, K.H. and MacLean, P.D. (1953). Neuronographic analysis of medial and basal cerebral cortex. II. Monkey. *J. Neurophysiol.*, **16**, 324–340.

Rose, M. (1926). Über das histogenetische Prinzip der Einteilung der Großhirnrinde. *J. Psychol. Neurol.*, **32**, 97–160.

Sanides, F. (1969). Comparative architectonics of the neocortex of mammals and their evolutionary interpretation. *Ann. NY Acad. Sci.*, **16**, 404–423.

Smith, G.E. (1901). Notes upon the natural subdivision of the cerebral hemisphere. *J. Anat. Physiol.*, **35**, 431–454.

Smith, G.E. (1919). The significance of the cerebral cortex (Croonian Lectures). *Br. Med. J.*, **1**, 796–797; **2**, 11–12.

Van Hoesen, G.W. and Pandya, D.N. (1975). Some connections of the entorhinal (area 28) and perirhinal (area 35) cortices of the rhesus monkey. I. Temporal lobe afferents. *Brain Res.*, **95**, 1–24.

Vogt, B.A. and Gabriel, M. (Eds) (1992). *The Neurobiology of the Cingulate Cortex and Limbic Thalamus*, Birkhäuser, Boston, in press.

The Temporal Lobes and the Limbic System
Edited by M.R. Trimble and T.G. Bolwig

2

Excitatory Hippocampal Synapses: Functional Properties and Regulation

PER ANDERSEN
Institute of Neurophysiology, University of Oslo, Norway

INTRODUCTION

The hippocampal cortex serves as a useful model for the study of properties of central synapses. First, due to considerable research interest over the past 100 years, our histological knowledge about this structure is extensive. Secondly, largely due to the hippocampal slice technique there has been a large number of detailed investigations on the properties of hippocampal neurons, mostly the pyramidal cells. In this chapter, I shall attempt to describe the major properties of excitatory synaptic transmission in this structure, both as expressed at individual synapses and as the effect of a concerted action of several synapses. Finally, I shall discuss how their efficiency may change with use.

EXCITATORY SYNAPTIC POTENTIAL AND CURRENT

With intracellular recording, stimulation of a group of afferent fibres to hippocampal pyramidal cells leads to a depolarizing potential, an excitatory post-synaptic potential (EPSP). As with most other neurons, its amplitude depends upon the number of afferent fibres stimulated. The relation between the number of afferent fibres and the size of the EPSP is nearly linear. The time course is relatively slow, having a rise-time of 3–10 ms and a half-decay of 10–15 ms (Fig. 1). The slow rise-time is a real property of the synapses and not due to attenuation and slowing because of cable properties of the dendrites. Whole-cell recording has documented that the excitatory post-

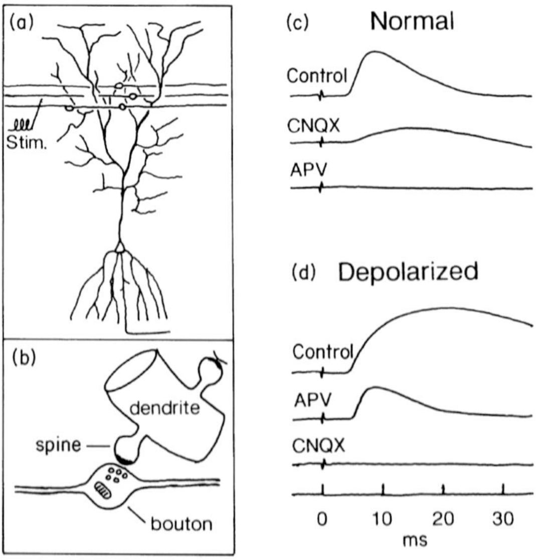

Figure 1. (a) Diagram of a CA1 pyramidal cell with a group of afferent fibres being stimulated (Stim). (b) A dendritic synapse with a spine as an important element. (c) The fast component of the EPSP is removed by CNQX (6-cyano-2,3-dihydroxy-7-nitroquinoxaline) and the remainder disappears on addition of APV (2-amino-5-phosphonovalerate). (d) In a depolarized state, the EPSP is prolonged. The main component is APV-sensitive, exposing the fast component which is CNQX-sensitive.

synaptic current (EPSC) is composed of two components with different time courses (Hestrin *et al.*, 1990).

THE TRANSMITTER AT EXCITATORY SYNAPSES

Based upon immunocytochemical and neurochemical evidence, glutamate is the most likely transmitter at excitatory hippocampal synapses (Storm-Mathisen, 1977; Storm-Mathisen and Ottersen, 1988). Following application of the AMPA receptor blocker, 6-cyano-2,3-dihydroxy-7-nitroquinoxaline (CNQX) (Honoré *et al.*, 1988), the major portion of the EPSP is blocked, leaving a slower and smaller component (Fig. 1(c)). Conversely, when 2-amino-5-phosphonovalerate (APV), an N-methyl-D-aspartate (NMDA) blocker, is added a small late fraction of the EPSP is reduced, particularly when the cell is depolarized (Dingledine, 1983; Andreasen *et al.*, 1989; Hablitz and Langmoen, 1986). These data make it likely that glutamate binds to two different receptors, each giving rise to a specific component of the EPSP.

The evidence for glutamate as the excitatory transmitter stems from its presence in the tissue, the existence of synthesizing enzymes, and of uptake machinery (Storm-Mathisen and Iversen, 1979). Furthermore, following afferent stimulation, release has been seen in slices (Nadler *et al.*, 1976) and *in vivo* using a push–pull canula following stimulation of afferent fibres (Bliss, *et al.*, 1986). Aspartate, which for a long time was regarded as a likely candidate, is probably not a quickly acting transmitter because of its neurochemical behaviour (Nicholls, 1989).

RECEPTOR STUDIES

Four different types

Many different types of receptors for glutamate have been found in hippocampal tissue. The first of these is the AMPA-receptor (named after the agonist α-amino-3-hydroxy-5-methyl-isoxazole-4-propionate, earlier called the quiscalate receptor. This is efficiently blocked by CNQX, and is responsible for the fast, major portion of the EPSP (Hestrin *et al.*, 1990). This receptor is responsible for most of the synaptically mediated impulse traffic within the structure (Fig. 2(a)).

The second receptor is called NMDA after its agonist N-methyl-D-aspartate. This receptor is responsible for the slow part of the EPSP, and increases in relative importance with depolarization of the post-synaptic cell due to a release of an Mg^{2+} blockade (Nowak *et al.*, 1984; Mayer *et al.*, 1984). The receptor, which is effectively blocked by APV, is responsible for calcium influx after synaptic activation (Fig. 2(b)), a feature which is important for plastic changes and excito-toxic reactions (MacDermott *et al.*, 1986). The AMPA and NMDA receptors are co-localized at hippocampal synapses (Bekkers and Stevens, 1990).

The third receptor is the metabotropic receptor (Sugiyama *et al.*, 1987; Masu *et al.*, 1991) where glutamate (and quisqualate) binds to the receptor (Fig. 2(c)). By way of a G-protein the enzyme phospholipase C is activated. This procedure splits the substrate phosphoinositol-serine into two components, diacylglycerol (DAG) and inositol-diphosphate. The latter is further phosphorylated in the cytosol to produce 1,4,5-inositol-triphosphate, a major secondary messenger. The metabotropic receptor causes a slow depolarization due to interference with an outward potassium leakage. It also reduces the slow after-hyperpolarization and causes a small increase in the duration of the action potentials (Hu and Storm, 1992).

The fourth receptor is located presynaptically and named L-AP4. This receptor is probably involved in autoregulation, by reducing the amount of glutamate released from the presynaptic terminal.

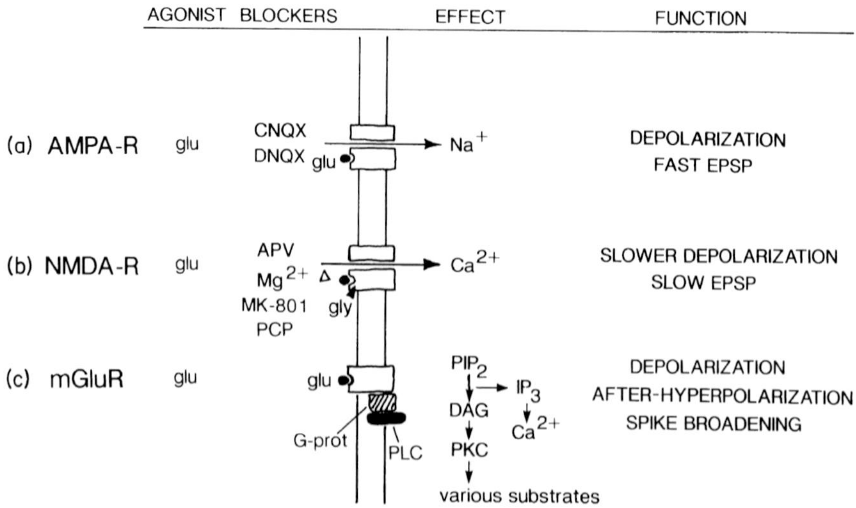

Figure 2. Diagram of (a) the AMPA receptor, (b) the NMDA receptor and (c) the metabotropic glutamate receptor with agonists, blockers, their immediate effect and their main function. glu, glutamate; DNQX, 6,7-dinitroquinoxaline-2,3-dione; PCP, phencyclidine; G-prot, GTP binding protein; PLC, phospholipase C; PIP2, phosphoinositolserine diphosphate; DAG, diacylglycerol, PKC, protein kinase C; IP_3, inositoltriphosphate.

Whether a fifth receptor for kainate forms a separate, functional entity is debated. It is possible that the effect of kainic acid, giving a large excito-toxic reaction, is mediated by the AMPA receptor itself or that the AMPA/kainate receptors form a closely related family.

Molecular studies

Recently, two groups have independently cloned and sequenced a family of AMPA receptors (Hollmann *et al.*, 1989; Keinänen *et al.*, 1990). Heinemann's group, who first sequenced these receptors, named them GluR-1 to GluR-4. In addition, his group recently found two more subunits, GluR-5, apparently coupled to synapse function, and GluR-6 which is specifically activated by kainic acid in CA3 cells. Each of the subunits is formed from about 900 amino acids with a molecular weight of about 100 000. The cloned sequences suggest four transmembrane domains, similar to other ligand-operated ion channels (Fig. 3(a)). There is a large N-terminal, probably extracellularly located due to the high number of NH_2-linked glycosylation sites. Both the N-terminal and the equally large C-terminal tail showed varying, but generally high degrees of conservation between the different subunits. Between

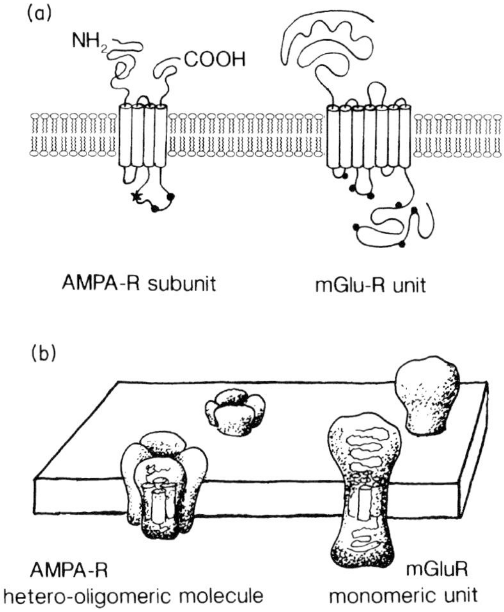

Figure 3. (a) Diagram of a subunit of the AMPA receptor (left) and the metabotropic glutamate receptor (right). Filled circles give serine phosphorylation sites for protein kinase C, star gives possible phosphorylation site for calcium/calmodulin-dependent protein kinase II. (b) Diagrammatic representation of an exposed AMPA receptor in front, composed of four subunits. Behind, a similar receptor is seen inserted into the membrane. To the right, similar displays are seen for two metabotropic receptor molecules.

the transmembrane regions (TM) 3 and 4 there is a relatively large loop with at least three possible serine phosphorylation sites. Expression of mRNA for the different subunits in frog oocytes has given current-to-voltage relationships for several of the subunits when expressed alone, e.g. GluR-1 or GluR-3 in isolation. However, when either GluR-1 and GluR-2 or GluR-2 and GluR-3 are expressed together, the current-to-voltage relationship becomes linear, like the native channel, indicative of a normal response to glutamate application. Interestingly, Seeburg's group has found that in all subunits a short stretch between TM 3 and TM 4 can exist in two versions with different amino acid sequences. These stretches have been named *flip* and *flop* expression type (Sommer *et al.*, 1990). The versions are encoded by neighbouring exons of the gene and convey different properties on glu-induced responses. *In situ* hybridization techniques have shown that all four subunits (GluR-1–4) can be expressed in the hippocampal tissue in both the *flip* and *flop* form. However, there is a segregation of these forms since some parts of the hippocampal formation express more of one variety than the others. This suggests that although glutamate is the transmitter at various synapses, its effect may differ due to an alternative complement of receptor types.

A reasonable view is that the AMPA receptor exists as an hetero-oligomer of different subunits (Fig. 3(b)). Injection of mRNA for these units indicates that GluR-2 always has to be present to form a glutamate-activated channel with near-normal kinetics. However, either GluR-1 or GluR-2 has to be added in order to give current–voltage relationships seen in intact receptors.

Because of the possible serine phosphorylation sites, it is highly likely that the large possibly intracellular loop is subject to phosphorylation by various protein kinases. Recently, both cAMP-dependent protein kinase (PKA), calcium-calmodulin-dependent protein kinase (CaMPK II), diacylglycerol-dependent protein kinase (PKC) and tyrosin kinase have been shown to have large modulatory effects on hippocampal synaptic transmission (Malinow and Tsien, 1990), particularly during long-term potentiation (see below). With so many kinases being able to change the receptor configuration, it will be interesting to see the result from recently started experiments in which the phosphatase level has been modified.

The metabotropic receptor has a different configuration. It consists of a single polypeptide with seven transmembrane segments. In both the very large extracellular amino terminal and in the carboxy terminal there are large hydrophilic sequences, making it different from other G-protein coupled receptors.

PROPERTIES OF A SINGLE SYNAPSE

Many groups have attempted to identify the functional contribution of an individual synapse. Such studies are important, not only to study the relative contribution of different synapses and, thereby, the necessity for concerted action of many synapses, but also as a background for the study of enhanced or decreased synaptic efficiency. Such studies can throw light on learning and memory processes on the one hand and dementias and other cases of impaired cortical activity on the other. Until recently, no method existed for reliable activation of one single afferent fibre. Instead, weak stimulation activating a small number of fibres, but not necessarily the same in every trial, was used. The amplitude histograms of the consequent EPSPs were analysed with the deconvolution method. With such techniques, the individual synapses were found to vary from 85–275 μV with a mean of 130 μV (Sayer *et al.*, 1989; Friedlander *et al.*, 1990). A considerable improvement was introduced by the whole-cell patching technique (Edwards *et al.*, 1989; Blanton *et al.*, 1989). With this technique, individual currents can be seen under a voltage clamp in response to stimulation of afferent fibres (Fig.

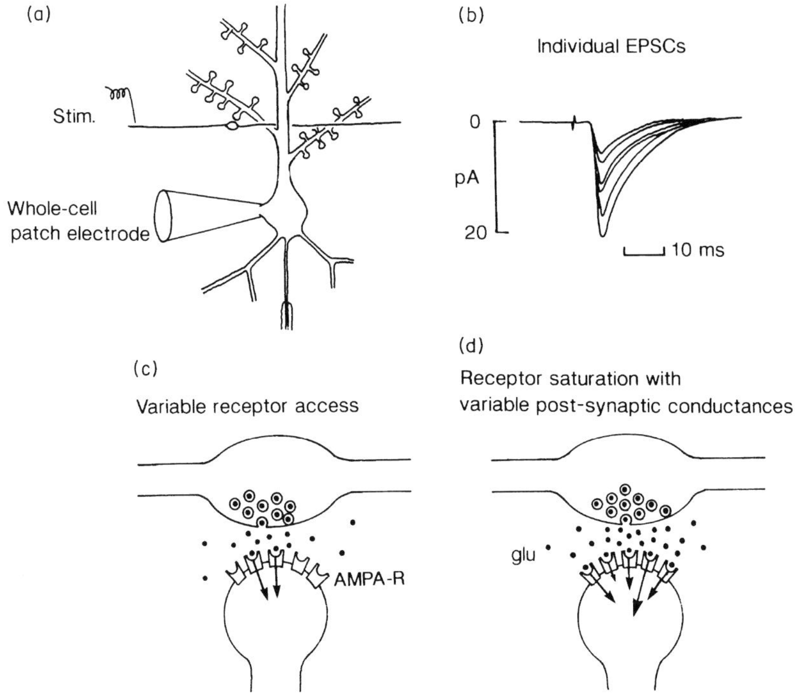

Figure 4. (a) Diagram of a CA1 pyramidal cell with stimulation of a single afferent fibre, and a patch electrode attached to the cell body. (b) Variably sized excitatory post-synaptic currents (EPSCs) in response to stimulation of a single fibre. (c) and (d) illustrate two possible explanations for the EPSC variability. Arrows symbolize the amplitude of the inward synaptic currents.

4(a),(b)). By stimulation of a single fibre in hippocampal culture, the variability was considerable (Bekkers and Stevens, 1990). With stimulation of a small number of fibres (Fig. 4(b)), individual excitatory post-synaptic currents (EPSCs) were seen to range from 1–20 pA. With a mean EPSC value of 6 pA (Raastad *et al.*, 1992) and a mean value of the input resistance of the hippocampal CA1 neurones of about 200 MΩ, the average voltage contribution at a single synapse would be 1.2 mV, about 10 times higher than the previous estimate of 0.13 mV. Recently, Raastad (1991) has developed a technique by which he reliably can activate a single afferent fibre. With this technique, the individual EPSCs are still showing the same range of 1–20 pA, and with an identical time course. These EPSCs are fully blocked by CNQX. Interestingly, the evoked EPSCs have exactly the same variability as those provoked by hyperosmolar solution or the ruthenium red. At the neuromuscular junction, these procedures are known to increase the release of individual acetylcholine quanta. Thus, it appears that the individual currents seen following electrical stimulation are composed of individual transmitter 'quanta'. With double stimulation, the second response is facilitated, as seen by a reduced failure rate. However, the facilitated EPSCs showed the same large variability but the same mean amplitude as the response to the first stimulus. Consequently, the facilitated response is not due to an enhanced number of released transmitter quanta but a higher probability that a unitary release will take place. These data are compatible with a single transmitter 'dose' being released per impulse per synapse. This contribution provides an inward current of great variability with a mean value of 6 pA. The reason for the large variability is difficult to ascertain. A similar, but smaller variability was suggested by Bekkers *et al.* (1990) to be due to the variability of the vesicle size. However, the large variability in hippocampal synapses *in vivo* would require a variation of the vesicle diameter of more than 100%, an observation which is in contrast to electron microscopic evidence. Alternatively, the variability could be due to a different degree of binding of the transmitter to the receptor molecules, so that a variable fraction of the latter will be reached by the transmitter released at successive trials (Fig. 4(c)). Alternatively, if the transmitter reaches all available receptors every time, the variability could be due to activation of different receptor-types having different physiological conductances and/or kinetics (Fig. 4(d)). This could be due to a different arrangement of hetero-oligomers of subunits as suggested by the cloning experiments refered to above. Due to the large variability, quantal release studies are complicated.

Thus, an individual synapse may provide only a single transmitter quantum. The effect of this single quantum varies from one impulse to the next. Each impulse, although releasing a single quantum only, will, however, have a considerable effect on the post-synaptic cell, providing a depolarization in the order of 1.2 mV. The low probability of release is interesting in relation to plastic changes in that the most likely mechanism for enhancement is an increased probability of release of the transmitter, and not an enhanced number of released transmitter molecules.

INTERACTION BETWEEN SEVERAL SYNAPSES

Minimum number of synapses to cause cell discharge

Naturally, with the relatively small contribution from an individual synapse, concerted action or coactivation of several synapses is needed to make the cell discharge. To arrive at an estimate of the required number of coactivated synapses, several methods are available. First, the number of afferent fibres can be reduced by lesions in the tissue. The proportion of remaining fibres

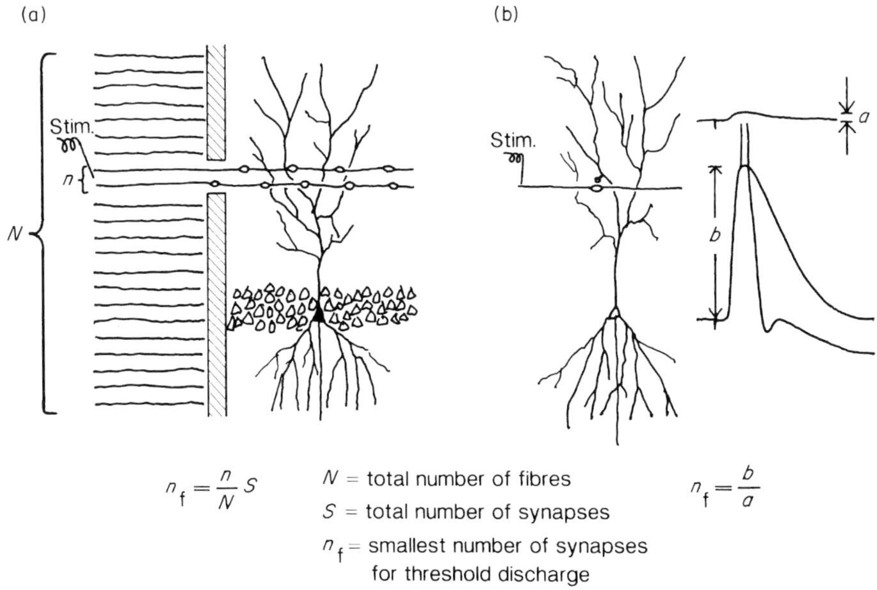

Figure 5. Two methods for estimation of the number of afferent fibres necessary to give cell discharge. (a) A lesion cuts most of the afferent fibres normally synapsing with the target cell (*N*). The smallest number (*n*) of activated fibres still able to discharge the cell is given by the gap between the two lesions. *S* is the total number of synapses, estimated from the number of spines. (b) The top trace shows the size of the EPSP in response to stimulation of a single fibre. The lower traces are a suprathreshold EPSP and action potential superimposed upon a just subthreshold EPSP (*b*), composed of the summation of a number of single fibre EPSPs (*a*).

can be estimated in the smallest amount of tissue, stimulation of which supports activation of the post-synaptic cell (Andersen *et al.*, 1980b). With this technique, less than 1% of the total complement of fibres to a CA1 cell seemed to be needed (Fig. 5(a)). Thus, about 100 synchronously active fibres appeared necessary to drive the cell. A different method, which gave a similar result, consists of comparing the single fibre EPSPs which follow the stimulation of a small bundle of fibres and deconvolution of the amplitude histogram obtained from a large number of trials. When the value of 130 μV (Friedlander *et al.*, 1990), was compared with the size of the EPSP required to produce an action potential discharge, (normally around 12–15 mV), again about 100 fibres were found (Fig. 5(b)). However, with the recently available voltage clamping with whole-cell recording, the contribution from individual synapses was estimated to lie around 1.2 mV and even higher for younger cells (Raastad *et al.*, 1992). With this large contribution, only 10 fibres appear necessary to provide the depolarization needed to reach the discharge threshold. Since the activated EPSPs sum linearly and also show the same amplitude irrespective of this synaptic position in the dendritic tree, the principle of equipotentiality of excitatory synapses was proposed (Andersen *et al.*, 1980b). This means that the same complement of afferent fibres (now estimated to be about 10) could be effective whether they are located close to the soma or further out on the dendrites. Only the very terminal portion of the dendrites seems to be different since stimulation of afferent fibres to this region was never able to discharge cells.

Afferent impulse frequency

Not only the activated number but also the frequency of activation of the afferent fibres is an important input factor for these calculations. Thus, if an individual fibre is producing a set of EPSPs which summate to a depolarized level through repetitive activation of AMPA receptors, simultaneous, or immediately subsequent activation of NMDA receptors would create a larger additional depolarization than at lower afferent impulse frequency. In another situation, repetitive activation of one fibre would cause a slightly reduced efficiency of the AMPA-component of the synaptic potential due to a neighbouring fibre, due to the reduced driving force for the EPSC. On the other hand, the NMDA component of the second input would be enhanced due to the depolarization produced by the first input (Fig. 7(d)). Experiments with tetanic activation seem to provide evidence that these two processes are fairly well balanced since long lasting plateau-like potentials can be created by tetanic activation (Herron *et al.*, 1986; Hvalby and Andersen, 1988).

Location of dendritic synapses

Another important factor controlling the efficiency of synaptic transmission is the distribution of synapses in the dendritic tree. Because of the equipotentiality principle, a distally located synapse has largely the same contribution as one located more proximally. Perhaps more important is whether the activating synapses are located on the same or different dendritic branches. Virtually all excitatory synapses are located on spines (Andersen *et al.*, 1966). The physiological implications of these structures are not known with certainty. The cable-theoretical implications of the dense spine coverage of dendrites have been recently analysed by Jaslove (1992). By a realistic modelling of dendritic structures with various coverage of spines, he found that the weighting factor given by the input resistance of the spine neck is less important than hitherto thought. However, due to the large expansion of the total surface area, the capacity of that portion of the dendrite is enhanced when compared with a naked dendrite. This enhanced capacity gives a reduced input resistance of the dendrite as a whole because of the

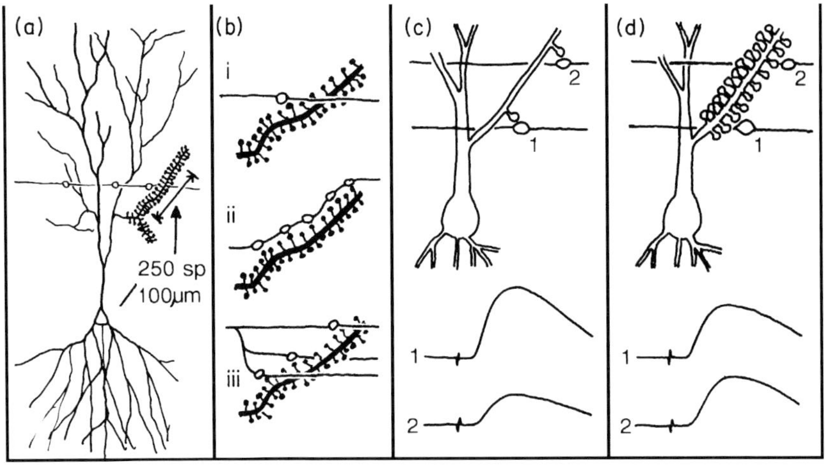

Figure 6. (a) Diagram of a CA1 pyramidal cell, highlighting the density of spines on secondary dendrites. (b) illustrates three possible contact patterns for afferent fibres. (c) and (d) illustrate possible effects of a changing number of spines on the EPSP amplitude.

relatively small contribution of the resistance of the spine neck due to its short length. In consequence, the lowered input resistance of the spine-covered dendrite would tend to reduce the contribution from each individual synapse, while at the same time making their effect more equal (Fig. 6(c),(d)). This feature is probably a major reason behind the equipotentiality of synapses located at different distances from the soma.

Following these observations, it will be of the utmost importance to know whether an afferent fibre makes only one or several contacts with a given dendritic branch. Since the fibres traverse the dendritic tree at right angles to its main axis and taking the spacing of the boutons in relation to the dimensions of the dendritic tree, Andersen (1990) estimated that on average each fibre has a single contact with a pyramidal cell. However, it is conceivable that an afferent fibre could have its boutons contacting several dendritic branches belonging to the same target cell. The daunting developmental task of achieving this connectivity could possibly be arranged by way of a conjunction paradigm. After the first synapse has activated the target cell, the consequent depolarization would spread to neighbouring portions of the dendritic tree, thus open for the possibility that a grazing synapse could be converted to an active and efficient one by conjoint activity. If this arrangement does occur, then each axon would contact a subset of pyramidal cells, leaving others to be contacted by other fibres (Fig. 6(a)). This organization would create a larger diversity than can be inferred by simple inspection of the average fibre distribution in normal histological preparations. Alternatively, a fibre could course alongside a dendritic branch, having several of its boutons connected to the same dendrite (Fig. 6(b)). In this way one would get a much more efficient input, explaining some of the EPSP variability that one can see by activating different single fibres.

ACTIVITY-DEPENDENT SYNAPTIC CHANGES

Short-lasting changes

Important synaptic changes occur during and after previous activation. A single activation is followed by a period of facilitation. In contrast to the neuromuscular junction where this process lasts only a few hundred milliseconds (Magleby, 1973), the facilitation process in hippocampal synapses may last up to 20–30 s (Hvalby and Andersen, 1988). It is this facilitation process which probably is a major cause of the great enhancement seen during tetanic stimulation, the so-called frequency potentiation (Andersen and Lømo, 1966). Whether augmentation (Magleby and Zengel, 1976), a facilitation lasting several seconds after a short tetanic activation, exists in hippocampal synapses is not clear. However, post-tetanic potentiation is readily elicited in hippocampal synapses, showing a fast decaying facilitation with a total duration of about 2–3 min. Long-term potentiation is a process lasting considerably longer, from several hours in an isolated slice to several weeks in intact animals (Barnes, 1979; Racine *et al.*, 1983).

Long-term potentiation

Long-term potentiation (LTP) has been proposed as a model for cellular learning and memory because of its long duration and fast induction, using physiologically acceptable signal patterns (Swanson *et al.*, 1982; Andersen, 1987). In appropriate areas, LTP may be elicited by tetanic stimulation of an afferent pathway to a group of target cells (Bliss and Lømo, 1973). Effective stimulation regimes may be a single tetanus (10–20 Hz) for a few seconds, or a series of shorter (100–500 ms) high frequency trains (100–500 Hz), repeated with intervals of a few seconds. The LTP effect is cumulative with repeated tetani.

LTP criteria

The expression of LTP appears as an increased release of synaptic transmitter (glutamate) and an enhanced synaptic transmission seen as a larger EPSP and an increased spike probability or as an increased extracellular population spike with reduced latency. To be called LTP, the effect should last more than 1 h. Neither recurrent nor forward inhibition is changed (Haas and Rose, 1982).

LTP induction

The requirement for induction is a sufficient regional (dendritic) post-synaptic depolarization paired with a local synaptic input (Wigström *et al.*, 1986; Gustafsson *et al.*, 1987). Normally, the post-synaptic depolarization is caused by the summing of the EPSPs caused by the tetanic stimulation (Fig. 7(d)), which also serves as the second required event, the synaptic activation. Under physiological conditions, one set of fibres (Fig. 7(a),(c); T = 'teacher') delivers the required summating EPSPs, while other fibres (P = 'pupil') provide the coincident synaptic activation. This *coactivation* is a central point in LTP induction. In addition, synapses having a dendritic location near the tetanized input are potentiated more than remotely placed synapses (Andersen *et al.*, 1980a). A central rule is, therefore, that potentiation requires *coactivation in time and space*. The original explanation was that a certain number of afferent fibres had to be activated, referred to as *cooperativity* (McNaughton *et al.*, 1978). In usual experimental situations, LTP is *input-specific*, or homosynaptic, in that it only develops in tetanized afferents

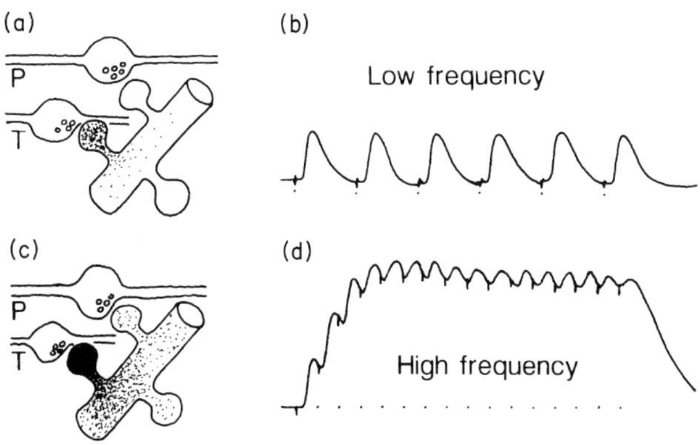

Figure 7. Induction rule for long-term potentiation (LTP). (a) Diagram of two fibres in synaptic contact with neighbouring spines on the same dendrite. The low frequency activation of the T ('teacher') fibre gives weak depolarization of the spine (dots), not sufficient to spread to the neighbouring spine. (c) With high frequency stimulation (d), the teacher fibre gives much stronger depolarization so that the neighbouring spine is depolarized. With coactivation of the P ('pupil') fibre, the latter may have LTP induced.

(Andersen *et al.*, 1977). Calcium ions are necessary for LTP to develop (Dunwiddie and Lynch, 1979; Wigström *et al.*, 1979; Lynch *et al.*, 1983).

Finally, blockade of the N-methyl-D-aspartate (NMDA) receptor with 2-amino-5-phosphono-valerate (APV) completely abolishes LTP production in spite of an unchanged synaptic transmission to single volleys (Collingridge *et al.*, 1983). The inductive depolarization allows the NMDA receptor channel to be relieved of its Mg^{2+}-blockade (Nowak *et al.*, 1984; Mayer *et al.*, 1984) with influx of Ca^{2+} as a result (MacDermott *et al.*, 1986).

Work with blockers of the QA and the NMDA receptors has suggested that although the NMDA receptor is essential for LTP induction, long-lasting LTP expression is exclusively mediated by the AMPA receptor (Kauer *et al.*, 1988; Muller *et al.*, 1988). Important facilitatory effects are produced by adrenergic afferents (Bliss *et al.*, 1983). Cholinergic facilitatory effects have not yet been convincingly demonstrated.

LTP expression

The nature of the cellular changes is not fully known. Four basic mechanisms could cause the sustained increase in synaptic efficiency characterizing LTP: (i) increased release of transmitter (Fig. 8(c,i)); (ii) changed number or properties of receptors (Fig. 8(c,ii)); (iii) local post-synaptic excitability changes; and, finally, (iv) morphological changes (Fig. 8(c,iii)). The different aspects need not be isolated events, but could represent a string of processes, coupled together in a cascade. The extent to which the cascade will develop is likely to depend upon the pattern and strength of the inducing stimuli and the degree of repetition (Fig. 8(a),(b)).

Presynaptically, the increased transmitter release seems coupled to an augmented level of Ca^{2+}, like other cases of plasticity. Following LTP induction there is an increased resting release of aspartate and glutamate to afferent stimuli in CA1 (Skrede and Malthe-Sørenssen, 1981) and in the dentate area (Dolphin *et al.*, 1982; Bliss *et al.*, 1986). The presynaptic changes could either be triggered by a retrograde signal from the post-synaptic cell, or by a parallel activation of presynaptic and post-synaptic receptors by the released glutamate (Fig. 8(c,i)).

Presynaptically, there is an elevated turnover of phospho-inositides (Lynch *et al.*, 1988) and enhanced phosphorylation of protein F1, also called B50 or GAP43, (Bär *et al.*, 1984; Akers *et al.*, 1986) which is associated with growth of axonal processes. Taken together with an observed translocation of diacylglycerol (DAG)-dependent protein kinase (protein kinase C, PKC) in synaptosomal membranes (Lovinger *et al.*, 1986), a role for PKC in the presynaptic LTP changes seems highly probable.

Unfortunately, attempts at quantal analysis of transmitter release during LTP in dentate or CA1 synapses have been hampered by the large variability

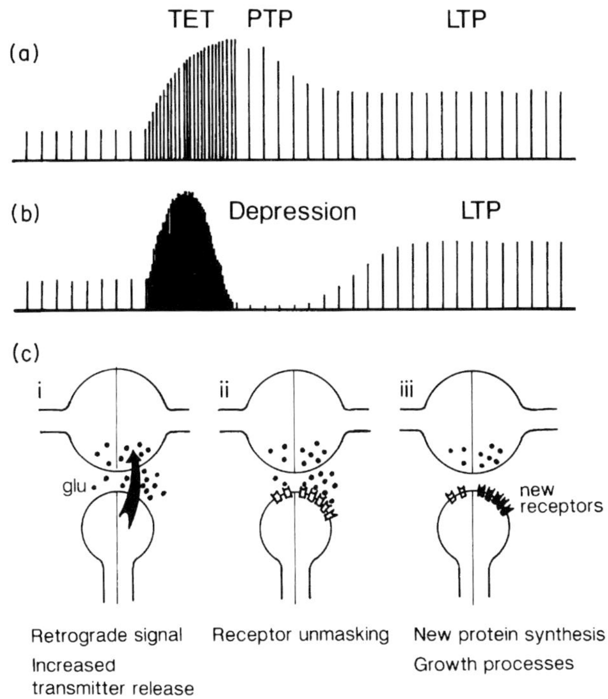

Figure 8. (a) and (b) Patterns of LTP and depression induced by various stimulation patterns. TET = tetanic stimulation; PTP = post-tetanic potentiation. (c) Three possible mechanisms involved in LTP induction and expression. In each panel, the left side gives the situation before, the right side the situation after LTP induction.

of elementary excitatory synaptic currents activated by single fibre input or by hyperosmolar chemical stimulation. This may explain some of the conflicting results obtained (Bekkers and Stevens, 1990; Malinow and Tsien, 1990; Foster and McNaughton, 1991; Raastad *et al.*, 1992). Such studies should, however, be possible for the mossy fibre synapses since the situation seems clearer here. Yamamoto *et al.* (1987) found that the mean quantal content increased after phorbol ester application while the mean quantal size remained unchanged or diminished.

Post-synaptic LTP effects may be several: unmasking of dormant receptors (Fig. 8(c,ii)), allosteric changes of receptors, closure of specific, phorbol ester-sensitive ionic channels, aggregation of ionic channels to dendritic spines, insertion of new or an increased number of ionic channels, and morphological changes at or close to the dendritic synapses (Fig. 8(c,iii)). Assuming a passive dendritic membrane, local resistance changes, such as a reduction in Cl-conductance, would give a larger and more prolonged synaptic depolarization locally, thus providing both enhanced synaptic potentials and improved electrotonic propagation to central parts of the neurone. Both factors would increase the probability of spike discharge. An even more radical proposal involves the presence of active dendritic processes, which could undergo plastic changes during LTP.

Lynch and Baudry (1984) proposed that LTP could be associated with an unmasking of a covert population of glutamate receptors, thereby giving a sustained improvement in synaptic efficiency. After early negative results, Davies *et al.* (1989) reported that responses to iontophoretic application of AMPA showed a durable increase, although after a substantial latency.

An important mediator for the post-synaptic changes may be the metabotropic glutamate receptor, mGluR (Sugiyama *et al.*, 1987). Activation of mGluR by glutamate increases 1,4,5-inositol triphosphate and diacylglycerol (DAG), which in turn activates PKC. Changes identical to LTP follow application of phorbol esters (Malenka *et al.*, 1986) and injection of PKC (Hu *et al.*, 1987), and LTP can be prevented by inhibitors of PKC, and calcium-calmodulin dependent protein kinase (Malinow *et al.*, 1988), and of tyrosine kinase (O'Dell *et al.*, 1991). One caveat is that the inhibitors so far used are relatively unspecific. Candidate substrates for PKC involve both ionic channels as alluded to above, but also proton pump mechanisms and growth-associated enzyme activation.

Morphological correlates of LTP

The synaptic efficiency might be controlled by activity-dependent changes in morphology. Cytoskeletal proteins, for example actin and fodrin, could provide a machinery for early rapid changes in shape (for a review see Fifkova, 1985), while the slower changes would require protein synthesis.

Since the initial reports by Fifkova (Fifkova and van Harreveld, 1977; Fifkova and Anderson, 1981), a variety of morphological changes has been reported to be correlated to LTP in the hippocampus.

First, changes in the shape of the spine head have been reported (Lee *et al.*, 1980), and changes in spine number and shape on dentate granule cells (Desmond and Levy, 1983; Chang and Greenough, 1984). Three-dimensional reconstructions of excitatory synaptic structures on dentate granule cells, taken from areas where LTP had been recorded, revealed significantly more spines per dendritic length, and more bifurcating spines than in control material (Trommald *et al.*, 1990). A subset of spines had somewhat thicker necks. Because the material was fixed between 40 and 45 min after induction of LTP, these morphological studies suggest that surprisingly fast growth processes are associated with LTP.

CONCLUSIONS

This chapter has considered some activity-dependent changes of hippocampal neurones. It seems they may be more dramatic and develop faster than we used to think. In pathological states one might expect changes in both directions; reduction and enhancement of the number of spines and their associated synapses might well take place. Such beneficial plastic synaptic changes may well be at the base of several clinical events, including the recovery of cognitive functions which many stroke patients enjoy with training.

REFERENCES

Akers, R.F., Lovinger, D.M., Colley, P.A., Linden, D.J. and Routtenberg, A. (1986). Translocation of protein kinase C activity may mediate hippocampal long-term potentiation. *Science*, **231**, 587–589.

Andersen, P. (1987). Long-term potentiation—outstanding problems. In: Changeux, J.P. and Konishi, M. (Eds), *The Neural and Molecular Basis of Learning*, Wiley, Chichester, pp. 239–262.

Andersen, P. (1990). Synaptic integration in hippocampal CA1 pyramids. In: Storm-Mathisen, J., Zimmer, J. and Ottersen, O.P. (Eds), *Understanding the Brain through the Hippocampus. Prog. Brain Res.*, **83**, 215–222.

Andersen, P. and Lømo, T. (1966). Mode of activation of hippocampal pyramidal cells by excitatory synapses on dendrites. *Exp. Brain Res.*, **2**, 247–260.

Andersen, P., Blackstad, T.W. and Lømo, T. (1966). Location and identification of excitatory synapses on hippocampal pyramidal cells. *Exp. Brain Res.*, **1**, 236–248.

Andersen, P., Sundberg, S.H., Sveen, O. and Wigström, H. (1977). Specific long-lasting potentiation of synaptic transmission in hippocampal slices. *Nature (London)*, **266**, 736–737.

Andersen, P., Sundberg, S.H., Sveen, O., Swann, J.W. and Wigström, H. (1980a). Possible mechanisms for long-lasting potentiation of synaptic transmission in hippocampal slices from guinea pigs. *J. Physiol. (London)*, **302**, 463–482.

Andersen, P., Silfvenius, H., Sundberg, S.H. & Sveen, O. (1980b). A comparison of distal and proximal dendritic synapses on CA1 pyramids in guinea-pig hippocampal slices *in vitro*. *J. Physiol. (London)*, **307**, 273–299.

Andreasen, M., Lambert, J.D.C. and Skovgaard Jensen, M. (1989). Effects of new non-N-methyl-D-aspartate antagonists on synaptic transmission in the *in vitro* rat hippocampus. *J. Physiol. (London)*, **414**, 317–336.

Bär, P.R., Wiegant, F., Lopes da Silva, F.H. and Gispen, W.H. (1984). Tetanic stimulation affects the metabolism of phosphoinositides in hippocampal slices. *Brain Res.*, **321**, 381–385.

Barnes, C. (1979). Memory deficits associated with senescence: a neurophysiological and behavioral study in the rat. *J. Comp. Physiol. Psychol.*, **93**, 74–104.

Bekkers, J. and Stevens, C.F. (1989). NMDA and non-NMDA receptors are co-localized at individual excitatory synapses in cultured rat hippocampus. *Nature (London)*, **341**, 230–233.

Bekkers, J. and Stevens, C.F. (1990). Presynaptic mechanisms for long-term potentiation in the hippocampus. *Nature (London)*, **346**, 724–729.

Bekkers, J., Richerson, G.B. and Stevens, C.F. (1990). Origin of variability in quantal size in cultured hippocampal neurons and hippocampal slices. *Proc. Natl Acad. Sci. USA*, **87**, 5359–5362.

Blanton, M.G., LoTurco, J.J. and Kriegstein, A.R. (1989). Whole cell recording from neurons in slices of reptilian and mammalian cerebral cortex. *J. Neurosci. Meth.*, **30**, 203–210.

Bliss, T.V.P. and Lømo, T. (1973). Long-lasting potentiation of synaptic transmission in the dentate area of the anaesthetized rabbit following stimulation of the perforant path. *J. Physiol. (London)*, **232**, 331–356.

Bliss, T.V.P., Goddard, G.V. and Riives, M. (1983). Reduction of long-term potentiation in the dentate gyrus of the rat following selective depletion of monoamines. *J. Physiol. (London)*, **334**, 475–491.

Bliss, T.V.P., Douglas, R.M., Errington, M.L. and Lynch, M.A. (1986). Correlation between long-term potentiation and release of endogenous amino acids from dentate gyrus of anaesthetized rats. *J. Physiol. (London)*, **377**, 391–408.

Chang, F.-L.F. and Greenough, W.T. (1984). Transient and enduring morphological correlates of synaptic activity and efficacy change in the rat hippocampal slice. *Brain Res.*, **309**, 35–46.

Collingridge, G.L., Kehl, S.J. and McLennan, H. (1983). Excitatory amino acids in synaptic transmission in the Schaffer collateral-commissural pathway of the rat hippocampus. *J. Physiol. (London)*, **334**, 33–46.

Davies, S.N., Lester, R.A.J., Reymann, K.G. and Collingridge, G.L. (1989). Temporally distinct pre- and post-synaptic mechanisms maintain long-term potentiation. *Nature (London)*, **338**, 500–503.

Desmond, N.L. and Levy, W.B. (1983). Synaptic correlates of associative potentiation/depression: an ultrastructural study in the hippocampus. *Brain Res.*, **265**, 21–30.

Dingledine, R. (1983). N-methyl-aspartate activates voltage-dependent calcium conductance in rat hippocampal pyramidal cells. *J. Physiol. (London)*, **343**, 385–405.

Dolphin, A.C., Errington, M.L. and Bliss, T.V.P. (1982). Long-term potentiation of the perforant path *in vivo* is associated with increased glutamate release. *Nature (London)*, **297**, 496–498.

Dunwiddie, T.V. and Lynch, G. (1979). The relationship between extracellular calcium concentrations and the induction of hippocampal long-term potentiation. *Brain Res.*, **169**, 103–110.

Edwards, F.A., Konnerth, A., Sakmann, B. and Takahashi, T. (1989). A thin slice preparation for patch clamp recordings from neurones of the mammalian central nervous system. *Pflügers Arch.*, **414**, 600–612.

Fifkova, E. (1985). A possible mechanism of morphometric changes in dendritic spines induced by stimulation. *Cell. Mol. Neurobiol.*, **5**, 47–63.

Fifkova, E. and Anderson, C.L. (1981). Stimulation-induced changes in dimensions of stalks of dendritic spines in the dentate molecular layer. *Exp. Neurol.*, **74**, 621–627.

Fifkova, E. and van Harreveld, A. (1977). Long-lasting morphological changes in dendritic spines of dentate granular cells following stimulation of the entorhinal area. *J. Neurocytol.*, **6**, 211–230.

Foster, T.C. and McNaughton, B.L. (1991). Long-term enhancement of CA1 synaptic transmission is due to increased quantal size, not quantal content. *Hippocampus*, **1**, 79–91.

Friedlander, M., Sayer, R.J. and Redman, S.J. (1990). Evaluation of long-term potentiation of small compound and unitary EPSPs at the hippocampal CA3-CA1 synapse. *J. Neurosci.*, **10**, 814–825.

Gustafsson, B., Wigström, H., Abraham, W.C. and Huang, Y.-Y. (1987). Long-term potentiation in the hippocampus using depolarizing current pulses as the conditioning stimulus to single volley synaptic potentials. *J. Neurosci.*, **7**, 774–780.

Haas, H.L. and Rose, G. (1982). Long-term potentiation of excitatory synaptic transmission in the rat hippocampus: the role of inhibitory processes. *J. Physiol. (London)*, **329**, 541–552.

Hablitz, J.J. and Langmoen, I.A. (1986). N-methyl-D-aspartate receptor antagonists reduce synaptic excitation in the hippocampus. *J. Neurosci.*, **6**, 102–106.

Herron, C.E., Lester, R.A.J., Coan, E.J. and Collingridge, G.L. (1986). Frequency-dependent involvement of NMDA-receptors in the hippocampus: a novel synaptic mechanism. *Nature (London)*, **322**, 265–268.

Hestrin, S., Nicoll, R.A., Perkel, D.J. and Sah, P. (1990). Analysis of excitatory synaptic action in pyramidal cells using whole-cell recording from rat hippocampal slices. *J. Physiol. (London)*, **422**, 203–225.

Hollmann, M., O'Shea-Greenfield, A., Rogers, S.W. and Heinemann, S. (1989). Cloning by functional expression of a member of the glutamate receptor family. *Nature (London)*, **342**, 643–648.

Honoré, T., Davies, S.N., Drejer, J., Fletcher, E.J., Jacobsen, P., Lodge, D. and Nielsen, F.E. (1988). Quinoxalinediones: potent competitive non-NMDA glutamate receptor antagonists. *Science*, **241**, 701–703.

Hu, G.-Y. and Storm, J.F. (1992). Excitatory amino acids acting on metabotropic glutamate receptors broaden the action potential in hippocampal neurons. *Brain Res.*, in press.

Hu, G.-Y., Hvalby, Ø., Walaas, S.I., Albert, K.A., Skjeflo, P., Andersen, P. and Greengard, P. (1987). Protein kinase C injection into hippocampal pyramidal cells elicits features of long term potentiation. *Nature (London)*, **328**, 426–429.

Hvalby, Ø. and Andersen, P. (1988). Properties of EPSP plateaus necessary for induction of long term potentiation of hippocampal synapses. *Eur. J. Neurosci.*, **1** (Suppl.), 312.

Jaslove, S.W. (1992). The integrative properties of spiny distal dendrites. *Neuroscience*, **41**, in press.

Kauer, J.A., Malenka, R.C. and Nicoll, R.A. (1988). A persistent postsynaptic modification mediates long-term potentiation in the hippocampus. *Neuron*, **1**, 911–917.

Keinänen, K., Wisden, W., Sommer, B., Werner, P., Herb, A., Verdoorn, T.A., Sakmann, B. and Seeburg, P.H. (1990). A family of AMPA-selective glutamate receptors. *Science*, **249**, 556–560.

Lee, K.S., Schottler, F., Oliver, M. and Lynch, G. (1980). Brief bursts of high frequency stimulation produce two types of structural change in rat hippocampus. *J. Neurophysiol.*, **44**, 247–258.

Lovinger, D.M., Colley, P.A., Akers, R.F., Nelson, R.B. and Routtenberg, A. (1986). Direct relation of long-term potentiation to phosphorylation of membrane protein F1, a substrate for membrane protein kinase C. *Brain Res.*, **399**, 205–211.

Lynch, G. and Baudry, M. (1984). The biochemistry of memory: a new and specific hypothesis. *Science*, **224**, 1057–1063.

Lynch, G., Larson, J., Kelso, S., Barrionuevo, G. and Schottler, F. (1983). Intracellular injections of EGTA block induction of hippocampal long-term potentiation. *Nature (London)*, **305**, 719–721.

Lynch, M.A., Clements, M.P., Errington, M.L. and Bliss, T.V.P. (1988). Increased hydrolysis of phosphatidylinositol-4,5-biphosphate in long-term potentiation. *Neurosci. Lett.*, **84**, 291–296.

MacDermott, A.B., Mayer, M.L., Westbrook, G.L., Smith, S.J. and Barker, J.L.

(1986). NMDA-receptor activation increases cytoplasmic calcium concentration in cultured spinal cord neurones. *Nature (London)*, **321**, 519–522.

McNaughton, B.L., Douglas, R.M. and Goddard, G.V. (1978). Synaptic enhancement in fascia dentata: cooperativity among coactive afferents. *Brain Res.*, **157**, 277–293.

Magleby, K.L. (1973). The effect of repetitive stimulation on facilitation of transmitter release at the frog neuromuscular junction. *J. Physiol. (London)*, **234**, 327–352.

Magleby, K.L. and Zengel, J.E. (1976). Augmentation: a process that acts to increase transmitter release at the frog neuromuscular junction. *J. Physiol. (London)*, **257**, 449–470.

Malenka, R.C., Madison, D.V. and Nicoll, R.A. (1986). Potentiation of synaptic transmission in the hippocampus by phorbol esters. *Nature (London)*, **321**, 175–177.

Malinow, R. and Tsien, R.W. (1990). Presynaptic enhancement shown by whole-cell recordings of long-term potentiation in hippocampal slices. *Nature (London)*, **346**, 177–180.

Malinow, R., Madison, D.V. and Tsien, R.W. (1988). Persistent protein kinase activity underlying long-term potentiation. *Nature (London)*, **335**, 821–824.

Masu, M., Tanabe, Y., Tsuchida, K., Shigemoto, R. and Nakanishi, S. (1991). Sequence and expression of a metabotropic glutamate receptor. *Nature (London)*, **349**, 760–765.

Mayer, M.L., Westbrook, G.L. and Guthrie, P.B. (1984). Voltage-dependent block by Mg^{2+} of NMDA responses in spinal cord neurones. *Nature (London)*, **309**, 261–263.

Muller, D., Joly, M. and Lynch, G. (1988). Contributions of quisqualate and NMDA receptors to the induction and expression of LTP. *Science*, **242**, 1694–1697.

Nadler, J.V., Vaca, K.W., White, W.F., Lynch, G.S. and Cotman, C.W. (1976). Aspartate and glutamate as possible transmitters of excitatory hippocampal afferents. *Nature (London)*, **260**, 538–540.

Nicholls, D.G. (1989). Release of glutamate, apartate and γ-aminobutyric acid from isolated nerve terminals. *J. Neurochem.*, **52**, 331–341.

Nowak, L., Bregestovski, P., Ascher, P., Herbet, A. and Prochiantz, A. (1984). Magnesium gates glutamate-activated channels in mouse central neurones. *Nature (London)*, **307**, 462–465.

O'Dell, T.J., Kandel, E.R. and Grant, S.G.N. (1991). Long-term potentiation in the hippocampus is blocked by tyrosine kinase inhibitors. *Nature (London)*, **353**, 558–560.

Raastad, M. (1991). A method for reliable activation of a single excitatory synapse in CA1 pyramidal cells. *Soc. Neurosci. Abstr.*, **17**, 1486.

Raastad, M., Storm, J.F. and Andersen, P. (1992). Putative single quantum and single fibre excitatory postsynaptic currents show similar amplitude range and variability in rat hippocampal slices. *Eur. J. Neurosci.*, **4**, in press.

Racine, R.J., Milgram, N.W. and Hafner, S. (1983). Long-term potentiation phenomena in the rat limbic forebrain. *Brain Res.*, **260**, 217–231.

Sayer, R.J., Redman, S.J. and Andersen, P. (1989). Amplitude fluctuations in small EPSPs recorded from CA1 pyramidal cells in the guinea pig hippocampal slice. *J. Neurosci.*, **9**, 840–850.

Skrede, K.K. and Malthe-Sørenssen, D. (1981). Increased resting and evoked release of transmitter following repetitive electrical tetanization in hippocampus: a biochemical correlate to long-lasting synaptic potentiation. *Brain Res.*, **208**, 436–441.

Sommer, B., Keinänen, K., Verdoorn, T.A., Wisden, W., Burnashev, N., Herb, A., Köhler, M., Takagi, T., Sakmann, B. and Seeburg, P.H. (1990). Flip and flop: a cell-specific functional switch in glutamate-operated channels of the CNS. *Science*, **249**, 1580–1585.

Storm-Mathisen, J. (1977). Glutamic acid and excitatory nerve endings: reduction of glutamic acid uptake after axotomy. *Brain Res.*, **120**, 379–386.

Storm-Mathisen, J. and Iversen, L.L. (1979). Uptake of [^{3}H]glutamic acid in excitatory nerve endings: light and electronmicroscopic observations in the hippocampal formation of the rat. *Neuroscience*, **4**, 1237–1253.

Storm-Mathisen, J. and Ottersen O.-P. (1988). Localization of excitatory amino acid transmitters. In: Lodge, D. (Ed.), *Excitatory Amino Acids in Health and Disease*, Wiley, Chichester, pp. 107–141.

Sugiyama, H., Ito, I. and Hirono, C. (1987). A new type of glutamate receptor linked to inositol phospholipid metabolism. *Nature (London)*, **325**, 531–533.

Swanson, L.W., Teyler, T.J. and Thompson, R.F. (1982). Hippocampal long-term potentiation: mechanisms and implications for memory. *Neurosci. Res. Prog. Bull.*, **20**, 611–769.

Trommald, M., Line Vaaland, J., Blackstad, T.W. and Andersen, P. (1990). Dendritic spine changes in rat dentate granule cells associated with long-term potentiation. In: Guidotti, A. (Ed.), *Neurotoxicity of Excitatory Amino Acids.* Fidia Research Foundation Symposium Series 4, Raven Press, New York, pp. 163–174.

Wigström, H., Swann, J.W. and Andersen, P. (1979). Calcium dependency of synaptic long-lasting potentiation in the hippocampal slice. *Acta Physiol. Scand.*, **105**, 126–128.

Wigström, H., Gustafsson, B., Huang, Y.-Y. and Abraham, W.C. (1986). Hippocampal long-term potentiation is induced by pairing single afferent volleys with intracellularly injected depolarizing current pulses. *Acta Physiol. Scand.*, **126**, 317–319.

Yamamoto, C., Higashima, M. and Sawada, S. (1987). Quantal analysis of potentiating action of phorbol ester on synaptic transmission in the hippocampus. *Neurosci. Res.*, **5**, 28–38.

The Temporal Lobes and the Limbic System
Edited by M.R. Trimble and T.G. Bolwig

3

Organizational Principles of Hippocampal Connections

MENNO P. WITTER and HENK J. GROENEWEGEN
Department of Anatomy and Embryology, Vrije University, Amsterdam, The Netherlands

INTRODUCTION

Structurally, the hippocampal formation is composed of the most simple cortex, yet it appears to be involved in the most complex cognitive functions. A striking feature of the connectivity of the hippocampal formation is that it has its major cortical connections with only a single cortical area, the entorhinal cortex, which itself is a link in numerous multisensory corticocortical networks (Witter *et al.*, 1989). The hippocampal formation is also connected with a variety of subcortical structures, each of which has been suggested to be part of a functionally different system. These connectional characteristics may in part explain why such a variety of functions have been attributed to the hippocampal formation and why malfunctioning of this structure has been proposed in such diverse neurological and psychiatric disorders as amnesia, epilepsy, and schizophrenia.

The quest for an understanding of the functional role of the hippocampal formation has resulted in a variety of models which take various levels of complexity of the organization of the hippocampal formation into account. A comparison of models dealing with different presumed hippocampal functions leads to an interesting observation. Whereas they share some basic aspects such as hippocampal-septal connections, in each model different and quite specific afferent and efferent pathways of the hippocampal formation are selectively incorporated. For example, in models describing the memory aspects of hippocampal function, the connection between the hippocampal formation and the adjacent parahippocampal and temporal association cortex figure prominently (Squire, 1986; Van Hoesen, 1982). Other models, stressing the importance of the hippocampal formation in processes like conditioning and stimulus association, emphasize the connections of the hippocampal formation with the cingulate cortex and the anterior thalamic complex (Gabriel *et al.*, 1986). Models that deal with the motor aspects of hippocampal functioning either focus on the projections of the hippocampal formation to the ventral striatum as an entry into the basal ganglia/extrapyramidal system (Lopes da Silva *et al.*, 1985) or on its projections to the cingulate cortex as an access to the motor system (Gray, 1982; Vilenski and Van Hoesen, 1981).

Many models have in common that they propose that the hippocampal formation functions as a comparator. Although differences exist between the kind of information that is thought to be analysed through such a comparator, like comparing a novel stimulus with a stored stimulus (Vinogradova, 1975), a novel stimulus with a predicted or expected stimulus (Gray, 1982), the contents of a temporary register with working memory (Olton, 1978), or fragments of patterns with the complete pattern (Rolls, 1989), the resulting actions are generally considered to be conveyed into different output channels. Recent insights in the anatomical organization of the hippocampal network, that will be summarized in this chapter, lead us to propose that the organization of the hippocampal formation indeed provides the means to select between various output channels. Through hard-wired channels, the results of hippocampal processing can selectively be distributed to functionally different targets like the entorhinal cortex and the retrosplenial cortex. This does not imply, however, that each channel specifically directs its output to only one target. Some projections, for example those to the ventral striatum and the entorhinal cortex, arise from the same population of subicular neurons (Witter *et al.*, 1990). Based on a comparison of the connections between non-hippocampal areas and the entorhinal cortex and the ventral striatum, on the one hand and the retrosplenial cortex on the other, we will argue that the former two structures share functional properties that are different from those of the retrosplenial cortex.

THE ENTORHINAL-HIPPOCAMPAL NETWORK

The basic features of the hippocampal organization have been described by numerous authors (Fig. 1). The entorhinal cortex gives rise to a powerful excitatory projection, called the perforant pathway, to the dentate gyrus and to additional projections to CA3, CA1, and the subiculum (Andersen *et al.*, 1971; Hjorth-Simonsen and Jeune, 1972; Steward, 1976; Steward and Scoville, 1976; Witter and Amaral, 1991; Witter *et al.*, 1988a,b; Wyss, 1981). The intrinsic wiring of the hippocampal formation consists largely of unidirectional connections. The granular cells of the dentate gyrus send 'mossy fibre'

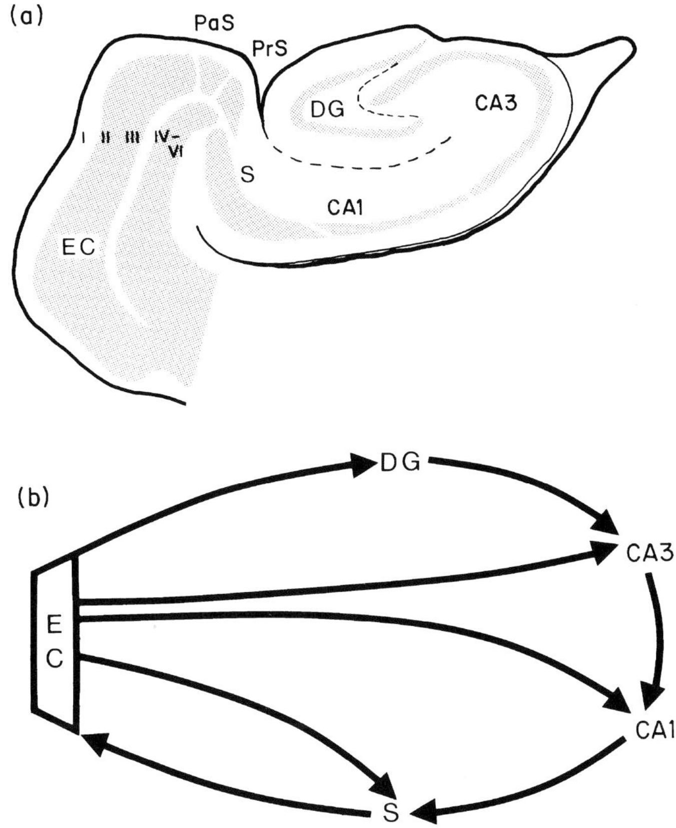

Figure 1. (a) Schematic representation of a transverse section, i.e. taken perpendicular to the long axis, of the hippocampal formation and parahippocampal region of the rat. The hippocampal formation comprizes three distinct cytoarchitectonic regions: the dentate gyrus (DG), the Ammon's horn, which is divided into fields CA3, CA2 (not indicated), and CA1, and the subiculum (S). The divisions of the parahippocampal region are the presubiculum (PrS), the parasubiculum (PaS), and the entorhinal cortex (EC). I–VI, layers of the entorhinal cortex. (b) Simplified representation of the largely unidirectional projections in the hippocampal circuitry and the distribution of the perforant pathway to the hippocampal components (a more detailed summary of these connections is shown in Fig. 2).

projections to CA3. Subsequently, pyramidal cells in CA3 give rise to collateralized axons of which the so-called Schaffer collaterals provide a major input to CA1. Finally, pyramidal cells of CA1 project to the subiculum which constitutes the major output structure of the hippocampal formation. At first glance, this organization does not support the notion of a selection between different output channels. However, it has been argued that even within a diffusely organized system, such as the hippocampal formation, selection processes may result in the specific activation of restricted sets of neurons, implying the selection of different channels (Buzsaki *et al.*, 1990; Edelman, 1989). The results of recent anatomical studies also indicate that the wiring enables the entorhinal-hippocampal network to select specific pathways.

Pathway differentiation at the level of the entorhinal cortex and the perforant path

The perforant path arises predominantly from the superficial layers of the entorhinal cortex. These layers receive inputs from the sensory association areas of the temporal lobe, conveying visual, auditory, somatosensory, gustatory, nociceptive, and olfactory signals (Insausti *et al.*, 1987; Room and Groenewegen, 1986; Van Hoesen and Pandya, 1975; Van Hoesen *et al.*, 1975). These inputs are distributed along the rostrocaudal extent of the entorhinal cortex with the olfactory inputs occupying the most rostral part. The intrinsic network of the entorhinal cortex combines a preponderance of longitudinal fibres with a restricted lateral-to-medial connectivity (cf. Witter *et al.*, 1986, 1989). This arrangement has two consequences. First, in a particular rostrocaudally oriented zone integration of all inputs that enter this zone may take place along the longitudinal axis. Although it is not yet clear whether and how such integration occurs, it may be assumed that the superficial layers of the entorhinal cortex supply the hippocampal formation with highly processed multimodal sensory information. An argument in favour of this is the absence in the entorhinal cortex and the hippocampal formation of neuronal responses to specific features of sensory stimuli (cf. Lopes da Silva *et al.*, 1990). Secondly, since several of the major inputs of the entorhinal cortex show a restricted lateral-to-medial distribution, it can be hypothesized that lateral-to-medial zones of the entorhinal cortex convey different types of information to the hippocampal formation. Since a lateral-to-medial gradient in the entorhinal cortex corresponds to a dorsal-to-ventral gradient in the hippocampal formation (Witter and Groenewegen, 1984; Witter *et al.*, 1989; see also in the monkey: Witter and Amaral, 1991), it may be concluded that the dorsal and ventral parts of the hippocampal formation receive different kinds of information. This suggests different functional roles for the dorsal and ventral hippocampal formation (cf. Witter, 1986; Witter *et al.*, 1989).

In addition to the lateral-to-medial differentiation within the entorhinal cortex, there is also a differentiation between layers II and III that form the origin of the perforant path. Fibres from layer II distribute almost exclusively to the dentate gyrus and CA3, whereas the projections that arise from cells in layer III project exclusively to CA1 and the subiculum. Moreover, these two components differ with respect to their distribution in the molecular layer of their targets. Whether layers II and III transmit different information to the hippocampal system is not clear. There is some anatomical evidence that, for example, afferents from the presubiculum may selectively innervate cells in layer III of the entorhinal cortex, whereas fibres from the parasubiculum may selectively terminate on layer II cells (Köhler, 1985; Caballero Bleda and Witter, unpublished observations).

The diffuse 'Dentate-CA3' system

The perforant pathway

The projections from cells in layer II of the entorhinal cortex to the dentate gyrus and CA3 show a terminal distribution that is related to their site of origin. Fibres from the lateral entorhinal area terminate exclusively in the outer one-third of the dentate stratum moleculare or lacunosum-moleculare (CA3), whereas those from the medial entorhinal area reach the middle one-third of this layer (Fig. 2(a)). This organization suggests that information from the lateral and medial parts of the entorhinal cortex is transmitted diffusely over the entire population of cells of both the dentate gyrus and CA3. It should be pointed out that the difference between the terminal fields of the lateral and medial components of the layer II projections is most marked in the rat (Steward, 1976; Witter *et al.*, 1989), whereas in the monkey this pattern is only vaguely present (Witter and Amaral, 1991). Although this may point to an important distinction between rodents and primates, the elegant physiological experiments of Andersen (Andersen *et al.*, 1980) have shown that the proximodistal position of a synapse on CA1 pyramidal cells has no influence on its effect at the level of the soma. The two pathways are chemically distinct, at least in rodents (Fredens *et al.*, 1984; Stengaard-Pedersen *et al.*, 1983), and accordingly they respond differently to pharmacological manipulation (Bramham *et al.*, 1988; Dahl, 1987). Therefore, it may be assumed that they also exert different effects onto their target cells, a suggestion that is supported by physiological data (Dahl *et al.*, 1990; McNaughton, 1980; Tielen *et al.*, 1981).

The mossy fibre projection

The dentate granule cells give rise to mossy fibres that distribute to the entire transverse or proximo-distal extent of CA3 (Fig. 2(b)). The dentate gyrus may thus be considered to transfer its input from the entorhinal cortex equally to all CA3 pyramidals. In contrast to the relatively abundant distribution of the perforant pathway along the long axis of the hippocampal formation, the mossy fibres distribute only to a restricted lamella of CA3 at the level of the origin of the fibres (Claiborne *et al.*, 1986; Blackstad *et al.*, 1970; Swanson *et al.*, 1978).

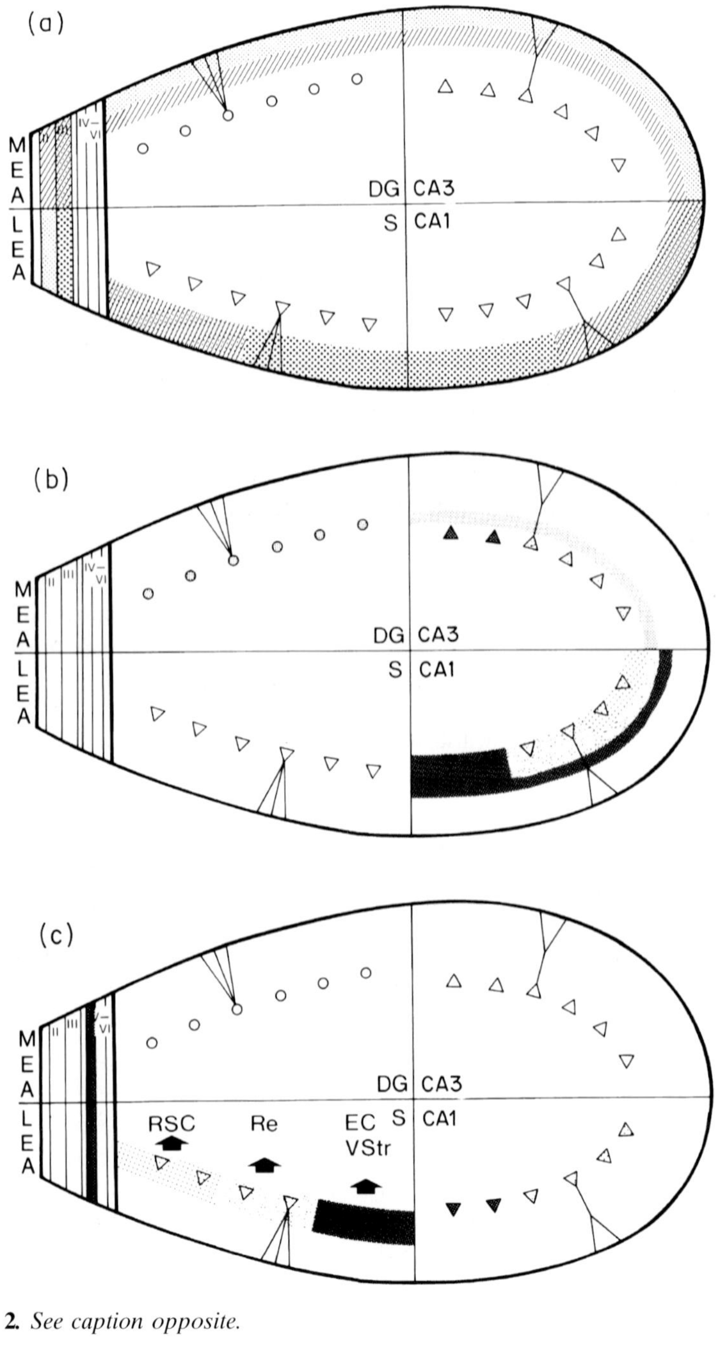

Figure 2. *See caption opposite.*

Transition from diffuse to selective: the Schaffer collateral projection from CA3 to CA1

The first clear indication of selectivity along the transverse axis of the hippocampal formation is provided by the organization of the Schaffer collaterals. As described in detail by Ishizuka *et al.* (1990), fibres from cells located proximally in CA3 issue projections that, at least at the level of their origin, terminate predominantly in the distal portion of CA1, i.e. close to the border with the subiculum. In contrast, CA3 projections from cells located distally in CA3 terminate most heavily in the proximal portion of CA1, i.e. close to the CA2 border (Fig. 2(b)). In addition to this transverse differentiation, the system also exhibits a laminar arrangement such that fibres directed at the proximal part of CA1 preferentially distribute over the proximal portions of the apical dendrites as well as to the cell somata and the basal dendritic domains. More distally in CA1, the fibres from CA3 terminate on the more distal portion of the dendrites. Ishizuka *et al.* (1990) confirmed and extended previous observations that the Schaffer collaterals have an extensive spread along the long axis of the hippocampal formation (see also Amaral and Witter, 1989).

Figure 2. Schematic illustration of the organization of several of the connections of the entorhinal-hippocampal circuits along the transverse axis of the hippocampal formation. (a) The differential distribution of the perforant path components originating in layers II and III of both the lateral (LEA) and medial (MEA) entorhinal area are indicated. Cells in layer II of both LEA and MEA project to the molecular layer of the dentate gyrus and CA3. MEA layer II cells project to the middle one-third of the molecular layer, whereas LEA layer II cells project to the outer one-third. Layer III cells project exclusively to CA1 and the subiculum. MEA layer III cells distribute fibres to the proximal portions of CA1 and the distal portions of the subiculum (S), whereas LEA layer III cells give rise to projections that distribute in a complementary way to the distal portions of CA1 and the proximal portion of the subiculum (S). (b) The granule cells in the dentate gyrus give rise to a diffuse projection that reaches all cells throughout the transverse extent of CA3. From this point on, the organization of the hippocampal connections is related to the transverse position of the cells of origin. Cells located in the proximal portion of CA3 (indicated by dark stippling) preferentially project to cells in the distal portion of CA1. In contrast, more distally located CA3 cells preferentially project to more proximal portions of CA1. (c) The topographic organization of the projections from CA1 to the subiculum (S) are indicated showing a transverse organization similar to that described for the CA3 to CA1 projections, such that for example cells in the distal portion of CA1 project preferentially to proximal portions of S. The topographic relationship between cells of orgin in the subiculum and some of the extra-hippocampal structures that receive subicular projections, such as the entorhinal cortex (EC) and the ventral striatum (VStr), the nucleus reuniens thalami (Re) and the retrosplenial cortex (RSC) are also illustrated in this diagram.

The selective CA1-subiculum system

The perforant pathway

As mentioned above, both CA1 and the subiculum are reached by fibres from layer III of the entorhinal cortex. In contrast to the projections from layer II to the dentate gyrus and CA3, the layer III system distributes differentially along the transverse axis of its target fields. Interestingly, this distribution of the layer III component can be observed both in the rat and the monkey (Witter *et al.*, 1989; Witter and Amaral, 1991). Fibres from the lateral entorhinal cortex distribute to the distal portion of CA1, whereas those from the medial entorhinal cortex connect to the proximal part of CA1. An inverted terminal distribution along the transverse axis is present in the subiculum (Fig. 2(a)). In this way, specific populations of cells in the entorhinal cortex may transmit different types of information to restricted populations of cells both in CA1 and the subiculum.

The CA1-subiculum projection

The organization of the projections from CA1 to the subiculum has recently been described in great detail in the rat (Amaral *et al.*, 1991). Cells located in the proximal portion of CA1 project preferentially to the distal portion of the subiculum, i.e. close to the presubiculum. Neurons in the distal portion of CA1 distribute their axons to the adjacent proximal portion of the subiculum. Cells in a mid-transverse position in CA1 send their fibres to similarly positioned cells in the subiculum (Fig. 2(c)). Amaral *et al.* (1991) conclude that the transverse width of each of the terminal fields equals approximately one-third of the total transverse axis of the subiculum. Similar conclusions were derived from an intracellular study on the CA1-subicular projections (Tamamaki *et al.*, 1987). It was further observed by Amaral *et al.* (1991) that the CA1-subiculum projection shows extensive longitudinal spread, covering approximately one-third of the long axis of the hippocampal formation which is comparable with the longitudinal spread of the perforant pathway.

The subiculum as 'selective' output structure

The observation by Amaral *et al.* (1991) that the CA1-subiculum projections divide the subiculum into three slabs of cells is of interest in view of the fact that the outputs of the subiculum are comparably organized (Fig. 2(c)); Witter *et al.*, 1990; Witter and Groenewegen, 1990). We could demonstrate that cells in the proximal portion of the subiculum preferentially project to, for example, the entorhinal cortex, the nucleus accumbens and the lateral septal complex, whereas cells in the distal portion of the subiculum preferentially project to the retrosplenial cortex, the presubiculum and possibly also to the anterior thalamus. The projections from the subiculum to structures in the midline thalamus, such as the nucleus reuniens, originate almost exclusively from the mid-transverse portion of the subiculum. Each of the three cellular slabs represents a width of approximately one-third of the total transverse width of the subiculum and thus appears to coincide with the slabs characterized by the CA1 inputs. It should be noted that not all of the subiculum projections respect the same organizational principle, since, for example, the projections to the mammillary nuclei originate from the entire transverse extent of the subiculum (Witter *et al.*, 1990).

Summarizing the organizational features of the entorhinal-hippocampal network, it thus appears that cells in the dentate gyrus and CA3 may be privy to a common entorhinal input. The organization of the remaining hippocampal network enables a subsequent segregation of the flow of information. In this way, subsets of information can be directed to different targets of the hippocampal formation. Although clear physiological evidence for such a selection is lacking, the observation by Buzsaki *et al.* (1990) that stimulation of the incoming entorhinal fibres, despite relatively uniform activation of the granular cell population, results in an active focus in CA1 seems to be in line with the present proposition.

FUNCTIONAL RELEVANCE OF HIPPOCAMPAL ORGANIZATION

An intriguing question that remains to be answered is why the subicular output organization is selective for some but not all target structures? We propose that structures that receive hippocampal input from the same population of subicular cells receive similar sets of information and are thus functionally related. The projections to the entorhinal cortex and the ventral striatum, both of which originate from the proximal slab of subicular neurons, will be used to provide support for this notion. In order to do so, we will first outline the organization of these two subicular projections and relate this to the functionally different networks in which the entorhinal cortex and the ventral striatum participate.

The hippocampal-entorhinal projection as part of a memory system

The reciprocating projections from the proximal portion of the subiculum to the entorhinal cortex predominantly reach the deep layers of this area. The intrinsic network of the entorhinal cortex preferentially connects deep to superficial layers (Köhler, 1985; Witter *et al.*, 1989). This arrangement may provide a substrate for interactions between the reentrant hippocampal signals and the superficial layers that supply the cortical input to the hippocampal formation (Buzsaki *et al.*, 1990; Lopes da Silva *et al.*, 1990). It is still unclear whether the entorhinal-hippocampal network functions in a reverberatory way, i.e. whether signals are transmitted from one area to another and are reflected back to the area of origin in such a way that a certain state of activity may be preserved after a short stimulus. Such circuits may work as temporary memory storage devices. Experimental evidence for the existence of reverberatory circuits in the entorhinal-hippocampal network is scarce, but reports of multiple responses in the dentate gyrus to a single stimulus applied to the entorhinal cortex (Deadwyler *et al.* 1975; Buzsaki *et al.*, 1990; Curtis *et al.*, 1991) may be considered suggestive in this context. Since the deep layers of the entorhinal cortex also give rise to projections that reciprocate most if not all of the inputs from the sensory areas to the superficial layers, this offers the possibility that the results of entorhinal-hippocampal processing are conveyed back to the sensory areas. This processed information may result in the strengthening or weakening of already existing activation patterns in the cortex. Such a process may be instrumental in long-lasting and selective memory formation (Posner, 1984; Rolls, 1989). Although little is known about the effects of interactions at the level of the entorhinal cortex, there is clear evidence that cholinergic inputs from the septum as well as dopaminergic inputs that arise from the mesencephalon modulate synaptic activity of the major entorhinal circuits (see below).

The hippocampal-striatal pathway as a motor pathway

A substantial projection of the hippocampal formation reaches, via the precommissural fornix, the ventral part of the striatum. These fibres mainly originate in the proximal portion of the subiculum. They terminate predominantly in the outer 'shell' region of the nucleus accumbens with offsets to the striatal elements of the olfactory tubercle, the central 'core' region of the nucleus accumbens, and the adjacent ventral parts of the caudate-putamen complex. Relatively weak hippocampal projections also reach more caudal parts of the caudate-putamen complex (Groenewegen *et al.*, 1982, 1987; Kelley and Domesick, 1982). The hippocampal inputs to the ventral striatum are topographically organized such that a ventral-to-dorsal gradient in the hippocampus corresponds to a caudomedial-to-rostrolateral gradient in the nucleus accumbens (Groenewegen *et al.*, 1987). Taking into account the functional differences that have been suggested for the dorsal and ventral hippocampus (see above; Witter *et al.*, 1989), this points to a functional differentiation within the ventral striatum. Such a notion is supported by a comparable topographical arrangement of a number of other cortical and subcortical inputs to the ventral striatum (Groenewegen *et al.*, 1982, 1991; Phillipson and Griffiths, 1985).

The presently held view of the organization of the basal ganglia circuits emphasizes that the inputs and outputs of basal ganglia are arranged in a

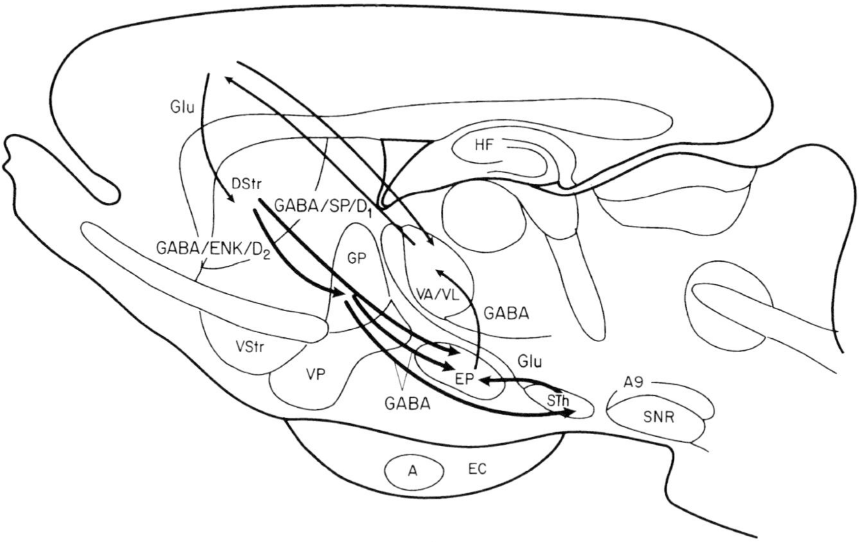

Figure 3. Schematic representation of a mid-sagittal view of the rat brain, illustrating the major connections of the cortico-striato-pallido-thalamic-cortical circuit of the dorsal striatum. Glutamatergic (Glu) projections from the cortex distribute to the dorsal striatum (DStr) that in turn give rise to GABAergic, *direct* and *indirect* projections to the internal segment of the globus pallidus (in the rat the entopeduncular nucleus, EP). The *direct* pathway also contains substance P (SP) and the cells of origin express the D_1 receptor. The *indirect* pathway also contains enkephalin (ENK) and the cells of origin express the D_2 receptor. This projection reaches the external globus pallidus (GP) which in turn gives rise to a GABAergic projection to the subthalamic nucleus (STh). The latter distributes a glutamatergic projection to the entopedunduar nucleus. The *direct* and the *indirect* pathway thus exert opposite effects on the cells in the entopeduncular nucleus and, through the projections to the ventral complex of the thalamus (VA/VL), on the thalamo-cortical connections. Projections from the striatum and the pallidum to the substantia nigra (SNR) are not indicated.

number of parallel circuits of which each involves a particular cortical area (Alexander *et al.*, 1986, 1990; Alexander and Crutcher, 1990; DeLong and Georgopoulos, 1981; Groenewegen *et al.*, 1990). Thus, pathways from functionally different parts of the frontal cortex lead through distinct parts of the striatum, the pallidonigral complex and the thalamus back to the frontal cortical area of origin (Fig. 3). According to this concept, the output of the basal ganglia, via parallel, functionally segregated basal ganglia-thalamocortical circuits, is directed to the motor, the supplementary motor, the premotor, and the prefrontal cortical areas. At the level of the striatum, inputs from several other cortical and subcortical sources feed into the circuits. For instance, the dopaminergic system, by its massive input to the

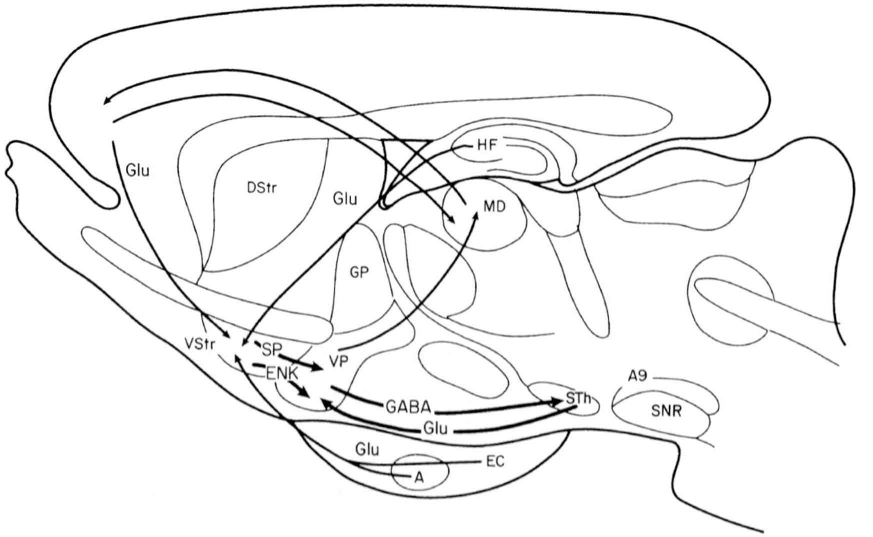

Figure 4. Schematic representation of a mid-sagittal view of the rat brain, illustrating the major connections of cortico-striato-pallido-thalamic-cortical circuit involving the ventral striatum. Glutamatergic (Glu) projections from the prefrontal and entorhinal cortices (EC), the amygdala (A), and the hippocampal formation (HF) reach the ventral striatum (VStr) which in turn gives rise to enkephalin- (ENK) and substance P- (SP) containing projections to the ventral pallidum. The ventral pallidum is reciprocally connected with the medial part of the subthalamic nucleus (STh). A differentiation between external and internal segments of the ventral pallidum cannot be made. The ventral pallidum influences the thalamo-cortical circuits through projections to the mediodorsal nucleus (MD). Projections to the ventral mesencephalon, including the substantia nigra are not indicated (compare with Fig. 5). SNR, substantia nigra pars reticulata.

striatal complex, plays an important role in the gating of the flow of information through the different circuits.

The ventral striatum is involved in a 'limbic loop' which leads from particular parts of the prefrontal cortex via the ventral striatum, the ventral pallidum and the mediodorsal thalamic nucleus back to the prefrontal cortex (Fig. 4; Alexander *et al.*, 1990; Haber *et al.*, 1985; Heimer *et al.*, 1982). Information from limbic structures, such as the hippocampus, the entorhinal cortex, and the basolateral amygdaloid nucleus, enters this limbic circuit at both the striatal and the prefrontal cortical levels (Groenewegen *et al.*, 1990; Jay and Witter, 1991; Kita and Kitai, 1990; Witter *et al.*, 1989).

Basic features of the basal ganglia circuits involving the dorsal striatum are the excitatory glutamatergic nature of the corticostriatal projections and the inhibitory, GABAergic character of the pathways from the internal pallidal segment (entopeduncular nucleus in the rat) and the reticular part of the substantia nigra to the thalamus (Fig. 3). The pallidonigral complex is influenced in an opposing manner by two parallel organized striatal output pathways (Alexander and Crutcher, 1990). A *direct* channel is formed by the inhibitory GABAergic striatopallidal and striatonigral projections arising from striatal neurons that, in addition, contain substance P and express the dopamine D_1 receptor (Fig. 3; Gerfen and Young, 1988; Gerfen *et al.*, 1990; LeMoine *et al.*, 1991). In the *indirect* channel, the first link is formed by the striatal projections to the external segment of the globus pallidus. This pathway utilizes GABA and enkephalin as neurotransmitters, and the striatal cells of origin express the dopamine D_2 receptor (Fig. 3; Gerfen and Young, 1988; Gerfen *et al.*, 1990; LeMoine *et al.*, 1990). The external segment of the globus pallidus sends GABAergic fibres to the subthalamic nucleus which, in turn, via a glutamatergic pathway reaches the internal segment of the globus pallidus and the reticular part of the substantia nigra (Fig. 3; Alexander and Crutcher, 1990). The external pallidal segment has also a strong direct GABAergic input to the pars reticulata of the substantia nigra and the internal segment of the globus pallidus (not illustrated; Smith and Bolam, 1991). An important aspect of the physiology of the neurons in the internal pallidal segment and the pars reticulata of the substantia nigra is their spontaneous activity by which they tonically inhibit the thalamic target nuclei (Deniau and Chevalier, 1985).

The influence of the direct and the indirect channels from the striatum to the pallidum and the substantia nigra on the thalamocortical system may be described as follows. Through the direct channel an excitatory, glutamatergic input to the striatum, which may stem, for example, from the cortex, the thalamus or the amygdala, results in an inhibitory influence on the pallidonigral output neurons and a disinhibitory effect on the thalamic target nuclei. In contrast, a stimulating influence on the striatal neurons, that give origin to the indirect channel via the external segment of the globus pallidus, leads to a disinhibition of the subthalamic nucleus and, consequently, to an increased excitation of the pallidonigral output neurons (Alexander and Crutcher, 1990). In the same channel, inhibition of the external pallidal neurons produces, via the pathways bypassing the subthalamic nucleus, a disinhibition of the pallidonigral output neurons. The net result of an activation at the striatal level of both pathways in the indirect channel is an inhibition of the thalamic target nuclei. The ascending dopaminergic system may have an opposing effect on the two striatal output channels, i.e. a stimulating effect on the direct, substance P-containing pathway and an inhibitory effect on the indirect, enkephalin-containing pathway (Gerfen *et al.*, 1990). As indicated above, the former effect is mediated by the dopamine D_1 receptor and the latter by the dopamine D_2 receptor. This implies that one of the roles of dopamine in the striatum is to modulate the balance between the two output channels of the basal ganglia to the thalamocortical system in order to bring about normal intended movement (Gerfen *et al.*, 1990).

Whether the connections of the 'limbic' basal ganglia circuits are organized in the same way as described above, remains to be established, but some important similarities and dissimilarities may be noted (Fig. 4). First, the cortical, amygdaloid and thalamic inputs to the ventral striatum most probably contain excitatory amino acids as neurotransmitters (Fig. 4; Christie *et al.*, 1987; Fuller *et al.*, 1987). Ventral striatal projections reach the ventral pallidum, the lateral hypothalamus, the substantia nigra, and more caudal mesencephalic areas, including the mesencephalic locomotor area (Groenewegen and Russchen, 1984; Haber *et al.*, 1990; Heimer *et al.*, 1991; Nauta *et al.*, 1978). The presumptive GABAergic, ventral striatopallidal pathways consist of both substance P- and enkephalin-containing fibres, but a clear distinction in the ventral pallidum between an internal and an external segment cannot be made (Fig. 4; Haber and Nauta, 1983). The ventral pallidum and the medial part of the subthalamic nucleus have a strong reciprocal relationship (Fig. 4; Groenewegen and Berendse, 1990). However, it is

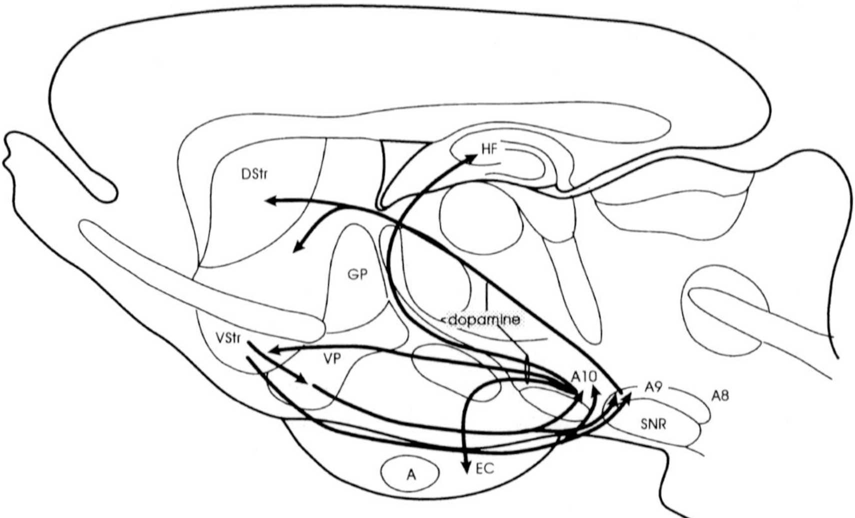

Figure 5. Schematic illustration of the descending projections from the ventral striatum (VStr)-ventral pallidum (VP) complex to the dopaminergic cell groups in the mesencephalon, through which the ventral striatum can modulate ascending dopaminergic projections to the dorsal (DStr) and ventral striatum (VStr), the hippocampal formation (HF), and the entorhinal cortex (EC). A8, retrorubral cell group; A9, pars compacta of the substantia nigra; A10, ventral tegmental area; SNR, substantia nigra pars reticulata.

not clear whether there are any direct and indirect pathways from the ventral striatum to the ventral pallidal neurons that project to the mediodorsal thalamic nucleus, in a way similar to the circuits involving the dorsal striatum. The ventral striatal projections to the ventral mesencephalon, on the one hand, parallel those from other parts of the striatum in that they terminate in the medial part of the substantia nigra pars reticulata (Groenewegen *et al.*, 1991; Nauta *et al.*, 1978) and thus have access to basal ganglia outputs to the thalamus and the deep layers of the superior colliculus. On the other hand, a substantial projection from the ventral striatum terminates in the dopaminergic cell groups A10, A9 and A8, respectively located in the ventral tegmental area of Tsai, the pars compacta of the substantia nigra, and the retrorubral cell group (Fig. 5; Groenewegen *et al.*, 1991; Heimer *et al.*, 1991; Nauta *et al.*, 1978). In this way, the ventral striatum can influence the ascending dopaminergic pathways to the entire striatum (Fig. 5; Groenewegen *et al.*, 1991; Nauta and Domesick, 1984). Through its projections to the ventral tegmental area, the ventral striatum may also influence dopaminergic neurons projecting to the prefrontal, entorhinal and hippocampal cortical areas (Fig. 5; Swanson, 1982; Swanson *et al.*, 1987; Verney *et al.*, 1985). In view of the recent findings of Smith and Bolam (1991) that the external segment of the globus pallidus projects heavily to GABAergic neurons in the pars reticulata of the substantia nigra, it is interesting to note that ventral pallidal terminals have similar arrangements with dopaminergic neurons (Groenewegen *et al.*, 1991).

The hippocampal-striatal pathway as output to the mesolimbic dopaminergic system: dopaminergic modulation of epileptic activity

On the basis of the hippocampal-striatal-nigral projections that influence the dopaminergic cells innervating the hippocampal formation and the adjacent parahippocampal and temporal cortices, it has been suggested that manipulations of the dopaminergic system will affect the occurrence and spread of seizures within the medial temporal lobe (cf. Patel *et al.*, 1988). The functional importance of the dopaminergic innervation of the hippocampal formation, although anatomically weak, has recently been reviewed by Bischoff (1986). In the entorhinal cortex, the dopaminergic innervation is more dense than in the hippocampal formation, most conspicuously in the superficial layers II and III of its rostrolateral portion (cf. Swanson *et al.*, 1987).

The obvious complexity of the dopaminergic innervation of the forebrain has resulted in many conflicting reports on the effects of manipulations of this system in epilepsy. It is beyond the scope of this chapter to summarize all these studies, but some of the above discussed insights in the organization of striatal connectivity and the related dopamine receptor specificity may explain the apparent experimental contradictions. From a comparison of the effects of various atypical neuroleptics on behaviour and specific binding to different types of dopamine receptors, Bischoff (1986) proposed that extrapyramidal effects, such as stereotyped behaviour, are specifically mediated through particular dopamine receptors in the dorsal striatum. In contrast, the antipsychotic effects are preferentially mediated through a different type of dopamine receptor that, although present in the striatum, is more abundant in the hippocampal formation. In recent studies, the relationship between dopamine receptor types and various response components has been addressed in more detail using selective D_1 and D_2 receptor agonists and antagonists. In the pilocarpine model, Turski *et al.* (1988) reported that a D_2 receptor agonist injected in the caudate-putamen of the rat exhibits marked anticonvulsant effects as measured by changes in the EEG. Injecting a D_1 receptor agonist into the dorsal striatum does not suppress pilocarpine-induced seizures, and injection of a preferential D_1 receptor antagonist does not enhance the susceptibility in this model. According to these authors, the suppression of seizures appears to be mediated by D_2 receptors, but not by D_1 receptors. In contrast, Barone *et al.* (1990) showed that in the rat low doses of pilocarpine induced limbic stereotypies but not convulsions or seizure-related brain damage. After systemic pretreatment with a D_1 receptor agonist, the same dose of pilocarpine resulted in convulsions and brain damage similar to that observed after higher doses of pilocarpine. In contrast, pretreatment with a D_2 receptor agonist did not have a marked effect on the induction of convulsions. They further reported that pretreatment with a D_1 receptor antagonist prevented the convulsive actions of pilocarpine alone or pilocarpine and a D_1 receptor agonist. Moreoever, neither dopamine receptor agonists nor antagonists altered the stereotypies induced by low doses of pilocarpine. Barone *et al.* (1990) addressed the apparent contradiction by suggesting (i) that the employed models are different in that the ways to induce seizure activity differ or that they employ convulsant versus non-convulsant doses of pilocarpine and (ii) that the two types of dopamine receptors may mediate functionally opposing roles. This suggestion appears consistent with the association of the two dopamine receptor types with different output channels of the striatum as outlined in the preceding paragraphs. Moreover, in view of the organizational complexity of the relationships between the dopaminergic system, the striatum and the hippocampal formation, part of the conflicting results might be related to effects on different components of this network. Since most studies report on the effects of systemic application of dopaminergic drugs, the site where these modulators exert their effects cannot be determined with certainty. Manipulations of the dopaminergic system will at least affect the transmission of sensory information through the hippocampal network, both at the level of entry in the entorhinal cortex as well as at the level of the hippocampal intrinsic network. Another possible site of action is the ventral striatum where dopamine may modulate the transmission of hippocampal activity to ventral striatal outputs. The resulting signal of the ventral striatum may in turn exert effects, both directly and indirectly via the ventral pallidum, on the cells in the ventral mesencephalon that give rise to the major dopamine-containing projections to the dorsal striatum and the cortex of both the medial temporal and the prefrontal lobes. One way to cut the Gordian knot is to systematically study the effects of manipulations of the dopamine system at the different way stations in these networks. Until such information is available, the construction of connectionists' models in order to understand the effects of dopamine on the generation and spread of epileptic activity will remain subject to fundamental criticism.

CONCLUDING REMARKS

In this chapter, we have shown that within the entorhinal-hippocampal network there is a substrate for selection between different output channels. We argued that since the targets of a particular channel receive the same copies of hippocampal activity, these targets should be functionally related. We subsequently summarized the organization of the pathways linking the hippocampal formation to the entorhinal-cortical and to the ventral striatum-basal ganglia networks. At this point, we have to return to our initial proposition and discuss whether these two pathways are functionally related and how they differ from targets of one of the other output channels, such as the retrosplenial cortex that receives projections from the distal subiculum. As already indicated, a common functional attribute of the hippocampal formation is that it functions as a comparator or participates in pattern completion. Depending on whether a stimulus is categorized as novel or familiar (matching to expectation or prediction; cf. Gray and Rawlins, 1986; Gabriel *et al.*, 1986) and whether the hippocampal formation is able or not able to complete a stored pattern of network activation, one of two possible output channels for the resulting activation will be selected. In case of a 'novel' or still incomplete activity pattern, the activity may selectively be transmitted through the proximal subicular channel to the entorhinal cortex and the ventral striatum (Fig. 6). In the entorhinal cortex, the hippocampal activity may result in the potentiation of previously activated neurons (cf. Buzsaki *et al.*, 1990; Lopes da Silva *et al.*, 1990), resulting in reverberation and temporal storage of the stimulus. Through repeated activation, the process may eventually result in transmission of the information into a more permanent register that presumably resides in the cortex (Squire, 1986). These ongoing processes in the entorhinal cortex are no doubt continuously dependent on incoming sensory information and ongoing hippocampal evaluation and may also be modulated through several major input systems such as the cholinergic and dopaminergic systems. At the

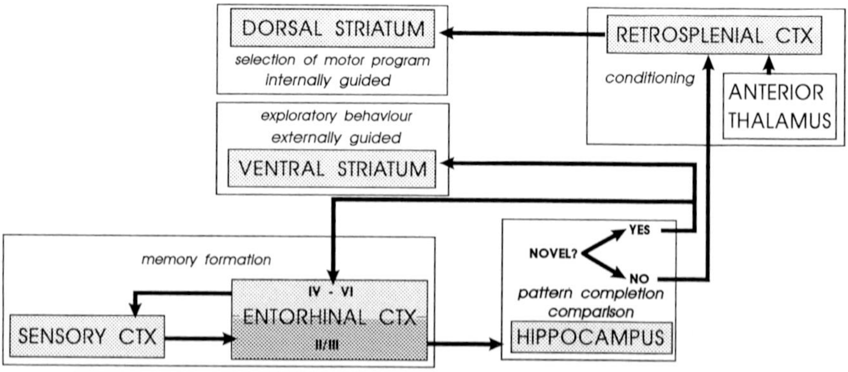

Figure 6. Schematic illustration of the functional connections between the hippocampal formation (HIPPOCAMPUS), the entorhinal and retrosplenial cortices, and the dorsal and ventral striatum, as proposed in the present study. Incoming sensory information is transmitted through the superficial layers of the entorhinal cortex to the hippocampus. The hippocampal formation performs comparison or pattern completion processes and, depending on the result or success of such processing in relation to the functional meaning of the stimulus, the resulting hippocampal activity is transmitted through morphologically segregated output channels either to the entorhinal cortex and the ventral striatum, or to the retrosplenial cortex. In each of the rectangles that surround anatomical structures or networks, functional attributes are indicated. See text for further details.

level of the ventral striatum, the hippocampal information may lead to the initiation and selection of appropriate behavioural strategies, such as increased exploratory behaviour in order to assess the relevance of the stimulus (Fig. 6). The incoming information during this exploration phase may be instrumental in the formation of a memory trace in case the stimulus is considered of interest, both in terms of reward or aversion. Alternatively, when a stimulus is categorized as not in need of further elaboration or completion and its associated attributes make it an important stimulus that requires a fixed or conditioned response, the resulting hippocampal activity will be gated to the retrosplenial cortex (Fig. 6). The latter cortex has been proposed to be involved in conditioned responses that are mediated through its direct connections with the mesencephalic premotor regions and the dorsal striatum. At the level of the retrosplenial cortex, the hippocampal output is thought to gate the transmission of information from the anterior complex of the thalamus to the dorsal striatum. In the latter structure, the selection of appropriate motor programs may take place (Gabriel *et al.*, 1986; Gray, 1982; Vogt, 1985).

One final remark should be made. The present proposal relies heavily on a functional differentiation between the dorsal and the ventral striatum. Arguments for such a differentiation have been put forward in detail in a recent review of the mesolimbic system (Scheel-Krüger and Willner, 1991). These authors review evidence that the ventral striatum is involved in switching behaviour under the control of external cues, whereas the dorsal striatum-prefrontal network is essential for the arbitrary internal selection of behaviour. In the latter process, ongoing available sensory information is not taken into account. It thus appears that the entorhinal cortex and the ventral striatum, where ongoing processing is responsive to external information, share the same hippocampal output channel. In contrast, the retrosplenial cortex which, in connection with the dorsal striatum, is involved in fixed response patterns, receives hippocampal information through another hippocampal output channel.

REFERENCES

Alexander, G.E. and Crutcher, M.D. (1990). Functional architecture of basal ganglia circuits: neural substrates of parallel processing. *Trends Neurosci.*, **13**, 266–271.

Alexander, G.E., DeLong, M.R. and Strick, P.L. (1986). Parallel organization of functionally segregated circuits linking basal ganglia and cortex. *Annu. Rev. Neurosci.*, **9**, 357–381.

Alexander, G.E., Crutcher, M.D. and DeLong, M.R. (1990). Basal ganglia-thalamocortical circuits: parallel substrates for motor, oculomotor, 'prefrontal' and 'limbic' functions. In: Uylings, H.B.M., Van Eden, C.G., De Bruin, J.P.C., Corner, M.A. and Feenstra, M.G.P. (Eds), *The Prefrontal Cortex: its Structure, Function, and Pathology*, *Prog. Brain Res.*, **85**, 119–146.

Amaral, D.G. and Witter, M.P. (1989). The three dimensional organization of the hippocampal formation: a review of anatomical data. *Neuroscience*, **31**, 571–591.

Amaral, D.G., Dolorfo, C. and Alvarez-Royo, P. (1991). Organization of CA1 projections to the subiculum: a PHA-L analysis in the rat. *Hippocampus*, **1**, 415–435.

Andersen, P., Bliss, T.V.P. and Skrede, K.K. (1971). Lamellar organization of hippocampal excitatory pathways. *Exp. Brain Res.*, **13**, 222–238.

Andersen, P., Silfvenius, H., Sundberg, S.H. and Sveen, O. (1980). A comparison of distal and proximal dendritic synapses on CA1 pyramids in hippocampal slices *in vitro*. *J. Physiol. (London)*, **307**, 273–299.

Barone, P., Parashos, S.A., Palma, V., Marin, C., Campanella, G. and Chase, T.N. (1990). Dopamine D_1 receptor modulation of pilocarpine-induced convulsions. *Neuroscience*, **34**, 209–217.

Bischoff, S. (1986). Mesohippocampal dopamine system. Characterization, functional and clinical implications. In: Isaacson, R.L. and Pribram, K.H. (Eds), *The Hippocampus, Vol. 3*, Plenum Press, New York, pp. 11–32.

Blackstad, T.W., Brink, K., Hem, J. and Jeune, B. (1970). Distribution of hippocampal mossy fibres in the rat. An experimental study with silver impregnation methods. *J. Comp. Neurol.*, **138**, 433–450.

Bramham, C.R., Errington, M.L. and Bliss, T.V.P. (1988). Naloxone blocks the induction of long-term potentiation in the lateral but not in the medial perforant pathway in the anesthetized rat. *Brain Res.*, **449**, 352–356.

Buzsaki, G., Chen, L.S. and Gage, F.H. (1990). Spatial organization of physiological activity in the hippocampal region: relevance to memory formation. In: Storm-Mathisen, J., Zimmer, J. and Ottersen, O.P. (Eds), *Understanding the Brain through the Hippocampus. The Hippocampal region as a Model for Studying the Brain Structure and Function, Progr. Brain Res.*, **83**, 257–268.

Christie, M.J., Summers, R.J., Stephenson, J.A., Cook C.J. and Beart, P.M. (1987). Excitatory amino acid projections to the nucleus accumbens septi in the rat: a retrograde transport study utilizing D[^{3}H]aspartate and [^{3}H]GABA. *Neuroscience*, **22**, 425–439.

Claiborne, B.J., Amaral, D.G. and Cowan, W.M. (1986). A light and electron microscopic analysis of the mossy fibres of the rat dentate gyrus. *J. Comp. Neurol.*, **246**, 453–458.

Curtis, M. de, Pare, D. and Llinas, R.R. (1991). The electrophysiology of the olfactory-hippocampal circuit in the isolated and perfused adult mammalian brain *in vitro. Hippocampus*, **1**, 341–354.

Dahl, D. (1987). Single pulse stimulation of the medial perforant pathway with concurrent administration of CCK-8-S appears to potentiate the rat dentate gyrus. *Soc. Neurosci. Abstr.*, **13**, 1667.

Dahl, D., Burgard, E.C. and Sarvey, J.M. (1990). NMDA receptor antagonists reduce medial, but not lateral perforant path-evoked EPSPs in dentate gyrus of rat hippocampal slice. *Exp. Brain Res.*, **83**, 172–177.

Deadwyler, S.A., West, J.R., Cotman, C.W. and Lynch, G. (1975). Physiological studies of the reciprocal connections between the hippocampus and the entorhinal cortex. *Exp. Neurol.*, **49**, 35–57.

DeLong, M.R. and Georgopoulos, A.P. (1981). Motor functions of the basal ganglia. In: Brookhart, J.M., Mountcastle, V.B. and Brooks, V.B. (Eds), *Handbook of Physiology. Section 1. The Nervous System, Vol. II, Part 2*, American Physiological Society, Bethesda, pp. 1017–1061.

Deniau, J.M. and Chevalier, G. (1985). Disinhibition as a basic process in the expression of striatal functions. II. The striatonigral influence on thalamocortical cells of the ventromedial thalamic nucleus. *Brain Res.*, **334**, 227–233.

Edelman, G.M. (1989). *The Remembered Present: a Biological Theory of Consciousness*, Basic Books Inc., New York.

Fredens, K., Stengaard-Pedersen, K. and Larsson, L.I. (1984). Localization of enkephalin and cholecystokinin immunoreactivities in the perforant path terminal fields of the rat hippocampal formation. *Brain Res.*, **304**, 255–263.

Fuller, T.A., Russchen, F.T. and Price, J.L. (1987). Sources of presumptive glutamergic/aspartergic afferents to the rat ventral striatopallidal region. *J. Comp. Neurol.*, **258**, 317–338.

Gabriel, M., Sparenborg, S.P. and Stolar, N. (1986). An executive function of the hippocampus: pathway selection for thalamic neuronal significance code. In: Isaacson, R.L. and Pribram, K.H. (Eds), *The Hippocampus, Vol. 4*, Plenum Press, New York, pp. 1–40.

Gerfen, C.R. and Young III, E.D. (1988). Distribution of striatonigral and striatopallidal peptidergic neurons in both patch and matrix compartments: an *in situ* hybridization histochemistry and fluorescent retrograde tracing study. *Brain Res.*, **460**, 161–167.

Gerfen, C.R., Engber, T.M., Mahan, L.C., Susel, Z., Chase, T.N., Monsma, F.J. and Sibley, D.R. (1990). D_1 and D_2 dopamine receptor-regulated gene expression of striatonigral and striatopallidal neurons. *Science*, **250**, 1429–1432.

Gray, J.A. (1982). *The Neuropsychology of Anxiety*, Oxford University Press, Oxford.

Gray, J.A. and Rawlins, J.P.N. (1986). Comparator and buffer memory: an attempt to integrate two models of hippocampal function. In: Isaacson, R.L. and Pribram, K.H. (Eds), *The Hippocampus, Vol. 4*, Plenum Press, New York, pp. 159–202.

Groenewegen, H.J. and Berendse, H.W. (1990). Connections of the subthalamic nucleus with ventral striatopallidal parts of the basal ganglia in the rat. *J. Comp. Neurol.*, **294**, 607–622.

Groenewegen, H.J. and Russchen, F.T. (1984). Organization of the efferent projections of the nucleus accumbens to pallidal, hypothalamic, and mesencephalic structures: a tracing and immunohistochemical study in the cat. *J. Comp. Neurol.*, **223**, 347–367.

Groenewegen, H.J., Room, P., Witter, M.P. and Lohman, A.H.M. (1982). Cortical afferents of the nucleus accumbens in the cat, studied with anterograde and retrograde transport techniques. *Neuroscience*, **7**, 977–996.

Groenewegen, H.J., Vermeulen-Van Der Zee, E., te Kortschot, A. and Witter, M.P. (1987). Organization of the projections from the subiculum to the ventral striatum in the rat. A study using anterograde transport of *Phaseolus vulgaris* leucoagglutinin. *Neuroscience*, **23**, 103–120.

Groenewegen, H.J., Berendse, H.W., Wolters, J.G. and Lohman, A.H.M. (1990). The anatomical relationship of the prefrontal cortex with the striatopallidal system, the thalamus and the amygdala: evidence for a parallel organization. In: Uylings, H.B.M., Van Eden, C.G., De Bruin, J.P.C., Corner, M.A. and Feenstra, M.G.P. (Eds), *The Prefrontal Cortex: Its Structure, Function, and Pathology*, *Prog. Brain Res.*, **85**, 95–118.

Groenewegen, H.J., Berendse, H.W., Meredith, G.E., Haber, S.N., Voorn, P., Wolters, J.G. and Lohman, A.H.M. (1991). Functional anatomy of the ventral, limbic system-innervated striatum. In: Willner, P. and Scheel-Krüger, J. (Eds), *The Mesolimbic Dopamine System: From Motivation to Action*, Wiley, Chichester, pp. 19–59.

Haber, S.N. and Nauta, W.J.H. (1983). Ramifications of the globus pallidus in the rat as indicated by patterns of immunohistochemistry. *Neuroscience*, **9**, 245–260.

Haber, S.N., Groenewegen, H.J., Grove, E.A. and Nauta, W.J.H. (1985). Efferent connections of the ventral pallidum: evidence of a dual striato-pallidofugal pathway. *J. Comp. Neurol.*, **235**, 322–335.

Haber, S.N., Lynd, E., Klein, C. and Groenewegen, H.J. (1990). Topographic organization of the ventral striatal efferent projections in the rhesus monkey: an anterograde tracing study. *J. Comp. Neurol.*, **293**, 282–298.

Heimer, L., Switzer, R.D. and Van Hoesen, G.W. (1982). Ventral striatum and ventral pallidum. Components of the motor system? *Trends Neurosci.*, **5**, 83–87.

Heimer, L., Zahm, D.S., Churchill, L., Kalivas, P.W. and Wohltman, C. (1991). Specificity in the projection patterns of accumbal core and shell in the rat. *Neuroscience*, **41**, 89–125.

Hjorth-Simonsen, A. and Jeune, B. (1972). Origin and termination of the hippocampal perforant path in the rat studied by silver impregnation. *J. Comp. Neurol.*, **144**, 215–232.

Insausti, R., Amaral, D.G. and Cowan, W.M. (1987). The entorhinal cortex of the monkey II. Cortical afferents. *J. Comp. Neurol.*, **264**, 356–395.

Ishizuka, N., Weber, J. and Amaral, D.G. (1990). Organization of intrahippocampal projections originating from CA3 pyramidal cells in the rat. *J. Comp. Neurol.*, **295**, 580–623.

Jay, T.M. and Witter, M.P. (1991). Distribution of the hippocampal CA1 and subicular efferents in the prefrontal cortex of the rat studied by means of anterograde transport of *Phaseolus vulgaris*-leucoagglutinin. *J. Comp. Neurol.*, **313**, 574–586.

Kelley, A.E. and Domesick, V.B. (1982). The distribution of the projection from the hippocampal formation to the nucleus accumbens in the rat: an anterograde- and retrograde-horseradish peroxidase study. *Neuroscience*, **7**, 2321–2335.

Kita, H. and Kitai, S.T. (1990). Amygdalostriatal projections to the frontal cortex and the striatum in the rat. *J. Comp. Neurol.*, **298**, 40–49.

Köhler, C. (1985). Intrinsic projections of the retrohippocampal region in the rat brain. I. The subicular complex. *J. Comp. Neurol.*, **236**, 504–522.

LeMoine, C., Normand, E., Guitteny, A.F., Fouque, B., Teoule, R. and Bloch, B. (1990). Dopamine receptor gene expression by enkephalin neurons in rat forebrain. *Proc. Natl. Acad. Sci. USA*, **87**, 230–234.

LeMoine, C., Normand, E. and Bloch, B. (1991). Phenotypical characterization of the striatal neurons expressing the D_1 receptor gene. *Proc. Natl. Acad. Sci. USA*, **88**, 4205–4209.

Lopes da Silva, F.H., Groenewegen, H.J., Holsheimer, J., Room, P., Witter, M.P., Van Groen, Th. and Wadman, W.J. (1985). The hippocampus as a set of partially overlapping segments with a topographically organized system of inputs and outputs: the entorhinal cortex as a sensory gate, the medial septum as a gain-setting system and the ventral striatum as a motor interface. In: Buzsaki, G. and Vanderwolf, C.H. (Eds), *Electrical Activity of the Archicortex*. Akademiai Kiado, Budapest, pp. 83–106.

Lopes da Silva, F.H., Witter, M.P., Boeijinga, P.H. and Lohman, A.H.M. (1990). Anatomic organization and physiology of the limbic cortex. *Physiol. Rev.*, **70**, 453–511.

McNaughton, B.L. (1980). Evidence for two physiologically distinct perforant pathways to the fascia dentata. *Brain Res.*, **199**, 1–19.

Nauta, W.J.H. and Domesick, V.B. (1984). Afferent and efferent relationships of the basal ganglia. In: Evered, D., O'Connor, M. (Eds), *Functions of the Basal Ganglia* (Ciba Foundation Symposium 107), Pitman, London, pp. 3–29.

Nauta, W.J.H., Smith, G.P., Faull, R.L.M. and Domesick, V.B. (1978). Efferent connections and nigral afferents of the nucleus accumbens septi in the rat. *Neuroscience*, **3**, 385–401.

Olton, D.S. (1978). Characteristics of spatial memory. In: Hulse, S.H., Fowler, H. and Honig, W.K. (Eds). *Cognitive Processes in Animal Behavior*, Erlbaum, Hillsdale, pp. 341–373.

Patel, S., De Sarro, G.B. and Meldrum, B.S. (1988). Regulation of seizure threshold by excitatory amino acids in the striatum and entopeduncular nucleus of rats. *Neuroscience*, **27**, 837–850.

Phillipson, O.T. and Griffiths, A.C. (1985). The topographic order of inputs to nucleus accumbens in the rat. *Neuroscience*, **16**, 275–296.

Posner, M.I. (1984). Selective attention and the storage of information. In: Lynch, G., McGaugh, J.L. and Weinberger, N.M. (Eds), *Neurobiology of Learning and Memory*, Guilford Press, New York, pp. 89–101.

Rolls, E.T. (1989). Parallel distributed processing in the brain: implications of the functional architecture of neuronal networks in the hippocampus. In: Morris, R.G.M. (Ed.), *Parallel Distributed Processing. Implications for Psychology and Neurobiology*, Clarendon Press, Oxford, pp. 286–308.

Room, P. and Groenewegen, H.J. (1986). Connections of the parahippocampal cortex in the cat. I. Cortical afferents. *J. Comp. Neurol.*, **251**, 415–450.

Scheel-Kruger, J. and Willner, P. (1991). The mesolimbic system: principles of operation. In: Willner, P. and Scheel-Kruger, J. (Eds), *The Mesolimbic Dopamine System: From Motivation to Action*, Wiley, New York, pp. 559–597.

Smith, Y. and Bolam, J.P. (1991). Convergence of synaptic inputs from the striatum and the globus pallidus onto identified nigrocollicular cells in the rat: a double anterograde labelling study. *Neuroscience*, **44**, 45–74.

Squire, L.R. (1986). Mechanisms of memory. *Science*, **232**, 1612–1619.

Stengaard-Pedersen, K., Fredens, K. and Larsson, L.I. (1983). Comparative localization of enkephalin and cholecystokinin immunoreactivities and heavy metals in the hippocampus. *Brain Res.*, **273**, 81–96.

Steward, O. (1976). Topographic organization of the projections from the entorhinal area to the hippocampal formation in the rat. *J. Comp. Neurol.*, **167**, 285–314.

Steward, O. and Scoville, S.A. (1976). Cells of origin of entorhinal cortical afferents to the hippocampus and fascia dentata of the rat. *J. Comp. Neurol.*, **169**, 347–370.

Swanson, L.W. (1982). The projections of the ventral tegmental area and adjacent regions: a combined fluorescent retrograde tracer and immunofluorescence study in the rat. *Brain Res. Bull.*, **9**, 321–353.

Swanson, L.W., Wyss, J.M. and Cowan, W.M. (1978). An autoradiographic study of the organization of intrahippocampal association pathways in the rat. *J. Comp. Neurol.*, **181**, 681–716.

Swanson, L.W., Köhler, C. and Björklund, A. (1987). The limbic region. I: The septohippocampal system. In: Björklund, A., Hökfelt, T. and Swanson, L.W. (Eds), *Handbook of Chemical Neuroanatomy, Vol. 5: Integrated Systems of the CNS, Part 1*, Elsevier, Amsterdam, pp. 125–2771.

Tamamaki, N., Abe, K. and Nojyo, Y. (1987). Columnar organization in the subiculum formed by axon branches originating from single CA1 pyramidal neurons in the rat hippocampus. *Brain Res.*, **412**, 156–160.

Tielen, A.M., Lopes da Silva, F.H., Mollevanger, W.J. and de Jonge, F.H. (1981). Differential effects of enkephalin within hippocampal areas. *Exp. Brain Res.*, **44**, 343–346.

Turski, L., Cavalheiro, E.A., Bortootto, Z.A., Ikonomidou-Turski, C., Kleinrok, Z. and Turski, W.A. (1988). Dopamine-sensitive anticonvulsant site in the rat striatum. *J. Neurosci.*, **8**, 4027–4037.

Van Hoesen, G.W. (1982). The parahippocampal gyrus. New observations regarding its cortical connections in the monkey. *Trends Neurosci.*, **5**, 345–350.

Van Hoesen, G.W. and Pandya, D.N. (1975). Some connections of the entorhinal (area 28) and perirhinal (area 35) cortices of the rhesus monkey. I. Temporal lobe afferents. *Brain Res.*, **95**, 1–24.

Van Hoesen, G.W., Pandya, D.N. and Butters, N. (1975). Some connections of the entorhinal (area 28) and perirhinal (area 35) cortices of the rhesus monkey. II. Frontal lobe afferents. *Brain Res.*, **95**, 25–38.

Verney, C., Baulac, M., Berger, B., Alvarez, C., Vigny, A. and Helle, K.B. (1985). Morphological evidence for a dopaminergic terminal field in the hippocampal formation of young and adult rat. *Neuroscience*, **14**, 1039–1052.

Vilenski, J.A. and Van Hoesen, G.W. (1981). Corticopontine projections from the cingulate cortex in the rhesus monkey. *Brain Res.*, **205**, 391–395.

Vinogradova, O.S. (1975). Functional organization of the limbic system in the process of registration of information: facts and hypotheses. In: Isaacson, R.L. and Pribram, K.H. (Eds), *The Hippocampus, Vol. 2*, Plenum Press, New York, pp. 1–70.

Vogt, B.A. (1985). Cingulate cortex. In: Jones, E.G. and Peters, A. (Eds), *Cerebral Cortex*, Plenum Press, New York, pp. 89–149.

Witter, M.P. (1986). A survey of the anatomy of the hippocampal formation, with emphasis on the septotemporal organization of its intrinsic and extrinsic connections. In: Schwarcz, R. and Ben-Ari, Y. (Eds), *Excitatory Amino Acids and Epilepsy*, *Adv. Exp. Med. Biol.*, **23**, 67–82.

Witter, M.P. and Amaral, D.G. (1991). Entorhinal cortex of the monkey: V.

Projections to the dentate gyrus, hippocampus and subicular complex. *J. Comp. Neurol.*, **307**, 437–459.

Witter, M.P. and Groenewegen, H.J. (1984). Laminar origin and septotemporal distribution of entorhinal and perirhinal projections to the hippocampus in the cat. *J. Comp. Neurol.*, **224**, 371–385.

Witter, M.P. and Groenewegen, H.J. (1990). The subiculum: cytoarchitectonically a simple structure, but hodologically complex. In: Storm-Mathisen, J., Zimmer, J. and Ottersen, O.P. (Eds), *Understanding the Brain through the Hippocampus, Progr. Brain Res.*, **83**, 47–58.

Witter, M.P., Room, P., Groenewegen, H.J. and Lohman, A.H.M. (1986). The connections of the parahippocampal cortex in the cat. V. Intrinsic connections: comments on input/output connections with the hippocampus. *J. Comp. Neurol.*, **252**, 78–94.

Witter, M.P., Griffioen, A.W., Jorritsma-Byham, B. and Krijnen, J.L.M. (1988a). Entorhinal projections to the hippocampal CA1 region in the rat: an underestimated pathway. *Neurosci. Lett.*, **85**, 193–198.

Witter, M.P., Van Hoesen, G.W. and Amaral, D.G. (1988b). Topographical organization of the entorhinal projection to the dentate gyrus of the monkey. *J. Neurosci.*, **9**, 216–228.

Witter, M.P., Groenewegen, H.J., Lopes da Silva, F.H. and Lohman, A.H.M. (1989). Functional organization of the extrinsic and intrinsic circuitry of the parahippocampal region. *Progr. Neurobiol.*, **33**, 161–253.

Witter, M.P., Ostendorf, R.H. and Groenewegen, H.J. (1990). Heterogeneity in the dorsal subiculum of the rat. Distinct neuronal columns project to different cortical and subcortical targets. *Eur. J. Neurosci.*, **2**, 718–725.

Wyss, J.M. (1981). An autoradiographic study of the efferent connections of the entorhinal cortex in the rat. *J. Comp. Neurol.*, **199**, 495–512.

The Temporal Lobes and the Limbic System
Edited by M.R. Trimble and T.G. Bolwig

4

Excitotoxins, Limbic Pathology and Excitatory Amino Acid Antagonists

BRIAN S. MELDRUM
Department of Neurology, Institute of Psychiatry, De Crespigny Park, London, UK

INTRODUCTION

Glutamate is the principal fast excitatory neurotransmitter substance in the mammalian brain. It acts on three categories of receptors in post-synaptic membranes that open cationic channels (the NMDA, the AMPA/quisqualate and the kainate receptors). Glutamate and some structural analogues that act as agonists on excitatory amino acid receptors are toxic to neurons in culture and can cause an acute neuronal degeneration *in vivo.* Given systemically in high doses to infant rodents glutamate or aspartate produce lesions in various periventricular structures including the arcuate and paraventricular nuclei of the hypothalamus (Olney *et al.*, 1971). In contrast, kainate or domoate, which are excitotoxins derived from marine plants, when given systemically to rodents induce limbic seizures and a selective pattern of limbic system pathology (Ben Ari *et al.*, 1980; Olney *et al.*, 1974). Domoate poisoning in man also induces limbic seizures and limbic pathology. Microinjection into the brain of selective NMDA receptor agonists (such as NMDA or ibotenate or quinolinic acid) produces purely focal lesions (Köhler and Schwarcz, 1983). Injection of AMPA/quisqualate or kainate agonists produces local lesions and distant lesions, which appear to reflect spread of seizure activity (Menini *et al.*, 1980).

We shall discuss here whether the classical patterns of limbic pathology associated with epilepsy (or similar pathologies, associated with hypoglycaemia, ischaemia or viral infections) may arise through the action of exogenous or endogenous excitotoxins.

MESIAL TEMPORAL SCLEROSIS

The pattern of cell loss found in patients with intractable seizures has been repeatedly described since its first precise histological characterization by Sommer (1880). Some key features were described by Margerison and Corsellis (1966) in patients dying in a long stay institution and a morphometric analysis was provided by Dam (Dam, 1980; see also Chapter 9). A quantitative analysis of the pattern of cell loss within the hippocampus in neurosurgical material has been provided by Babb (Babb *et al.*, 1984; Babb, 1991). This confirms the predominant 'Sommer sector' pyramidal cell loss of the post-mortem studies (approximately 80% cell loss in CA1 and 70% loss in the prosubiculum, but also reveals a 50–65% cell loss in the dentate gyrus, (CA4, CA3 and CA2) as occurring in 65% of the patients as the sole pathology and in a further 10% in conjunction with heterotopia (developmentally displaced neurons or collections of glia).

Patients with a primary hamartoma or glioma show a much less severe cell loss but with a similar pattern. The term mesial temporal sclerosis refers to the fact that neuronal loss and gliosis may also be found in extrahippocampal structures such as the amygdala and pyriform cortex.

STATUS EPILEPTICUS: ACUTE PATHOLOGY IN MAN AND EXPERIMENTAL MODELS

Limbic pathology with a distribution similar to that occurring in patients with chronic epilepsy is found acutely in patients dying shortly after status epilepticus, most notably in children dying after prolonged febrile convulsions or asymmetric status epilepticus (Zimmerman, 1938; Norman, 1964). Many factors including systemic hypoxia or local reductions in CBF might contribute to such pathology. Experimental studies in rodents and primates have shown that similar pathology can be produced when continuous seizure activity is sustained for more than 90 min (Meldrum and Brierley, 1973; Meldrum *et al.*, 1973; Evans *et al.*, 1983). The acute cytopathology is characteristic of that found in excitotoxic cell damage (i.e. it is post-synaptic with focal swelling of dendrites, and somatic changes initially characterized by dilated mitochondria loaded with calcium, by swollen Golgi apparatus and endoplasmic reticulum, and eventually by condensed cytoplasmic structure with a pyknotic nucleus (Evans *et al.*, 1983; Griffiths *et al.*, 1983, 1984). Similar cytopathology is produced by a variety of chemical convulsants (bicuculline, kainate, allylglycine) and by sustained electrical stimulation of the excitatory afferent path to the hippocampus (Olney *et al.*, 1983; Sloviter, 1991). Multiple brief seizures within one day can also produce hippocampal pathology within CA1 and CA3 (Meldrum *et al.*, 1974). It is characteristic of the acute experimental models that pathology occurs selectively in either CA1, CA3 or hilar neurons or in some combination of these three sites. Different models may favour particular combinations of the pathologies.

The question arises whether the pathology found *post mortem* in patients with intractable epilepsy or surgically in temporal lobe epilepsy is a consequence of an episode of status epilepticus early in life, a consequence of repeated brief seizures or a consequence of some other event (perinatal hypoxia, viral encephalitis) that preceded and contributed to epileptogenesis. The lesser degree of cell loss in the temporal lobectomy specimens showing a glioma or hamartoma (a result also found by Kim *et al.*, 1990) suggests that repeated brief seizures may contribute to the cell loss but are not responsible for the more severe pathology of mesial temporal sclerosis. On the other hand the majority of patients showing mesial temporal sclerosis give a history of a severe prolonged convulsion in the first 2 years of life (Sagar and Oxbury, 1987) or of prolonged or repeated febrile convulsions in the first 5 years of life (Falconer, 1974; Kim *et al.*, 1990).

Viral infections can give rise to hippocampal sclerosis. This has recently been demonstrated experimentally in mice with a measles virus (Andersson *et al.*, 1991). The pattern of pyramidal cell loss in CA1 and CA3 was similar to that seen in epilepsy and was prevented by an NMDA antagonist (it is not clear whether this result implicates local seizure activity in the pathogenesis or whether, for example, quinolinate formed in response to the viral infection might be producing an excitotoxic effect).

Transient global cerebral ischaemia can also produce selective hippocampal pathology involving predominantly CA1 and CA3 pyramidal cells and some hilar interneurons. The excitotoxic action of glutamate appears to contribute to this pathology and some protection can be produced by NMDA and non-NMDA antagonists (Meldrum, 1990; Sheardown *et al.*, 1990). However perinatal hypoxia is an improbable explanation for the pathology found in chronic epilepsy as the hippocampus (apart from the dentate gyrus) is less vulnerable to hypoxia than the cortex, thalamus and striatum in the neonatal period, both experimentally (Ikonomidou *et al.*, 1989) and in man (Veith, 1970).

Profound hypoglycaemia can also cause hippocampal damage in experimental animals but this preferentially involves the dentate gyrus. It has been proposed that an excitotoxic action either of aspartate or of quinolinate may be involved (Westerberg *et al.*, 1990).

DOMOATE POISONING

In eastern Canada between November and December 1987, more than 100 people became acutely ill following consumption of blue mussels that contained domoic acid (derived from *Nitzschia pungens* or *Chondria armata*). Although the predominant symptoms were gastrointestinal, many of the patients showed acute neurological abnormalities including headache, disorientation, amnesia, purposeless chewing and grimacing and seizures (Perl *et al.*, 1990). Several patients showed severe anterograde memory deficits months after the intoxication. The severity of the disorder and the pathological outcome was more severe in elderly males. Post-mortem studies in four subjects dying 7 days to 3 months after the episode showed a consistent pattern of limbic system pathology within the hippocampus involving dentate granule cells and all pyramidal cell subfields but with relative sparing of CA2 (H2) (Teitelbaum *et al.*, 1990). The amygdaloid nucleus, secondary olfactory areas, claustrum and nucleus accumbens septi were involved as was the sixth cortical lamina in the insular and subfrontal cortex.

FOCAL HIPPOCAMPAL INJECTION OF EXCITOTOXINS

Various authors have reported the pathological effects of either the focal intrahippocampal injection of kainate or of NMDA selective agonists (NMDA, ibotenate, quinolinate) (Köhler and Schwarcz, 1983; Olney, 1983; Schwarcz *et al.*, 1984). Most such studies have employed single injections of relatively large volumes/concentration of the excitotoxins, which may not be ideal for assessing selectivity of action. There is broad agreement that kainate shows a preferential action on CA3 neurons, and to a lesser extent on CA1 and dentate granule cells. Kainate also induces distant damage, involving other limbic structures including amygdala, pyriform cortex, and sometimes various thalamic nuclei. In contrast NMDA selective agonists do not induce distal damage. Reports differ concerning the selectivity of NMDA agonists; NMDA and ibotenate apparently lack selectivity but some authors report a preferential excitotoxic action of quinolinate on CA1 pyramidal neurons.

We (Meldrum and Jarrard, 1991; Jarrard and Meldrum, unpublished) have used a procedure employing 13 microinjections into each hippocampus, such that all subfields are similarly exposed to the toxin (Jarrard, 1989). We have compared the effect of injections of NMDA, ibotenate, kainate and quisqualate, assessing local and distant pathology by cell stains and a silver stain (for degenerating neurons, axons and terminals). NMDA and ibotenate lesioned all hippocampal cell types (dentate gyrus granule cells, hilar interneurons, CA3, CA2 and CA1 pyramidal neurons) but not extrahippocampal structures. Quisqualate and kainate both preferentially lesioned hilar cells and CA3 pyramidal cells and to a lesser extent CA1 neurons. Extrahippocampal structures showing damage included the amygdala, some thalamic nuclei, the entorhinal cortex and laminae III, V and VI of ventral cortex. Intraperitoneal injection of the NMDA antagonist 3-(+)-2-carboxy-piperazin-4-yl-propyl-1-phosphonate (CPP) protected against the hippocampal pathology induced by NMDA or by ibotenate, indicating that their toxicity was most probably due to a direct action on NMDA receptors. CPP did not protect against the hippocampal cell loss following focal quisqualate or kainate, but it did prevent the distal damage. This supports the view that such damage is secondary to the limbic seizure activity, and involves the action of endogenous glutamate on NMDA receptors.

RELEASE OF GLUTAMATE AND ASPARTATE DURING SEIZURES

The application of the technique of *in vivo* microdialysis has revealed that transient global ischaemia is associated with a massive increase in the extracellular concentration of glutamate and aspartate (Benveniste *et al.*, 1984; Hagberg *et al.*, 1985). It may be supposed that the excessive synchronous discharges associated with seizures would also be accompanied by an increase in extracellular glutamate concentration. However a study of seizures induced in rabbits by bicuculline or kainate by Lehmann *et al.*, 1985 found no increase in the extracellular concentration of glutamate or aspartate. We have recently used intrahippocampal microdialysis probes in rats with on-line analysis of glutamate that gives a higher time resolution than previous studies to re-examine this question, producing seizures either by systemic injection of picrotoxin or focal injections of bicuculline in the pyriform cortex (Millan *et al.*, 1991). We find no increase in extracellular glutamate even when the uptake of glutamate is blocked by dihydrokainate or DIDS. It may be that the excitotoxic effect of endogenous neurotransmitters can be a product of synchronous release over many post-synaptic receptors or excitation unopposed by inhibition.

PROTECTION AGAINST PATHOLOGY WITH EXCITATORY AMINO ACID ANTAGONISTS

Excitatory amino acid antagonists acting either on NMDA or non-NMDA receptors can block seizures in experimental models of epilepsy (reflex seizures in rodents and primates, chemically and electrically-induced seizures in rodents; Meldrum, 1991; Chapman, 1991; Chapman *et al.*, 1991). They may be less effective at arresting status epilepticus. Nevertheless it is consistently reported that NMDA antagonists block the limbic system pathology normally found after prolonged limbic seizures induced by systemic kainate (Fariello *et al.*, 1989; Clifford *et al.*, 1990; Lerner-Natoli *et al.*, 1991) even though the seizure as judged by EEG recordings appears not to be modified. *In vitro* studies of intratracellular bursts with some forms of chemically induced seizures show that NMDA antagonists may shorten the depolarizing shifts without changing their frequency. Such an effect by reducing the calcium influx might reduce the toxic effect of sustained seizure activity.

VARIATIONS IN CALCIUM BUFFERING

Selective patterns of neuronal loss in the hippocampus appear to be only partially explicable in terms of the density of glutamate receptors. A further hypothesis has been proposed concerning variations in calcium buffering capacity provided by parvalbumin and calbindin-D28K (Sloviter, 1989). In the rat hippocampus dentate granule cells show prominent staining for calbindin, whereas CA3 pyramidal cells have neither calbindin nor parvalbumin. The hilar somatostatin/neuropeptide Y interneurons and hilar mossy cells which are vulnerable to epileptic activity also have neither calbindin nor parvalbumin. In the human hippocampus dentate granule cells and CA2 pyramidal neurons contain calbindin, whereas CA1 pyramidal neurons do not (Sloviter *et al.*, 1991). These correlations between selective vulnerability and the presence of calcium-buffering proteins suggests that calcium buffering may play a critical role in the excitotoxic process that follows seizure activity.

CONCLUSIONS

The patterns of selective cell loss found in the limbic system acutely after status epilepticus, and in temporal lobectomy specimens in patients with intractable seizures are a consequence of sustained excessive neuronal activity. Activation of NMDA and non-NMDA receptors by glutamate or other excitatory agents contributes importantly to the pathological process. The contribution to selectivity provided by variations in the intensity of the glutamatergic input or the density of NMDA and non-NMDA receptors or various intracellular protective mechanisms (calcium buffering, free radical quenching systems) has, as yet, not been adequately defined.

REFERENCES

Andersson, T., Schultzberg, M., Schwarcz, R., Löve, A., Wickman, C. and Kristensson, K. (1991). NMDA-receptor antagonist prevents measles virus-induced neurodegeneration. *Eur. J. Neurosci.*, **3**, 66–71.

Babb, T.L. (1991). Research on the anatomy and pathology of epileptic tissue. In: Luders, H. (Ed.), *Neurosurgery of Epilepsy*, Raven Press, New York, pp. 719–727.
Babb, T.L., Brown, W.J., Pretorius, J., Davenport, C., Lieb, J.P. and Crandall, P.H. (1984). Temporal lobe volumetric cell densities in temporal lobe epilepsy. *Epilepsia*, **25**, 729–740.
Ben-Ari, Y., Tremblay, E., Ottersen, O.P. and Meldrum, B.S. (1980). The role of epileptic activity in hippocampal and 'remote' cerebral lesions induced by kainic acid. *Brain Res.*, **191**, 79–97.
Benveniste, H., Drejer, J., Schousboe, A. and Diemer, N.H. (1984). Elevation of the extracellular concentrations of glutamate and aspartate in rat hippocampus during transient cerebral ischemia monitored by intracerebral microdialysis. *J. Neurochem.*, **43**, 1369–1374.
Chapman, A.G. (1991). Excitatory amino acid antagonists and therapy of epilepsy. In: Meldrum, B.S. (Ed.), *Excitatory Amino Acid Antagonists*, Blackwell Scientific Publications, Oxford, pp. 265–286.
Chapman, A.G., Smith, S.E. and Meldrum, B.S. (1991). The anticonvulsant effect of the non-NMDA antagonists, NBQX and GYKI 52466, in mice. *Epilepsy Res.*, **9**, 92–93.
Clifford, D.B., Olney, J.W., Benz, A.M., Fuller, T.A. and Zorumski, C.F. (1990). Ketamine, phencyclidine, and MK-801 protect against kainic acid-induced seizure-related brain damage. *Epilepsia*, **31**, 382–390.
Dam, A.M. (1980). Epilepsy and neuron loss in the hippocampus. *Epilepsia*, **21**, 617–629.
Evans, M., Griffiths, T. and Meldrum, B.S. (1983). Early changes in the rat hippocampus following seizures induced by bicuculline or L-allylglycine: a light and electron microscope study. *Neuropathol. Appl. Neurobiol.*, **9**, 39–52.
Falconer, M.A. (1974). Mesial temporal (Ammon's horn) sclerosis as a common cause of epilepsy. Aetiology, treatment and prevention. *Lancet*, **ii**, 767–770.
Fariello, R.G., Golden, G.T., Smith, G.G. and Reyes, P.F. (1989). Potentiation of kainic acid epileptogenicity and sparing from neuronal damage by an NMDA receptor antagonist. *Epilepsy Res.*, **3**, 206–213.
Griffiths, T., Evans, M.C. and Meldrum, B.S. (1983). Intracellular calcium accumulation in rat hippocampus during seizures induced by bicuculline or L-allylglycine. *Neuroscience*, **10**, 385–395.
Griffiths, T., Evans, M.C. and Meldrum, B.S. (1984). Status epilepticus: the reversibility of calcium loading and acute neuronal pathological changes in the rat hippocampus. *Neuroscience*, **12**, 557–567.
Hagberg, H., Lehmann, A., Sandberg, M., Nyström, B., Jacobson, I. and Hamberger, A. (1985). Ischemia-induced shift of inhibitory and excitatory amino acids from intra- to extracellular compartments. *J. Cereb. Blood Flow Metab.*, **5**, 413–419.
Ikonomidou, C., Price, M.T., Mosinger, J.L., Frierdich, G., Labruyere, J., Shahid Salles, K. and Olney, J.W. (1989). Hypobaric-ischemic conditions produce glutamate-like cytopathology in infant rat brain. *J. Neurosci.*, **9**, 1693–1700.
Jarrard, L.E. (1989). On the use of ibotenic acid to lesion selectively different components of the hippocampal formation. *J. Neurosci. Meth.*, **29**, 251–259.
Kim, J.H., Guimaraes, P.O., Shen, M.Y., Masukawa, L.M. and Spencer, D.D. (1990). Hippocampal neuronal density in temporal lobe epilepsy with and without gliomas. *Acta Neuropathol. (Berlin)*, **80**, 41–45.
Köhler, C. and Schwarcz, R. (1983). Comparison of ibotenate and kainate neurotoxicity in rat brain: a histological study. *Neuroscience*, **8**, 819–835.
Lehmann, A., Hagberg, H., Jacobson, I. and Hamberger, A. (1985). Effect of status

epilepticus on extracellular amino acids in the hippocampus. *Brain Res.*, **359**, 147–151.

Lerner-Natoli, M., Rondouin, G., Belaidi, M., Baldy-Moulinier, M. and Kamenka, J.M. (1991). N-[1-(2-thienyl)cyclohexyl]-piperidine (TCP) does not block kainic acid-induced status epilepticus but reduces secondary hippocampal damage. *Neurosci. Lett.*, **122**, 174–178.

Margerison, J.H. and Corsellis, J.A.N. (1966). Epilepsy and the temporal lobes. *Brain*, **89**, 499–530.

Meldrum, B.S. (1990). Protection against ischaemic neuronal damage by drugs acting on excitatory neurotransmission. *Cereb. Brain Metab. Rev.*, **2**, 27–57.

Meldrum, B.S. (1991). Excitatory amino acid neurotransmission in epilepsy and anticonvulsant therapy. In: Meldrum, B.S., Moroni, F., Simon, R.P. and Woods, J.H. (Eds), *Excitatory Amino Acids*, Raven Press, New York.

Meldrum, B.S. and Brierley, J.B. (1973). Prolonged epileptic seizures in primates: ischaemic cell change and its relation to ictal physiological events. *Arch. Neurol.*, **28**, 10–17.

Meldrum, B.S. and Jarrard, L.E. (1991). The role of excitotoxins in the mechanism of hippocampal damage. In: Yonezawa, T. (Ed.), *Proceedings of the XIth International Congress of Neuropathology. Neuropathology*, **4** (Suppl.), 215–218.

Meldrum, B.S., Vigoroux, R.A. and Brierley, J.B. (1973). Systemic factors and epileptic brain damage. Prolonged seizures in paralysed artificially ventilated baboons. *Arch. Neurol.*, **29**, 82–87.

Meldrum, B.S., Horton, R.W. and Brierley, J.B. (1974). Epileptic brain damage in adolescent baboons following seizures induced by allylglycine. *Brain*, **97**, 417–428.

Menini, C., Meldrum, B.S., Riche, D., Silva-Comte, C. and Stutzmann, J.M. (1980). Sustained limbic seizures induced by intraamygdaloid kainic acid in the baboon: symptomatology and neuropathological consequences. *Ann. Neurol.*, **8**, 501–509.

Millan, M.H., Obrenovitch, T.P., Sarna, G.S., Lok, S.Y., Symon, L. and Meldrum, B.S. (1991). Changes in rat brain extracellular glutamate concentration during seizures induced by systemic picrotoxin or focal bicuculline injection: an *in vivo* dialysis study with on-line enzymatic detection. *Epilepsy Res.*, **9**, 86–91.

Norman, R.M. (1964). The neuropathology of status epilepticus. *Medicine, Sci. Law*, **4**, 46–51.

Olney, J.W. (1983). Excitotoxins: an overview. In: Fuxe, K., Roberts, P. and Schwarcz, R. (Eds), *Excitotoxins*, Macmillan Press, London, pp. 82–96.

Olney, J.W., Ho, O.C. and Rhee, V. (1971). Cytotoxic effects of acidic and sulphur containing amino acids on the infant mouse central nervous system. *Exp. Brain Res.*, **14**, 61–76.

Olney, J.W., Rhee, V. and Ho, O.L. (1974). Kainic acid: a powerful neurotoxic analogue of glutamate. *Brain Res.*, **77**, 507.

Olney, J.W., de Gubareff, T. and Sloviter, R.S. (1983). 'Epileptic' brain damage in rats induced by sustained electrical stimulation of the perforant path. II Ultrastructural analysis of acute hippocampal pathology. *Brain Res. Bull.*, **10**, 699–712.

Perl, T.M., Bedard, L., Kosatsky, T., Hockin, J.C., Todd, E.C.D. and Remis, R.S. (1990). An outbreak of toxic encephalopathy caused by eating mussels contaminated with domoic acid. *N. Engl. J. Med.*, **322**, 1775–1780.

Sagar, H.J. and Oxbury, J.M. (1987). Hippocampal neuron loss in temporal lobe epilepsy: correlation with early childhood convulsions. *Ann. Neurol.*, **22**, 334–340.

Schwarcz, R., Brush, G.S., Foster, A.C. and French, E.D. (1984). Seizure activity and lesions after intrahippocampal quinolinic acid injection. *Exp. Neurol.*, **84**, 1–17.

Sheardown, M.J., Nielsen, E.O., Hansen, A.J., Jacobsen, P. and Honoré, T. (1990). 2,3-Dihydroxy-6-nitro-7-sulfamoyl-benzo (F)quinoxaline: a neuroprotectant for cerebral ischemia. *Science*, **247**, 571–574.

Sloviter, R.S. (1989). Calcium-binding protein (Calbindin-D28KO) and parvalbumin immunocytochemistry: localization in the rat hippocampus with specific reference to the selective vulnerability of hippocampal neurons to seizure activity. *J. Comp. Neurol.*, **280**, 183–196.

Sloviter, R.S. (1991). Permanently altered hippocampal structure, excitability, and inhibition after experimental status epilepticus in the rat: the 'dormant basket cell' hypothesis and its possible relevance to temporal lobe epilepsy. *Hippocampus*, **1**, 41–66.

Sloviter, R.S., Sollas, A.L., Barbaro, N.M. and Laxer, K.D. (1991). Calcium-binding protein (calbindin-D28K) and parvalbumin immunocytochemistry in the normal and epileptic human hippocampus. *J. Comp. Neurol.*, **308**, 381–396.

Sommer, W. (1880). Erkrankung des Ammonshornes als aetiologisches Moment der Epilepsie. *Arch. Psychiatr. Nervenkr.*, **10**, 631–675.

Teitelbaum, J.S., Zatorre, R.J., Carpenter, S., Gendron, D., Evans, A.C., Gjedde, A. and Cashman, N.R. (1990). Neurologic sequelae of domoic acid intoxication due to the ingestion of contaminated mussels. *N. Engl. J. Med.*, **322**, 1781–1787.

Veith, G. (1970). Anatomische Studien über die Ammonshornsklerose im Epileptikergehirn. *Dtsch. Z. Nervenheilk.*, **197**, 293–314.

Westerberg, E., Magnusson, K., Wieloch, T., Ungerstedt, U., Speciale, C. and Schwarcz, R. (1990). Extracellular levels of quinolinic acid are moderately increased in rat neostriatum following severe insulin-induced hypoglycaemia. *Acta Physiol. Scand.*, **138**, 417–422.

Zimmerman, H.M. (1938). The histopathology of convulsive disorders in children. *J. Pediatr.*, **13**, 859–890.

The Temporal Lobes and the Limbic System
Edited by M.R. Trimble and T.G. Bolwig

5

Hippocampal Kindling: Some Structure/Activity Relationships

TOM G. BOLWIG,* JØRN KRAGH* AND OLE STEEN JØRGENSEN**
*Laboratory for Experimental Neuropsychiatry, Department of Psychiatry, State University Hospital, Rigshospitalet, Copenhagen, and **Institute of Neuropsychiatry, University of Copenhagen, Denmark

INTRODUCTION

Since the first description of the kindling phenomenon by Goddard (Goddard, 1967; Goddard *et al.*, 1969) the number of research reports concerning aspects of this important neurophysiological phenomenon have been steadily increasing (Wada, 1986). The original observations and the early literature on kindling have emphasized seizures as an endpoint. Kindling requires the triggering of epileptiform discharge brought about by changes which in response appear to involve long-lasting change in brain function. Once the stimulation has started triggering motor seizures it will continue to produce these responses even after delays of several months.

Kindling has therefore been used abundantly to investigate the cellular mechanisms of epilepsy, and although it is not yet definitively proven that kindling can be established in humans, a number of similarities between laboratory findings of electrophysiological and behavioural phenomena and clinical observations of, especially, temporal lobe epilepsy with secondary generalization point to kindling as being a clinically highly relevant model for epilepsy.

Emphasizing the behavioural aspects in addition to the epileptic consequences, several investigators have viewed a number of conditions related to psychiatric syndromes in the light of the kindling paradigm. Kindling, while being an experimental model for epileptic disorders, may therefore have clinical relevance beyond epilepsy. Among conditions carefully studied we can mention briefly anxiety disorders (Adamec and Stark-Adamec, 1983), manic depressive illness (Post and Kopanda, 1976; Post and Weiss, 1989), schizophrenia (Stevens and Livermore, 1978), alcoholism (Ballenger and Post, 1978; Clemmesen and Hemmingsen, 1984; Clemmesen *et al.*, 1988), abuse of psychomotor stimulants (Ballenger and Post, 1989), tardive dyskinesia (Glenthøj *et al.*, 1990), and the psychopathology associated with epilepsy (Trimble, 1991). Some of these aspects have recently been reviewed (Bolwig and Trimble, 1989).

In this chapter some aspects of the kindling phenomenon with special reference to basic mechanisms concerning limbic structures will be presented.

THE KINDLING PHENOMENON

Kindling was first described in detail by Graham Goddard, who in an animal model demonstrated a phenomenon in which repeated administration of an initially subconvulsive electrical stimulus leads to a progressive intensification of seizure activity culminating in a generalized seizure. Following stimulation in the amygdala, the initial stimulus often elicits focal electrical seizure activity (after-discharge (AD) measured on EEG (Fig. 1)). Subsequent stimulation will induce the development of motor seizures, and when fully kindled, the animals for months will have full strength responses after one or two stimulations (Wada and Sato, 1974).

Anatomical substrates

In the earliest work Goddard *et al.* (1969) showed that the amygdala required the smallest number of stimulations to kindle, and there was a reasonable correlation between the number of stimulations required by other structures and their anatomical distance from the amygdala. Subsequent work has shown that among limbic system and related structures the olfactory bulb and pyriform cortex kindle with the smallest number of stimulations (McIntyre and Plant, 1989), while the dorsal hippocampus requires the greatest number of stimulations. These differences may be related to the fact that the amygdala/pyriform region has relatively strong connections with the motor systems or because the neurons in this area have especially reactive properties (Fig. 2).

Electrographic measures

The most characteristic change occurring during kindling is the increased propagation of the epileptiform electrical discharge to other sites and the possible recruitment of those sites into the discharge. The first spontaneous events often appear from the pyriform cortex, even if the kindling stimulation has been given at another site (Kairiss *et al.*, 1984). The evoked

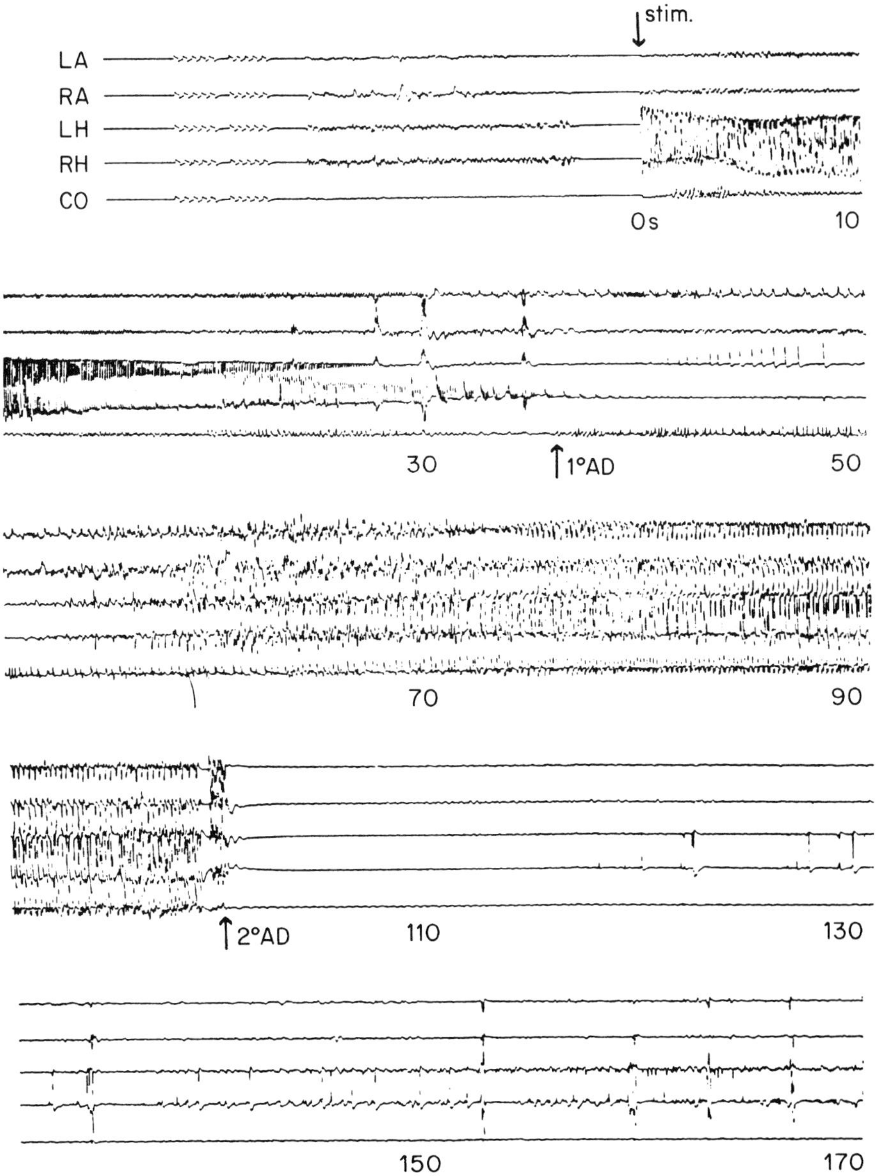

Figure 1. Typical EEG of a fully kindled rat. The five leads are, from top down: left and right amygdala, left and right hippocampus and motor cortex. Primary after-discharge (AD) starts with stimulation at time 0 s and lasts 36 s. A secondary after-discharge builds up and ends after 100 s.

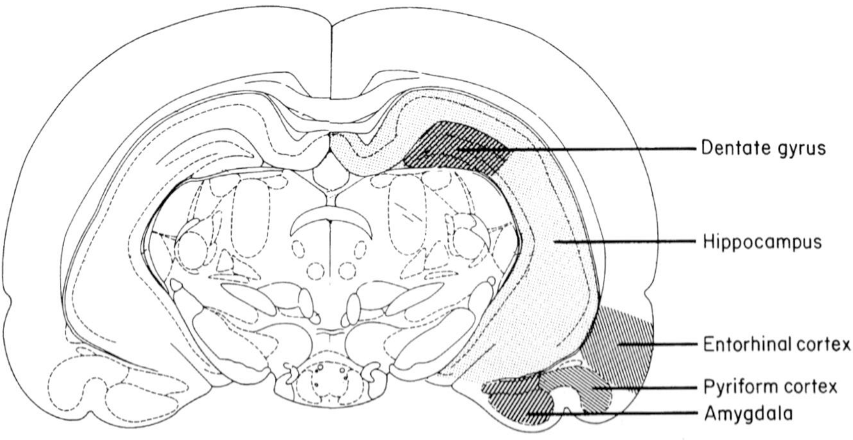

Figure 2. The structures of the rat brain relevant to this chapter are given in the hatched areas. (Modified from Paxinos and Watson, 1986.)

electrographic measure, namely the epileptiform after-discharge (AD) triggered by the local stimulation is typically about 10 s in duration with relatively weak propagation to anatomically related sites. With repetition of the stimulus, there is an increase in the discharge both with respect to duration, amplitude, and propagation; these changes are permanent. Thus if animals have been left for long periods of time a retest will show full strength electrographic responses.

Apart from the evoked responses kindling also comprizes the development of spontaneously occurring epileptiform events. Interictal spikes may appear after a few ADs have been evoked and following establishment of the fully kindled state they will last for several weeks. With continuation of daily kindling stimulations the animals will eventually begin to show spontaneous ictal events as well (Pinel, 1981).

Behavioural measures

Following the initial evoked discharge the typical response in the rat is an arrest followed by investigatory behaviour. With the progression of kindling there is a sequence of behavioural stages which have been described by Racine (1972). Stage 1 includes mouth movements, stage 2 clonic head movements, stage 3 forelimb clonus, stage 4 clonic rearing and stage 5 rearing and loss of postural control. Stages 4–5 are generally used as criteria for completion of kindling. If the animals are retested several months after they have been fully kindled, they have full strength behavioural responses (Wada and Sato, 1974). Of relevance for the behavioural (non-convulsive) aspects of kindling are reports that kindled animals were more reactive to certain stimuli when compared with non-kindled animals (Pinel *et al.*, 1977; Adamec and Stark-Adamec, 1983; Adamec, 1989).

Pharmacological kindling

The description of the kindling phenomenon given above relates to studies based on electrical stimulation of various limbic structure sites. Kindling, however, may be induced also pharmacologically by agonists of excitatory neurotransmitters, such as acetylcholine and possibly glutamate. As this chapter describes mainly findings from electrophysiological kindling studies, we shall only briefly mention that daily injections of the muscarinic agonist carbachol into the amygdala results in kindling as judged from the development of seizure activity ending with a truly epileptic state (Wasterlain and Jonec, 1983). Likewise, pharmacological kindling using other neurotransmitter agonists has been obtained in many, but not all situations studied. Actually only muscarinic kindling fulfils strict criteria for demonstration of pharmacological kindling (for a review, see Wasterlain *et al.*, 1989).

Repeated administration of the local anaesthetic lidocaine as well as of the mixed psychomotor stimulant and local anaesthetic cocaine eventually leads to seizures (Post *et al.*, 1984; Post and Weiss, 1989). In contrast to electrical kindling repeated administration of lidocaine evokes seizures in only less than half of the animals studied. These pharmacologically induced seizures have many behavioural similarities to those induced by electrical stimulation in the amygdala, and they show similar electrophysiological spiking. Further, animals which have had lidocaine-induced seizures respond faster than normal to electrical kindling of the amygdala (Post *et al.*, 1984). It is on the basis of these similarities between the effect of lidocaine treatment and kindling, that Post and coworkers (1987) and Ballenger and Post (1989) have hypothesized that abuse of stimulants and alcohol may result in a form of kindling (for a review, see Chapter 17, this volume). It can, however, not be excluded that altered pharmacokinetics may play a role for the development of seizures following repeated administration of those local anaesthetics (Hwai-Tzong Pan *et al.*, 1991). Sato and Okamoto (1981) showed that electrical kindling and its transfer to the contralateral site is inhibited by chronic pretreatment with cocaine and is facilitated by treatment with the dopamine antagonist pimozide. This points to cocaine or dopaminergic kindling having a quite different biological base than electrical kindling, and actually one that is rather antagonistic.

Status epilepticus can also be induced by local or systemic injection of the neurotoxin kainic acid (KA) (Ben-Ari, 1985). This model has several similarities with proper kindling, and the condition is most easily induced in animals already electrically kindled (McIntyre *et al.*, 1982). KA status epilepticus characteristically is accompanied by tissue damage which will lead to massive loss of neurons in various sites with increased prolongation of seizure activity (Ben-Ari *et al.*, 1981). It is noteworthy that like in electrical kindling the pyriform cortex is highly sensitive, but damage has also been demonstrated in the hippocampal formation (Milgram *et al.*, 1985).

ELECTRICAL KINDLING: SOME STUDIES OF MECHANISMS

Neurophysiological investigations

Following amygdala-stimulation, Racine *et al.* (1975) demonstrated a kindling-induced synaptic potentiation effect, and in 1983 showed potentiation effects within several pathways including the lateral olfactory tract and its target site, the pyriform cortex (Racine *et al.*, 1983). They formulated a synaptic potentiation hypothesis in which they viewed kindling as a memory model as well as an epilepsy model based upon the idea that kindling produced effects emerging from mechanisms similar to those underlying the 'long-term potentiation' (LTP) phenomenon. They later rejected this hypothesis (Racine *et al.*, 1986) mainly because of the difference in timing of the onset and saturation of LTP and that of the kindling phenomenon, as well as the difference observed in the rapid decay of LTP contrasting with the relative permanence of kindling; kindling and LTP also respond differently to pharmacological agents. Moreover, noradrenaline depletion by reserpine facilitates kindling, but has no effect on LTP. Finally, kindling, but not LTP, will induce development of spontaneous epileptiform events (interictal spikes (for a review, see Racine *et al.*, 1986).

If a decrease in strength takes place in the connection between cells at inhibitory synapses there might be a corresponding increase in excitatory drive. However using a paired pulse technique, whereby a second pulse will trigger a response during a period of inhibition, Tuff *et al.* (1983) found that inhibition actually was increased in the dentate gyrus following kindling. This phenomenon was also repeated by King *et al.* (1985) in studies of hippocampal slices, while conversely a decrease in inhibition has been reported in the hippocampal area CA1 by the same authors. Kindling may thus be associated with changes of both inhibitory and excitatory interactions.

An antagonistic interaction between the amygdala and hippocampus may play an important role. Thus, the first appearance of the convulsive response takes place after termination of the hippocampal AD when the electrical recording from that region becomes depressed and spiking from the amygdala reaches maximum amplitude (Racine *et al.*, 1977). Concurrent stimulation of the dorsal hippocampal region was shown by Burdette and

Dichter (1988) to weaken both electrographic response and convulsive activity elicited by amygdala-stimulation in amygdala kindled animals. There also seems to be facilitatory interactions between amygdala and hippocampus as exemplified by a reciprocal positive transfer of kindling between amygdala and hippocampus in cats (Sato, 1976). With alternately applied kindling stimulations in two different sites, one of them will dominate and kindle convulsions, while the other will show only a partial kindling effect (Burchfiel *et al.*, 1986). Taken together, these findings show that there seem to be inhibitory as well as excitatory interactions.

Metabolic labelling

Using the 2-deoxyglucose technique to measure metabolic activity in kindled brains during seizures several investigators have found enhanced glucose metabolism in several brain regions. Amygdala-kindled stage 1 and stage 2 seizures are accompanied by an increased metabolic activity in limbic regions: amygdala and its direct projection fields. In stage 1 and stage 5 seizures increased uptake of glucose is also observed in extra-limbic regions: substantia nigra, thalamic nuclei, globus pallidus, and neocortex (Engel *et al.*, 1978; Ackermann *et al.*, 1986). Thus the 2-deoxyglucose studies clearly demonstrate the propagation of the epileptiform activity throughout the brain during the kindling process; findings which are consistent with the changes seen in different brain sites during the evolution of after-discharge or interictal spikes independent of the primary kindled site (Wada and Sato, 1974). However, the electrically kindled state is not, in itself, accompanied by an increase in baseline glucose utilization (Engel *et al.*, 1978; Blackwood *et al.*, 1981).

c-fos Induction

The proto-oncogene *c-fos* produces a phosphoprotein Fos which regulates gene transcription processes. Fos has been proposed to couple synaptic transmission to changes in gene expression by acting in the cell nucleus in concert with other proteins to form complexes in the AP1 recognition site on enhancers of target genes. *c-fos* activation may thus be important for the study of various types of neural plasticity. *c-fos* activation has been demonstrated in kindled brain tissue with the most reactive areas being the pyriform cortex and the dentate gyrus (Dragunow and Robertson, 1987; Dragunow *et al.*, 1988). The relevance for kindling of *c-fos* is described elsewhere in this volume (Chapter 17).

Neurochemical studies

A great number of investigations have been conducted to elucidate the neurochemistry of epileptiform activity, but they have yielded partly conflicting results. This is probably due to the fact that a multitude of events take place when epileptiform activity is induced, and a lot of the observations which can be made are likely to be secondary phenomena. Pertinent reviews are given by MacNamara (1984), Corcoran (1986) and Burnham (1988). Of special relevance for the electrophysiological studies of a possible synaptic potentiation mechanism for kindling are investigations concerning the NMDA receptor, which seems to be involved in the phenomenon of LTP (Collingridge and Bliss, 1987). NMDA receptor antagonists have been shown to retard kindling at doses that fully blocked LTP, suggesting a special role of NMDA receptor activation in the induction of kindling. Further, a kindling-induced upregulation of the NMDA receptor-channel complex has been demonstrated (Yeh *et al.*, 1989). The studies of Morimoto (1989) in the kindling model of epilepsy point to activation and subsequent collapse of GABA-mediated inhibition in combination with activation of the NMDA receptor complex being critical for the development of kindling.

It seems evident that at least three inhibitory systems modulate seizure activity and are relevant for kindling: GABA, thyrotropin releasing hormone (TRH) and noradrenaline (NA). GABA and TRH, in relation to the role of inhibitory synapses in the kindling process, have recently been described in a review by Sato *et al.* (1990). In our laboratory the role of NA in hippocampal kindling has been studied and therefore this seizure-inhibiting neurotransmitter will be described in more detail below.

Noradrenaline and kindling

Depletion or blockade of NA systems in the brain (Arnold *et al.*, 1973; McIntyre *et al.*, 1979) potentiates amygdala-kindling in rats. Furthermore, α_2-adrenergic receptor binding in the amygdala and pyriform cortex is reduced after kindling (Chen and MacNamara, 1988). The neurotoxin 6-hydroxydopamine (6-OHDA) injected into the ventricles will lead to a degeneration of the catacholaminergic nerve terminals accompanied by a permanent depletion of the NA content of the rat forebrain. The dopamine content is likewise reduced while contents of GABA and 5-HT remain normal (Björklund *et al.*, 1986). If such animals are kindled, they will develop seizures faster than normal animals, following stimulation of both the hippocampus and the amygdala (McIntyre and Racine, 1986). Using this animal model of epilepsy, Barry and coworkers (1987) took NA-rich tissue from the fetal locus coeruleus region and implanted it bilaterally into the hippocampus of NA-depleted, hyperexcitable rats. With this new strategy, it was found possible to retard the development of seizures in hippocampal kindling. The study indicated that even with extensive lesions of the entire forebrain NA and dopamine neuron systems, a graft-derived noradrenergic reinnervation of only a restricted area, namely the hippocampus, was able to

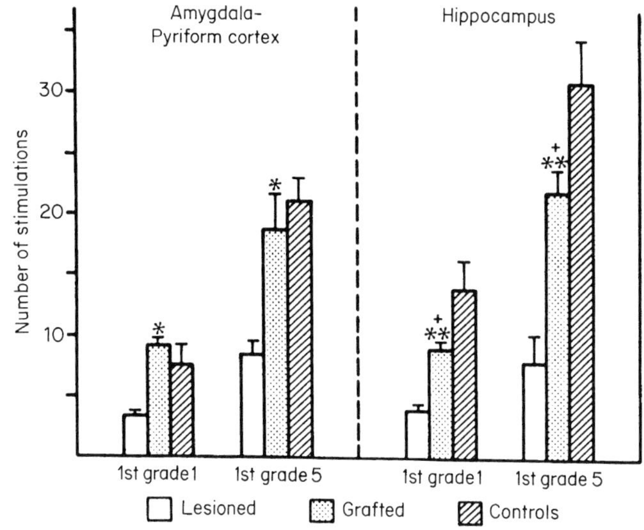

Figure 3. Number of daily stimulations to reach the first grade 1 and first grade 5 seizures in lesioned animals with sham grafts (glucose-saline), in grafted animals, and in normal controls. The figure compares the findings from the study with implantation of locus coeruleus tissue bilaterally into the amygdala-pyriform cortex (left) with the data obtained after grafting such tissue bilaterally into the hippocampus (right) (Barry *et al.*, 1987). Statistical differences were calculated using one-way analysis of variance (ANOVA) with post hoc Newman-Keuls' test. Grafted rats were significantly different from lesioned rats at *, $p < 0.05$ (amygdala-pyriform cortex group); or at **, $p < 0.01$ (hippocampus group; + grafted rats were significantly different from controls at $p < 0.05$. (Reproduced with permission, from Barry *et al.*, 1989.)

reverse the lesion-induced functional deficit, i.e. the facilitation of hippocampal kindling. Thus, functional recovery at least in this epilepsy model after 6-OHDA treatment does not seem to require reinstatement of noradrenergic neurotransmission in all denervated areas, but can be obtained by selective reinnervation of the stimulated structure, i.e. the site of epileptogenesis.

In a subsequent study (see Fig. 3) fetal locus coeruleus tissue was implanted either bilaterally into the amygdala-pyriform cortex (i.e. distant to the kindling site) or unilaterally into the hippocampus (close to the kindling site) (Barry *et al.*, 1989). Lesioned animals with either a sham graft or a control graft consisting of fetal striatal tissue showed a kindling rate faster than that of normal controls. The same applies to animals with locus coeruleus grafted unilaterally in hippocampus. In contrast, in rats with bilateral locus coeruleus grafts in the amygdala-pyriform cortex (implanted at three sites) the development of seizures was similar to that of controls and significantly slower than that in the lesioned animals with sham grafts. These findings indicate that grafting of fetal pontine tissue (rich in NA neurons) to a site distant to the stimulation focus, but important for the generalization and spread of seizures, can retard the seizure development in hippocampal kindling. Unilateral reinnervation of hippocampus did not normalize the kindling rate, and thus noradrenergic reinnervation of both hippocampi seems important for the seizure-suppressant action in hippocampal kindling. It should, however, be emphasized that such grafting has no influence on the severity or duration of established kindled seizures (Westerberg *et al.*, 1984). Furthermore, although kindling is associated with reduced NA inhibition of the limbic system (McIntyre and Racine, 1986) this does not result from inhibition of NA activity in the locus coeruleus, as the latter is normal during kindling (Bonhaus and MacNamara, 1987).

Neuronal and glial marker proteins

Current working hypotheses of kindling emphasize such changes in electrical properties of nerve cell membranes, which create hyper-responsive epileptic neurones (Racine *et al.*, 1986) and structural reorganization of neuronal connections (Geinisman *et al.*, 1988; Sutula *et al.*, 1988).

We shall describe recent investigations from our laboratory where we studied the possible role of synaptic remodelling in kindling by determining the concentration of a number of neuronal and glial marker proteins in the ventral and dorsal hippocampus, the pyriform cortex and the amygdala (Hansen *et al.*, 1990). As we planned to obtain information concerning especially the development of kindling we studied rats which were both partially and fully kindled. We stimulated electrically the limbic system through the ventro-caudal CA1/CA3 area of the hippocampus, which probably plays a minor role in the spread of seizure activity (Racine *et al.*, 1988), so as to avoid measuring any influence of direct mechanical damage to the amygdala which might result from the electrode placement.

Rats were subjected either to kindling (n=18) or sham-kindling (n=18), and they were given up to 44 single daily stimulations in the left hippocampus. Seizures were rated using the Racine severity scale. The animals were subdivided into a partially kindled group (n=6) having a single grade 2 seizure and a kindled group (n=12) defined as having had three grade 5 seizures. Following the experimental period, samples of hippocampus dentate gyrus and amygdala were collected. The cerebellum, which is not expected to be involved in the kindling process, served as a source of control tissue.

Using immunochemical methods the following neuronal marker proteins were investigated: NCAM, the neural cell adhesion molecule; D3-protein, a marker of synaptic membranes; and NSE, neurone specific enolase. The glial protein markers were GFAP, glial fibrillary acidic protein; S100, a soluble cytoplasmic protein, and GS, glutamine synthetase.

The main results of this series of experiments are given in the Figs 4 and 5, which show that in hippocampus, pyriform cortex and amygdala of fully kindled rats there was an increase in GFAP and in the glycolytic enzyme NSE. NSE, an enzyme catalysing one of the non-rate-limiting steps in the glycolytic pathway is an enolase isoenzyme specific for nerve cells (Bock and Dissing, 1975; Zomzely-Neurath, 1982). It is noteworthy that partial kindling had no significant effect on NSE whereas in the kindled rats NSE increased significantly bilaterally in all structures, mostly pronounced in the contralateral ventral hippocampus. This effect of full kindling on NSE is similar in direction but even more pronounced than that found following electroconvulsive stimulation in the rat (Jørgensen and Bolwig, 1979).

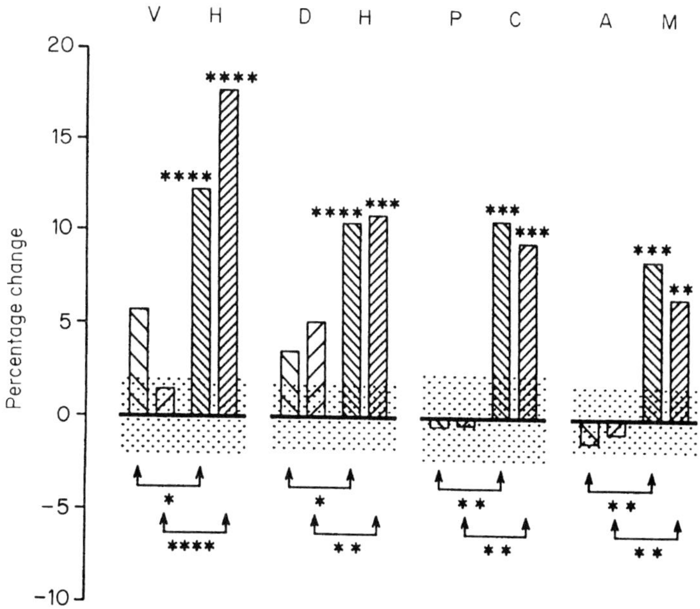

Figure 4. The concentration of NSE in four brain structures of partially kindled and kindled rats expressed as the percentage change from sham-kindled rats. From left to right: VH, ventral hippocampus; DH, dorsal hippocampus; PC, pyriform cortex; AM, amygdala. For each structure the four bars are: the ipsilateral hemisphere of the partially kindled group (broad stripes, slanting down), the contralateral hemisphere of the partially kindled group (broad stripes, slanting up), the ipsilateral hemisphere of the kindled group (narrow stripes, slanting down), and the contralateral hemisphere of the kindled group (narrow stripes, slanting up). Common SEM of group data is given by the dotted area along the baseline. *, $p < 0.05$; **, $p < 0.01$; ***, $p < 0.001$; ****, $p < 0.0001$. (Reproduced with permission, from Hansen *et al.*, 1990.)

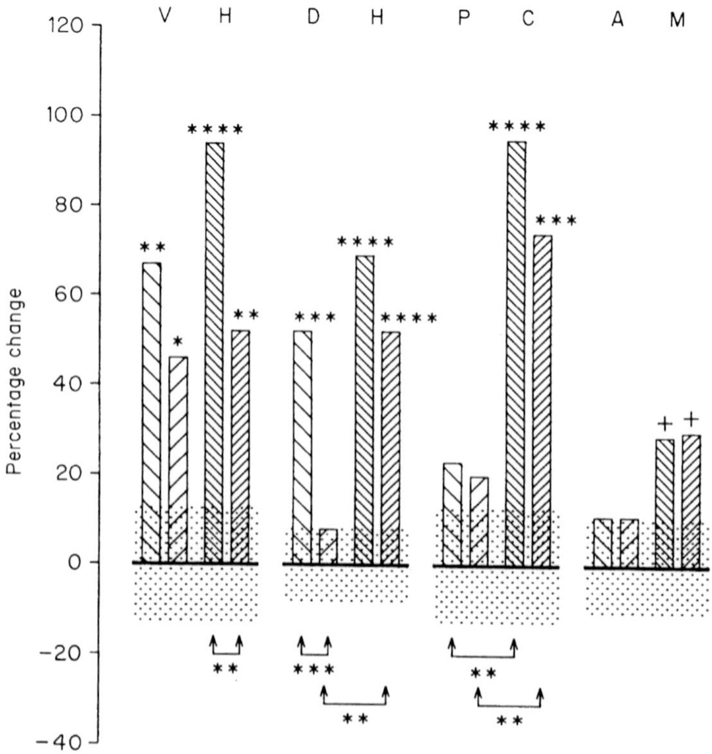

Figure 5. The concentration of GFAP in four brain structures of partially kindled and kindled rats expressed as the percentage change from sham-kindled rats. Symbols and abbreviations are as in Fig. 4 and +, $p < 0.02$. (Reproduced with permission, from Hansen *et al.*, 1990.)

GFAP, which is the major protein component of intermediate filaments in fibrous astrocytes is invariably synthesized when astrocytes are activated in response to injury or abnormally increased neuronal activity (Eng, 1988). The observed increase in GFAP in kindled rats is in good accordance with an as yet unpublished study mentioned in a recent review by Racine *et al.* (1989), who by immunohistochemistry demonstrated that amygdala-kindling results in astrogliosis in the amygdala and pyriform cortex. Our findings of increased GFAP and normal GS and S100 (Fig. 5) suggest that the GFAP increase in kindled rats is a result of astrocytes expressing more GFAP rather than an increased proliferation of glial cells. This increased GFAP is probably a consequence of a subtle neuronal degeneration or synaptic remodelling.

In a subsequent study (Hansen *et al.*, 1991) we investigated the concentration of GFAP over time in connection with hippocampal kindling. Again we

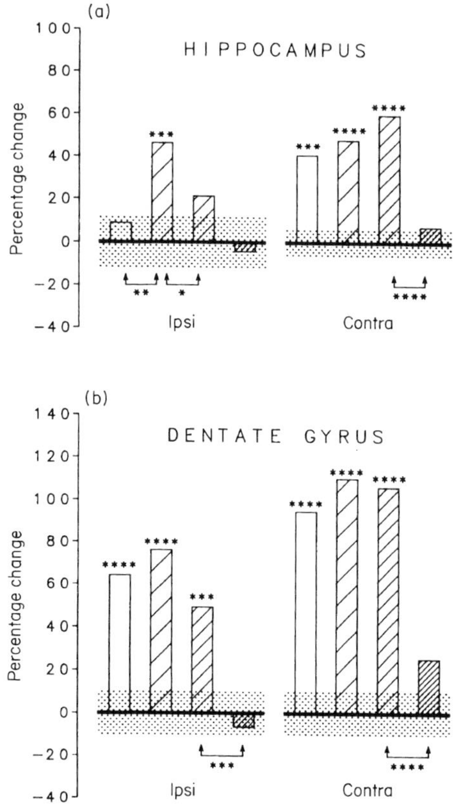

Figure 6. The concentration of GFAP, measured in arbitrary units, in the ipsilateral (stimulated) and contralateral hippocampus (a) and dentate gyrus (b) of kindled rats expressed as the percentage change from the mean value of the corresponding hemisphere of sham rats. The first bar in each set of four bars represents partially kindled rats; the second, (broad stripes), third (medium stripes), and fourth (narrow stripes) represent fully kindled rats with a post-kindling period of 24 h, 1 week, and 2 months, respectively. The dotted area along the baseline denotes the intergroup SEM estimate and is calculated from the intergroup variance component of the ANOVA analysis. *, $p < 0.05$; **, $p < 0.01$; ***, $p < 0.001$; ****, $p < 0.0001$. (Reproduced with permission, from Hansen *et al.*, 1991.)

studied partially and fully kindled rats after a post-kindling period of 24 h, 1 week and 2 months, respectively. In the limbic structures known to be involved in the kindling process, namely the hippocampus, the dentate gyrus, basolateral amygdala, pyriform cortex and entorhinal cortex the increase in GFAP concentration was maximal in the fully kindled animals studied after 24 h. In most brain areas the concentration was still elevated 1 week after

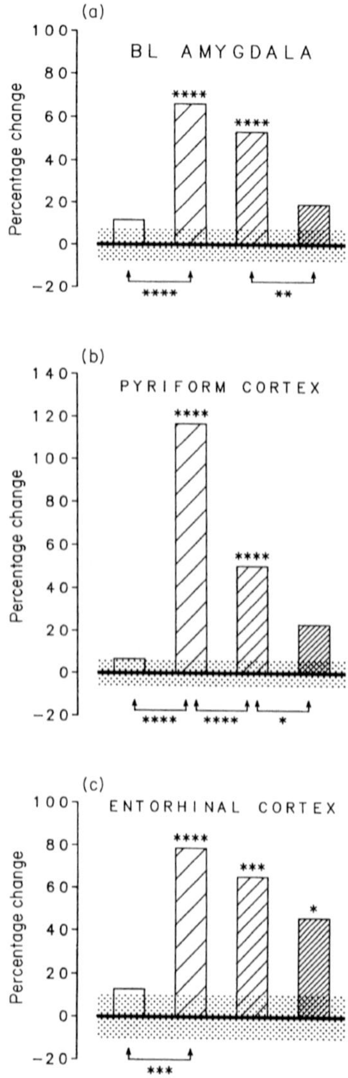

Figure 7. The concentration of GFAP, measured in arbitrary units, in the basolateral amygdala (a), pyriform cortex (b), and entorhinal cortex (c) of kindled rats expressed as the percentage change from the sham value. Values from the ipsilateral and contralateral hemispheres were not different and are therefore pooled. Bars are as Fig. 6. (Reproduced with permission, from Hansen *et al.*, 1991.)

kindling, but following 2 months post-kindling it had declined to control level. The GFAP increase appeared earlier in the hippocampus and dentate gyrus (i.e. in partially kindled animals) than in the other structures, probably because stimulation was applied to the CA1/CA3 area of the left hippocampus (Figs 6 and 7). It is noteworthy that the increase in the dentate gyrus was about twice that in the hippocampus proper, possibly indicating a greater sensitivity to kindling, a suggestion which is supported by the finding by Sutula *et al.* (1988) who found histological evidence that kindling induces synaptic reorganization in this area without any detectable neuronal loss. However, neuronal loss has actually been observed in the hilar polymorphic region of the dentate gyrus following brief seizures evoked by kindling (Cavazos and Sutula, 1990).

We find that the localization of the changed brain marker proteins fits well the working hypothesis for kindling proposed by Racine *et al.* (McIntyre and Racine, 1986; Racine *et al.*, 1986, 1988), which points to repeated activation of a forebrain site evoking an epileptiform discharge that will be transmitted to target areas of the stimulated structure, and thereby through abnormal discharge alter the response characteristic of neurons within the secondary sites as demonstrated by appearance of interictal spike activity and stronger ictal response. The limbic structures most susceptible to these changes are initially the amygdala/pyriform area and subsequently the entorhinal cortex and ventral hippocampus. In our study we observed an elevated GFAP concentration in these same areas, suggesting that activation of astrocytes is closely related to structures showing electrophysiological signs of independent epileptiform activity. As the elevation of GFAP concentration was not permanent, but began to decline after the electrical stimulation was stopped, GFAP does not appear to reflect directly the permanent change in brain function that characterizes kindling. We interpret this GFAP increase to be a transient kindling-induced activation of astrocytes triggered by subtle degeneration of neuronal processes and synapses.

Kindling is associated with neuronal degeneration

For many years it has been considered one of the attractions of the kindling model that it is free of much of the gross focal damage seen in the chemically induced models of epilepsy. Looking, however, at the induction of status epilepticus following injection with kainic acid (KA), the first indications of the cell damage produced may be quite subtle (Ben-Ari *et al.*, 1981), and such changes might also be induced during electrical kindling. The above-mentioned recent report by Cavazos and Sutula (1990) points to kindling as a mechanism which can induce histologically detectable neuronal loss, and our observation of an increase in the concentration of GFAP points to an activation of astrocytes indicative of degenerative changes in nearby neurons. Thus, not only during models of chemically induced epileptic status is there neural disruption, but degenerative changes also could be of importance in the development of electrical kindling.

CONCLUDING REMARKS

Since the first description of the kindling paradigm there has been a rapid increase in studies reflecting a multi-disciplinary pursuit of the mechanisms of kindling. Though a great number of hypothesis-generating studies have been conducted, no unitary theory for this highly relevant and intriguing process has so far been established. However, we find that the evidence of neuronal or synaptic degeneration is compelling. Certain structures within the limbic system are more important for the generation and maintenance of kindling than others, but experimental studies have yielded conflicting results. However, the recent development of our knowledge of kindling mechanisms produced through contributions from many research areas seems highly promising, and it is to be expected that within the next few years more light will be shed over some of the controversies which exist today.

The importance of the limbic system for our understanding of behaviour, affects and emotions, learning and memory, epilepsy and a number of neuropsychiatric syndromes has long been recognized. A better knowledge of the mechanisms underlying the kindling phenomenon may well be a bridge across one of the gaps which exist between basic and clinical research.

ACKNOWLEDGEMENTS

This study was supported by grants from the Danish Medical Research Council, Eli and Egon Larsen's Fund, and the Lundbeck Foundation.

REFERENCES

Ackermann, R.F., Chungani, H.T., Handforth, A., Moshé, S., Caldecott-Hazard, S. and Engel Jr, J. (1986). Autographic studies of cerebral metabolism and blood flow in rat amygdala kindling. In: Wada, J.A. (Ed.), *Kindling 3*, Raven Press, New York, pp. 73–90.

Adamec, R.E. (1989). Kindling, anxiety and personality. In: Bolwig, T.G. and Trimble, M.R. (Eds), *The Clinical Relevance of Kindling*, Wiley, Chichester, pp. 117–135.

Adamec, R.E. and Stark-Adamec, C. (1983). Limbic kindling and animal behaviour—implications for human psychopathology associated with complex partial seizures. *Biol. Psychiatry*, **18**, 269–293.

Arnold, P.S., Racine, R.J. and Wise, R.A. (1973). Effects of atropine, reserpine, 6-hydroxydopamine, and handling on seizure development in the rat. *Exp. Neurol.*, **40**, 457–470.

Ballenger, J.C. and Post, R.M. (1978). Potentiation of ethanol withdrawal by prior dependence. *Psychopharmacology*, **133**, 1–14.

Ballenger, J.C. and Post, R.M. (1989). Addictive behavior and kindling: relationship to alcohol withdrawal and cocaine. In: Bolwig, T.G. and Trimble, M.R. (Eds), *The Clinical Relevance of Kindling*, Wiley, Chichester, pp. 231–258.

Barry, D.I., Kikvadze, I., Brundin, P., Bolwig, T.G., Björklund, A. and Lindvall, O. (1987). Grafted noradrenergic neurons suppress seizure development in kindling-induced epilepsy. *Proc. Natl Acad. Sci. USA*, **84**, 8712–8715.

Barry, D.I., Wanscher, B., Kragh, J., Bolwig, T.G., Kokaia, M., Brundin, P., Björklund, A. and Lindvall, O. (1989). Grafts of fetal locus coeruleus neurons in rat amygdala-piriform cortex suppress seizure development in hippocampal kindling. *Exp. Neurobiol.*, **106**, 125–132.

Ben-Ari, Y. (1985). Limbic seizure and brain damage produced by kainic acid: mechanisms and relevance to human temporal lobe epilepsy. *Neuroscience*, **14**, 375–403.

Ben-Ari, Y., Trenblay, E., Riche, D., Ghilini, G. and Naquet, R. (1981) Electrographic, clinical and pathological alterations following systemic administration of kainic acid, bicuculline or pentetrazole: metabolic mapping using the deoxyglucose method with special reference to the pathology of epilepsy. *Neuroscience*, **6**, 1361–1391.

Björklund, A., Nornes, H. and Gage, F.H. (1986). Cell suspension grafts of noradrenergic locus coeruleus neurons in rat hippocampus and spinal cord: reinnervation and transmitter turnover. *Neuroscience*, **18**, 685–698.

Blackwood, D.H.R., Kapoor, V. and Martin, M.J. (1981). Regional changes in cerebral glucose utilization associated with amygdaloid kindling and electroshock in the rat. *Brain Res.*, **224**, 204–208.

Bock, E. and Dissing, J. (1975). Demonstrations of enolase activity connected to the brain-specific protein 14-3-2. *Scand. J. Immunol.*, **4** (Suppl. 2), 31–36.

Bolwig, T.G. and Trimble, M.R. (Eds) (1989). *The Clinical Relevance of Kindling*, Wiley, Chichester.

Bonhaus, D.W. and MacNamara, J.O. (1987). Activity of locus coeruleus neurons in amygdala kindled rats: role in the suppression of afterdischarge. *Brain Res.*, **407**, 102–109

Burchfiel, J.L., Applegate, C.D. and Konkol, R.J. (1986). Kindling antagonism: a role for norepinephrine in seizure suppression. In: Wada, J.A. (Ed.), *Kindling 3*, Raven Press, New York, pp. 213–229.

Burdette, L.J. and Dichter, M.A. (1988). Dorsal hippocampal stimulation suppresses amygdaloid kindled seizures. *Neurosci. Abstr.*, **14**, 1149.

Burnham, W.M. (1988). Receptor binding in the kindling model of epilepsy. In: Sen, A.K. and Lee, T. (Eds), *Receptors and Ligands in Neurological Disorders*, Cambridge University Press, Cambridge, pp. 171–210.

Cavazos, J. and Sutula, T. (1990). Progressive neuronal loss induced by kindling: a possible mechanism in mossy fibre reorganization and hippocampal sclerosis. *Brain Res.*, **527**, 1–6.

Chen, L.S. and MacNamara, J.O. (1988). Autographic localization of reduced α_2-adrenergic receptor binding in kindled rats. *Neurosci. Abstr.*, **14**, 1148.

Clemmesen, L. and Hemmingsen, R. (1984). Physical dependence on ethanol during multiple intoxication and withdrawal episodes in the rat: evidence of a potentiation. *Acta Pharmacol. Toxicol.*, **55**, 345–350.

Clemmesen, L., Ingvar, M., Hemmingsen, R. and Bolwig, T.G. (1988). Local cerebral glucose consumption during ethanol withdrawal in the rat: effects of single and multiple episodes and previous convulsive seizures. *Brain Res.*, **453**, 204–214.

Collingridge, G.L. and Bliss, T.V.P. (1987). NMDA receptors—their role in long-term potentiation. *Trends Neurosci.*, **10**, 288–293.

Corcoran, M.E. (1986). Studies of some neurochemicals and kindling. In: Wada, J.A. (Ed.), *Kindling 3*, Raven Press, New York, pp. 333–347.
Dragunow, M. and Robertson, H.A. (1987) Generalized seizures induce c-fos protein(s) in mammalian neurons. *Neurosci. Lett.*, **82**, 157–161.
Dragunow, M., Robertson, H.A. and Robertson, G.S. (1988). Amygdala kindling and c-fos protein(s). *Exp. Neurol.*, **102**, 261–263.
Eng, L.F. (1988). Regulation of glial intermediate filaments in astrogliosis. In: Norenberg, M.D., Hertz, L. and Schousboe, A. (Eds), *The Biochemical Pathology of Astrocytes*, Alan R. Liss, New York, pp. 79–90.
Engel Jr, J., Wolfson, L. and Brown, L. (1978). Anatomical correlates of electrical and behavioral events related to amygdaloid kindling. *Ann. Neurol.*, **86**, 483–492.
Geinisman, Y., Morrell, F. and Morrell, L.D. (1988). Remodeling of synaptic architecture during hippocampal 'kindling'. *Proc. Natl Acad. Sci. USA*, **85**, 3260–3264.
Glenthøj, B., Hemmingsen, R., Allerup, P. and Bolwig, T.G. (1990). Intermittent versus continuous neuroleptic treatment in a rat model. *Eur. J. Pharmacol.*, **190**, 275–286.
Goddard, G.V. (1967). Development of epileptic seizures through brain stimulation at low intensity. *Nature*, **214**, 1020–1021.
Goddard, G.V., McIntyre, D.C. and Leech, C.K. (1969). A permanent change in brain function resulting from daily electrical stimulation. *Exp. Neurol.*, **25**, 295–330.
Hansen, A., Jørgensen, O.S., Bolwig, T.G. and Barry, D.I. (1990). Hippocampal kindling alters the concentration of glial fibrillary acidic protein and other marker proteins in rat brain. *Brain Res.*, **531**, 307–311.
Hansen, A., Jørgensen, O.S., Bolwig, T.G. and Barry, D.I. (1991). Hippocampal kindling in the rat is associated with time-dependent increases in the concentration of glial fibrillary acidic protein. *J. Neurochem.*, **57**, 716–720.
Hwai-Tzong Pan, Menacherry, S. and Justice Jr, J.B. (1991). Differences in the pharmacokinetics of cocaine in naive and cocaine-experienced rats. *J. Neurochem.*, **56**, 1299–1306.
Jørgensen, O.S. and Bolwig, T.G. (1979). Synaptic proteins after electroconvulsive stimulation. *Science*, **205**, 705–707.
Kairiss, E.W., Racine, R.J. and Smith, G.K. (1984). Development of interictal spike during kindling in the rat. *Brain Res.*, **322**, 101–110.
King, G.L., Dingledine, R., Giacchino, J.L. and MacNamara, J.O. (1985). Abnormal neuronal excitability in hippocampal slices from kindled rats. *J. Physiol. (London)*, **54**, 1295–1304.
McIntyre, D.C. and Plant, J.R. (1989). Pyriform cortex involvement in kindling. *Neurosci. Biobehav. Rev.*, **13**, 177–280.
McIntyre, D.C. and Racine, R.J. (1986). Kindling mechanisms: current progress on an experimental epilepsy model. *Prog. Neurobiol.*, **27**, 1–12.
McIntyre, D.C., Saari, M. and Pappas, B.A. (1979). Potentiation of amygdala kindling in adult or infant rats by injection of 6-hydroxy-dopamine. *Exp. Neurol.*, **63**, 527–544.
McIntyre, D.C., Nathanson, D. and Edson, N. (1982). A new model of partial status epilepticus based on kindling. *Brain Res.*, **250**, 53–63.
MacNamara, J.O. (1984). Role of neurotransmitters in seizure mechanisms in the kindling model of epilepsy. *Fed. Proc. Fed. Am. Soc. Exp. Biol.*, **43**, 2516–2520.
Milgram, N.W., Green, I., Liberman, M., Riexinger, K. and Petit, T.L. (1985). Establishment of status epilepticus by limbic system stimulation in previously unstimulated rats. *Exp. Neurol.*, **88**, 253–264.
Morimoto, K. (1989). Seizure triggering mechanisms in the kindling model of epilepsy: collapse of GABA-mediated inhibition and activation of NMDA receptors. *Neurosci. Behav. Rev.*, **13**, 253–260.

Paxinos, G. and Watson, C. (1986). *The Rat Brain in Stereotaxic Coordinates*, Academic Press, Australia.
Pinel, J.P. (1981). Spontaneous kindled motor seizures in rats. In: Wada J.A. (Ed.), *Kindling 2*, Raven Press, New York, pp. 179–192.
Pinel, J.P.J., Treit, D. and Rowner, L.I. (1977). Temporal lobe aggression in rats. *Science*, **197**, 1088–1089.
Post, R.M. and Kopanda, R.T. (1976). Cocaine, kindling and psychosis. *Am. J. Psychiatry*, **133**, 627–634.
Post, R.M. and Weiss, S.R.B. (1989). Kindling and manic-depressive illness. In: Bolwig, T.G. and Trimble, M.R. (Eds), *The Clinical Relevance of Kindling*, Wiley, Chichester, pp. 209–230.
Post, R.M., Kennedy, C., Shinohara, M., Squillace, K., Miyaoka, M., Suda, S., Ingvar, D.H. and Sokoloff, L. (1984). Metabolic and behavioral consequences of lidocaine-kindled seizures. *Brain Res.*, **324**, 295–304.
Post, R.M., Weiss, S.R.B., Pert, A. and Uhde, T.W. (1987). Chronic cocaine administration: sensitization and kindling effects. In: Raskin, A. and Fisher, S. (Eds), *Cocaine: Clinical and Biobehavioral Aspects*, Oxford University Press, New York, pp. 109–173.
Racine, R.J. (1972). Modification of seizure activity by electrical stimulation. II. Motor seizure. *Electroencephalogr. Clin. Neurophysiol.*, **32**, 281–294.
Racine, R.J., Newberry, F. and Burnham, W.M. (1975). Post-activation potentiation and the kindling phenomenon. *Electroencephalogr. Clin. Neurophysiol.*, **39**, 261–271.
Racine, R.J., Rose, P.A. and Burnham, W.M. (1977). Afterdischarge thresholds and kindling rates in dorsal and central hippocampus and dentate gyrus. *Can. J. Neurol. Sci.*, **4**, 273–278.
Racine, R.J., Milgram, N.W. and Hafner, S. (1983). Long-term potentiation phenomena in the rat limbic forebrain. *Brain Res.*, **260**, 217–231.
Racine, R.J., Burnham, W.M., Gilbert, M. and Kairiss, E.W. (1986). Kindling mechanisms: I. Electrophysiological studies. In: Wada, J.A. (Ed.), *Kindling 3*, Raven Press, New York, pp. 263–282.
Racine, R.J., Paxinos, G., Mosher, J.M. and Kairiss, E.W. (1988). The effects of various lesions and knife-cuts on septal and amygdala kindling in the rat. *Brain Res.*, **454**, 264–274.
Racine, R.J., Ivy, G.O. and Milgram, N.W. (1989). Kindling: clinical relevance and anatomical substrate. In: Bolwig, T.G. and Trimble, M.R. (Eds), *The Clinical Relevance of Kindling*, Wiley, Chichester, pp. 15–34.
Sato, M. (1976). A study on psychomotor epilepsy with 'kindled' cat preparations. *Folia Psychiatr. Neurol. Jpn*, **30**, 426–434.
Sato, M. and Okamoto, M. (1981). Dopaminergic kindling and electrical kindling. In: Wada, J.A. (Ed.), *Kindling 2*, Raven Press, New York, pp. 105–121.
Sato, M., Racine, R.J. and McIntyre, D.C. (1990). Kindling: basic mechanisms and clinical validity. *Electroencephalogr. Clin. Neurophysiol.*, **76**, 459–472.
Stevens, J.R. and Livermore, A. (1978). Kindling in the mesolimbic dopamine system: animal model of psychosis. *Neurology*, **28**, 36–46.
Sutula, T., He, X.X., Cavazos, J. and Scott, G. (1988). Synaptic reorganization in the hippocampus induced by abnormal functional activity. *Science*, **239**, 1147–1150.
Trimble, M.R. (1991). *The Psychoses of Epilepsy*, Raven Press, New York.
Tuff, L.P., Racine, R.J. and Adamec, R. (1983). The effects of kindling on GABA-mediated inhibition in the dentate gyrus of the rat. I. Paired-pulse depression. *Brain Res.*, **277**, 79–90.

Wada, J.A. (1986). *Kindling 3*, Raven Press, New York.

Wada, J.A. and Sato, M. (1974). Generalized convulsive seizures induced by daily electrical stimulation of the amygdala in cats: correlative electrographic and behavioral features. *Neurology*, **24**, 565–574.

Wasterlain, C.G. and Jonec, V. (1983). Chemical kindling by muscarinic amygdaloid stimulation in the rat. *Brain Res.*, **271**, 311–323.

Wasterlain, C.G., Morin, A.M., Fujikawa, D.G. and Bronstein, J.M. (1989). Chemical kindling. In: Bolwig, T.G. and Trimble, M.R. (Eds), *The Clinical Relevance of Kindling*, Wiley, Chichester, pp. 35–53.

Westerberg, V., Lewis, J. and Corcoran, M.E. (1984). Depletion of noradrenaline fails to affect kindled seizures. *Exp. Neurol.*, **84**, 237–240.

Yeh, G.C., Bonhaus, D.W., Nadler, J.V. and MacNamara, J.O. (1989). N-methyl-D-aspartate receptor plasticity in kindling: quantitative–qualitative alterations in N-methyl-D-aspartate receptor-channel complex. *Proc. Natl Acad. Sci. USA*, **86**, 8157–8160.

Zomzely-Neurath, C.E. (1982). Nervous system—specific proteins: 14-3-2 protein, antigen alpha and neuron specific enolase. *Scand. J. Immunol.*, **15** (Suppl. 9), 1–40.

The Temporal Lobes and the Limbic System
Edited by M.R. Trimble and T.G. Bolwig

6

Antiepileptics and the Hippocampus

MARKUS SCHMUTZ, FELIX BRUGGER, HUGO BÜRKI, THOMAS FERRAT, ADELHEID HAUSDORF, KLAUS KLEBS, CHANTAL PORTET, MARIO POZZA, MARTIN STEINMANN AND HANS-RUDOLF OLPE
Research and Development Department, Pharmaceuticals Division, Ciba-Geigy Ltd, Basel, Switzerland

INTRODUCTION

Among the frequently occurring epilepsies, those involving the temporal lobe have the worst prognosis. Such patients tend to show a poor response to treatment and a higher incidence of psychiatric difficulties than patients suffering from most other forms of epilepsies (Rodin *et al.*, 1976). From an anatomical point of view, temporal epileptic seizures are associated with hippocampal sclerosis (Margerison and Corsellis, 1966; Sano and Malamud, 1953; Scheibel *et al.*, 1974). Therefore, spike-suppressing effects of drugs in hippocampal tissue may be indicative of therapeutic efficacy in (temporal lobe) epilepsies and, possibly, psychiatric disorders. From *in vitro* studies using rat hippocampal slices (Schmutz *et al.*, 1987) as well as from *in vivo* experiments in rats and cats with hippocampal stimulation (Kamei *et al.*, 1981; Schmutz *et al.*, 1981) it is known that antiepileptic drugs such as carbamazepine, phenytoin, phenobarbital, the benzodiazepines and valproate can suppress epileptic spiking. At present, the mechanisms underlying these effects are only partly understood.

In this chapter we want to concentrate on two drugs which are used in the epilepsies as well as in affective disorders, i.e. carbamazepine and valproate. Recently, some new findings on (mainly hippocampal) interactions of these compounds with dopamine, GABA, NMDA and ion channels have emerged, providing new insights into the putative modes of action of carbamazepine and valproate (Table 1; Figs 1 and 2). It is the goal of this chapter to review these findings. Two hypotheses dealing with mechanisms

Table 1. Summary of important effects of carbamazepine and valproate which may contribute to the modes of action of these drugs in epilepsies and affective disorders.

Effects	*Carbamazepine*	*Valproate*
Dopamine turnover	Reduced	Reduced
GABA turnover	Reduced	Reduced
GABA transmission	0	Increased
K^+ conductance	Increased	0
Na^+ channels	Blocked	Blocked

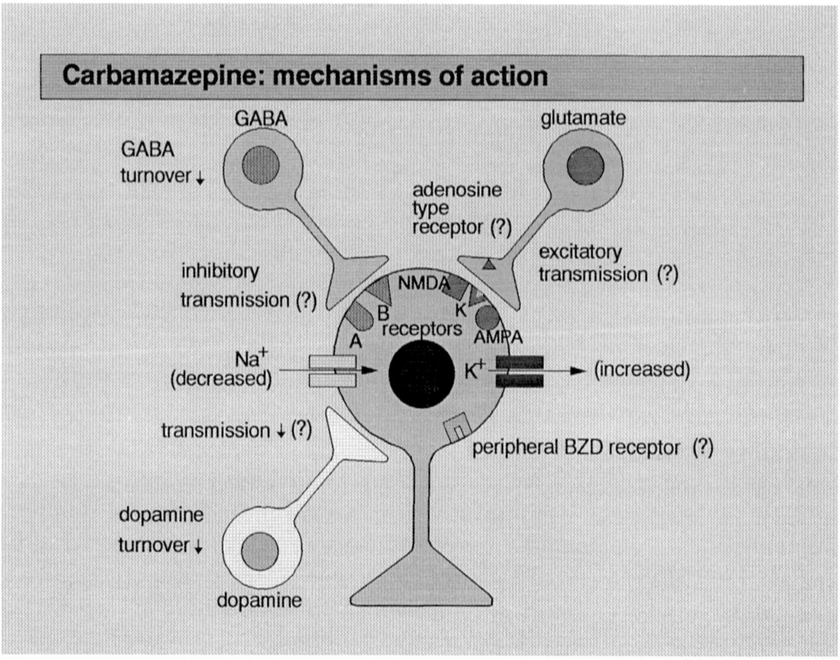

Figure 1. Putative mechanisms of action of carbamazepine. ? = Equivocal experimental results or doubtful clinical significance of the respective mode of action.

of actions of carbamazepine and valproate in affective disorders are discussed, followed by the other major pharmacological characteristics probably responsible for the drugs' antiepileptic effects. It should be mentioned, however, that the antiepileptic features could well contribute to the antimanic effects and vice versa.

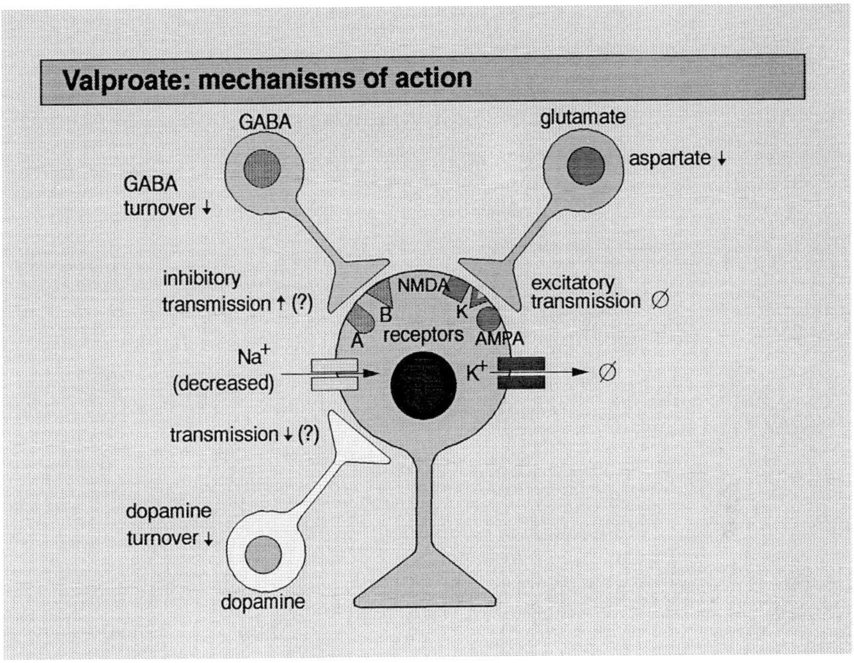

Figure 2. Putative mechanisms of action of valproate. ? = Equivocal experimental results or doubtful clinical significance of the respective mode of action.

PUTATIVE MODES OF ACTION OF CARBAMAZEPINE AND VALPROATE IN AFFECTIVE DISORDERS

Emrich *et al.* (1980) proposed the GABA-hypothesis of affective disorders. One of the pillars of this hypothesis was the observation that valproate and, at high doses, carbamazepine reduce the GABA turnover in rodents (see Bernasconi *et al.*, 1984a). This effect was interpreted to reflect the GABA-facilitating feature of the drugs, which in turn leads to a reduction in transmitter turnover. The molecular basis for these effects is not well understood. In the case of carbamazepine, electrophysiological studies have not demonstrated an acute effect on GABA transmission in the hippocampus (Hood *et al.*, 1983; Olpe *et al.*, 1985), and no affinity to the GABA receptor has been reported. It is therefore conceivable that the reduction of GABA turnover by carbamazepine results from an inactivation of Na^+ channels located on GABA cells, leading to limitation of neuronal cell firing (see below; Macdonald, 1988) and thus to a reduction of transmitter turnover. On the other hand, there is evidence for an interaction of valproate with GABA transmission. Schmutz *et al.* (1979) originally observed that valproate enhances exogenously applied GABA responses of cortical neurons *in vivo*. Subsequent investigations performed in hippocampal slices were controversial and only one study reported a potentiating effect at therapeutic concentrations (Olpe *et al.*, 1988).

In a more recent study we demonstrated (unpublished results) that valproate moderately potentiates GABA transmission *in vivo* in the CA1 area of the hippocampus. In chloral hydrate anaesthetized rats intravenously administered valproate, but not carbamazepine, potentiated paired-pulse inhibition of the population spike at doses of 30 and 100 mg/kg. Diazepam and phenobarbital elicited the same qualitative effect in the hippocampal CA1 area as valproate. This was most probably due to their affinity to the $GABA_A$ receptor–chloride channel complex.

About a decade ago Bunney and Garland (1982) published a modified version of the original catecholamine hypothesis of affective disorders. They postulated that an increase in central dopamine activity is linked with mania. This hypothesis is in keeping with the recent finding that carbamazepine and valproate exert a depressant effect on dopamine turnover (Waldmeier, 1987). Both drugs reduced dopamine synthesis dose-dependently, as measured by the accumulation of DOPA after inhibition of central decarboxylase. The biochemical basis for the drugs' depressant effect on dopamine turnover is unknown. It is conceivable, as in the case of the GABA hypothesis discussed above, that the primary site of action is at the level of the use- and voltage-dependent Na^+ channels (Macdonald, 1988). Since carbamazepine and valproate show anticonvulsant activity in some (but not all) kindling models (Kamei *et al.*, 1981; Post and Weiss, 1987; Schmutz, 1987; Schmutz and Klebs, 1989), it is of interest to note that limbic kindling may induce a lasting hyperdopaminergic function (see Adamec, 1990; Schmutz, 1987). This would be in line with the hypothesis that kindling-like processes may underly the evolution of psychiatric disorders in some settings and the observation that patients with temporal lobe epileptic seizures show a comparatively high incidence of psychiatric difficulties (Rodin *et al.*, 1976). However, at present there is relatively little evidence directly linking the anticonvulsant activity of carbamazepine and valproate in some of the kindling models to their therapeutic efficacy in affective disorders (Post and Weiss, 1987). In addition, the selective effectiveness of the drugs in some models of kindling and not others (Post and Weiss, 1987; Schmutz and Klebs, 1989) argues against the hypothesis that the drugs' therapeutic potential in any psychiatric disorder implicates a kindling-like mechanism in the disorder's pathophysiology. Moreover, in the case of carbamazepine and valproate the importance of temporal lobe dysfunction cannot be deduced, since both drugs are highly effective in convulsive syndromes not involving the temporal lobes (Post and Uhde, 1985).

PUTATIVE ANTIEPILEPTIC MODES OF ACTION OF CARBAMAZEPINE AND VALPROATE

Since no specific receptors have been described for carbamazepine or valproate, the most 'basic' known site of action was until recently the Na^+ channel. For instance, it was shown that at therapeutic concentrations, carbamazepine occupied about 50% of sites associated with Na^+ channels (Willow *et al.*, 1984). In addition, in electrophysiological investigations carbamazepine and valproate suppressed the Na^+ channel dependent high-frequency firing of cultured central neurons (Macdonald, 1988). These findings are in keeping with older studies on peripheral nerves (Honda and Allen, 1973) or voltage-clamped *Myxicola* axons (Schauf *et al.*, 1974). They are further supported from *in vitro* experiments on rat hippocampal slices where carbamazepine reduced Schaffer commissural fibre excitability at therapeutic concentrations, a property which is likely to result from blockade of Na^+ channels (Hood *et al.*, 1983; Olpe *et al.*, 1985). However, K^+ channels also may contribute to the antiepileptic effects of carbamazepine as discovered recently by two laboratories. Carbamazepine was shown to increase K^+ currents in rat cortical neurons at therapeutic concentrations (Zona *et al.*, 1990) and, in hippocampal slices made 'epileptic' by the exposure to penicillin, the spike-suppressing effect of carbamazepine was strongly attenuated by the K^+ channel blockers 4-aminopyridine and $BaCl_2$ (Olpe *et al.*, 1991). No effect on K^+ channels was observed in the case of valproate (Zona and Avoli, 1990). Given the important role of K^+ ions in the control of neuronal activity, these findings point to a possibly important function of K^+ channels in mediating the therapeutic effects of carbamazepine in epilepsy and/or affective disorders.

With regard to inhibitory neurotransmission, the interactions of valproate with GABA may well contribute to the drug's antiepileptic properties too, whereas there is much less evidence for such a relationship in the case of carbamazepine. Concerning excitatory neurotransmission, the hippocampal formation has proven to be a particularly suitable brain area for study since glutamate is thought to be the main neurotransmitter in the hippocampus. In biochemical investigations it was shown that carbamazepine reduces the (^{3}H)L-glutamate release with a threshold concentration of 10 μM, which is well within the therapeutic concentration range (Olpe *et al.*, 1985). Also in electrophysiological studies performed on hippocampal slices, carbamazepine has been shown to reduce excitatory transmission in the hippocampal formation when tested at this low concentration (Hood *et al.*, 1983; Olpe *et al.*, 1985). These findings are in agreement with previous *in vivo* investigations demonstrating that carbamazepine diminishes excitatory transmission in the cat trigeminal nucleus (Fromm *et al.*, 1982). On the other hand, carbamazepine does not bind to glutamate receptors and in a recent study the compound failed to affect the release of endogenous glutamate (Fagg and Thedinga, personal communication). The latter finding is supported by our recent observation (unpublished results) that in the CA1 area of the hippocampus therapeutic doses of carbamazepine did not attenuate extracellularly recorded EPSPs which were evoked by electrical stimulation of Schaffer commissural fibres. The important role of one of the subtypes of glutamate receptors, N-methyl-D-aspartate (NMDA), in mediating epileptic activity is well documented (e.g. Cavalheiro *et al.*, 1988), and it was recently reported that carbamazepine blocks NMDA-activated currents in cultured spinal neurons (Lampe and Bigalke, 1990). We verified this hypothesis, but failed to confirm the findings with carbamazepine (unpublished results). In the hemisected neonate rat spinal cord, carbamazepine at 40 μM had only a small nonselective depressant effect on responses evoked by NMDA, quisqualate and kainate. *In vivo*, the compound at the dose of 30 mg/kg i.p. was also without effect on the excitatory responses of hippocampal CA1 pyramidal neurons evoked by iontophoretically applied quisqualate, kainate or NMDA. Furthermore, turning behaviour induced in mice by subcutaneously administered NMDA was not antagonized by carbamazepine at doses of 10 and 60 mg/kg p.o. According to Zeise *et al.* (1991), valproate suppressed NMDA-evoked transient depolarizations in the rat neocortex *in vitro*. However, in preliminary, unpublished electrophysiological *in vitro* and *in vivo* studies we only observed weak effects of valproate on NMDA-induced responses in hippocampal tissue. In addition, NMDA-induced turning behaviour in mice was not affected by valproate at doses of 100 and 600 mg/kg p.o. (Portet and Jeker, personal communication.)

The effects of carbamazepine and/or valproate on GABA transmission, glutamate release, fibre excitability, high-frequency neuronal discharges and ion channels (Table 1; Figs 1 and 2) act synergistically in the direction of stabilizing hippocampal neuronal circuitry. This could be demonstrated *in vitro* in hippocampal slices (Schmutz *et al.*, 1987) as well as *in vivo* in awake cats provided with implanted hippocampal electrodes for stimulation and recording (Schmutz *et al.*, 1981). In close correlation with the aforementioned biochemical and neurophysiological findings, carbamazepine, and, to a lesser degree, valproate, suppressed penicillin-induced spiking *in vitro* and, under *in vivo* conditions, the evoked hippocampal after-discharges.

CONCLUSIONS

In conclusion, we have reviewed some of the recent findings on the mechanisms of action of carbamazepine and valproate bearing on their therapeutic effectiveness in diseases involving the hippocampus, i.e. temporal lobe epilepsy and, probably, affective disorders (see Table 1 and Figs 1 and 2). It is noteworthy that the list of pharmacological effects described for these two drugs includes additional features that have not been discussed in this paper (for reviews, see Bernasconi *et al.*, 1984b; Löscher, 1985; Post *et al.*, 1984; Schmutz, 1985; Schmutz *et al.*, 1987; Zieglgänsberger and Völger, 1987). The selection of pharmacological features highlighted here represents effects that we believe are currently considered to be particularly important.

It appears plausible that interference with voltage-sensitive Na^+ channels is one primary mode of action of both carbamazepine and valproate. In the case of carbamazepine, but not valproate, K^+ channel opening may represent another, 'basic' mechanism of action. The depressant action of both drugs on GABA and dopamine turnover and on repetitive neuronal firing could all possibly result from such interactions with ion channels. Whereas reduction of dopamine turnover could mainly contribute to the antimanic properties of the drugs, the Na^+ (carbamazepine and valproate) and K^+ channel interactions (carbamazepine only) as well as the reduction of GABA turnover (carbamazepine and valproate) and the potentiation of GABA transmission (valproate only) may well contribute to their therapeutic potential in epilepsies as well as affective disorders. The fact that only some of the reviewed actions are shared by both drugs, further demonstrates that the therapeutic effectiveness of different compounds in a given disorder may be based on different biological mechanisms.

REFERENCES

Adamec, R.E. (1990). Does kindling model anything clinically relevant? *Biol. Psychiatry*, **27**, 249–279.

Bernasconi, R., Schmutz, M., Martin, P. and Hauser, K. (1984a). GABA hypothesis for the mechanism of action of antiepileptic drugs: its usefulness and limitations. In: Fariello, R.G., Morselli, P.L., Lloyd, K.G., Quesney, L.F. and Engel Jr, J. (Eds), *Neurotransmitters, Seizures and Epilepsy II*, Raven Press, New York, pp. 95–107.

Bernasconi, R., Hauser, K., Martin, P. and Schmutz, M. (1984b). Biochemical aspects of the mechanism of action of valproate. In: Emrich, H.M., Okuma, T. and Müller, A.A. (Eds), *Anticonvulsants in Affective Disorders*, Elsevier Science Publishers, Amsterdam, pp. 14–32.

Bunney, W.E. and Garland, B.L. (1982). A second generation catecholamine hypothesis. *Pharmacopsychiatry*, **15**, 111–115.

Cavalheiro, E.A., Lehmann, J. and Turski, L. (1988). *Frontiers in Excitatory Amino Acid Research*, Liss, New York.

Emrich, H.M., Zerssen, D., Kissling, W., Möller, H.J. and Windorfer, A. (1980). Effect of sodium valproate on mania. *Arch. Psychiatr. Nervenkr.*, **229**, 1–6.

Fromm, G.H., Chattha, A.S., Terrence, C.F. and Glass, J.D. (1982). Do phenytoin and carbamazepine depress excitation and/or facilitate inhibition? *Eur. J. Pharmacol.*, **78**, 403–409.

Honda, H. and Allen, M.B. (1973). The effect of an imminostilbene derivative (G 32883) on peripheral nerves. *J. Med. Assoc. Ga.*, **62**, 38–42.

Hood, T.W., Siegfried, J. and Haas, H.L. (1983). Analysis of carbamazepine actions in hippocampal slices of the rat. *Cell. Mol. Neurobiol.*, **3**, 213–222.

Kamei, C., Oka, M., Masuda, Y. and Shimizu, M. (1981). Effects of 3-sulfamoylmethyl-1,2-benzisoxazole (AD-810) and some antiepileptics on the kindled seizures in the neocortex, hippocampus and amygdala in rats. *Arch. Int. Pharmacodyn. Ther.*, **249**, 164–176.

Lampe, H. and Bigalke, H. (1990). Carbamazepine blocks NMDA-activated currents in cultured spinal cord neurons. *Neuropharmacol. Neurotoxicol.*, **1**, 8–10.

Löscher, W. (1985). Valproic acid. In: Frey, H.-H. and Janz, D. (Eds), *Antiepileptic Drugs*, Springer Verlag, Berlin, pp. 507–536.

Macdonald, R.L. (1988). Anticonvulsant drug actions on neurons in cell culture. *J. Neural Transm.*, **72**, 173–183.

Margerison, J.H. and Corsellis, J.A. (1966). Epilepsy and the temporal lobes. *Brain*, **89**, 499–530.

Olpe, H.R., Baudry, M. and Jones, R.S.G. (1985). Electrophysiological and neurochemical investigations on the action of carbamazepine on the rat hippocampus. *Eur. J. Pharmacol.*, **110**, 71–80.

Olpe, H.R., Steinmann, M.W., Pozza, M.F., Brugger, F. and Schmutz, M. (1988). Valproate enhances GABA-A mediated inhibition of locus coeruleus neurones *in vitro. Naunyn-Schmiedeberg's Arch. Pharmacol.*, **338**, 655–657.

Olpe, H.R., Kolb, C.N., Hausdorf, A. and Haas, H.L. (1991). *Experientia*, **47**, 254–257.

Post, R.M. and Uhde, T.W. (1985). Are the psychotropic effects of carbamazepine in manic-depressive illness mediated through the limbic system? *Psychiatr. J. Univ. Ottawa*, **10**, 205–219.

Post, R.M., Uhde, T.W. and Ballenger, J.C. (1984). Efficacy of carbamazepine in affective disorders: implications for underlying physiological and biochemical substrates. In: Emrich, H.M., Okuma, T. and Müller, A.A. (Eds), *Anticonvulsants in Affective Disorders*, Elsevier Science Publishers, Amsterdam, pp. 93–115.

Post, R.M. and Weiss, S.R.B. (1987). Behavioral pharmacology of carbamazepine: differential effects on kindling. *Int. Clin. Psychopharmacol.*, **2** (Suppl. 1), 51–72.

Rodin, E.A., Katz, M. and Lennox, K. (1976). Differences between patients with temporal lobe seizures and those with other forms of epileptic attacks. *Epilepsia*, **17**, 313–320.

Sano, K. and Malamud, N. (1953). Clinical significance of sclerosis of cornu ammonis; ictal 'psychic phenomena'. *Arch. Neurol. Psychiatry*, **70**, 40–53.

Schauf, C.L., Davis, F.A. and Marder, V. (1974). Effect of carbamazepine on the ionic conductance of Myxicola giant axons. *J. Pharmacol. Exp. Ther.*, **189**, 538–543.

Scheibel, M.E., Crandall, P.H. and Scheibel, A.B. (1974). The hippocampal-dentate complex in temporal lobe epilepsy. *Epilepsia*, **15**, 55–80.

Schmutz, M. (1985). Carbamazepine. In: Frey H.-H. and Janz, D. (Eds), *Antiepileptic Drugs*, Springer Verlag, Berlin, pp. 479–506.

Schmutz, M. (1987). Relevance of kindling and related processes to human epileptogenesis. *Prog. Neuropsychopharmacol. Biol. Psychiatry*, **11**, 505–525.

Schmutz, M. and Klebs, K. (1989). Kindling and antiepileptic drugs. In: Bolwig, T.G. and Trimble, M.R. (Eds), *The Clinical Relevance of Kindling*, Wiley, Chichester, pp. 55–68.

Schmutz, M., Olpe, H.R. and Koella, W.P. (1979). Central actions of valproate sodium. *J. Pharm. Pharmacol.*, **31**, 413–414.

Schmutz, M., Bürki, H. and Koella, W.P. (1981). Electrically induced hippocampal after-discharge in the freely moving cat: an animal model of focal (possibly temporal lobe) epilepsy. In: Dam, M., Gram, L. and Penry, J.K. (Eds), *Advances in Epileptology*, Raven Press, New York, pp. 59–65.

Schmutz, M., Klebs, K., Mondadori, C. and Olpe, H.R. (1987). Das pharmakologische Profil des Carbamazepin. In: Krämer, G. and Hopf, H.Ch. (Eds), *Carbamazepin in der Neurologie*, Thieme Verlag, Stuttgart, pp. 4–13.

Waldmeier, P.C. (1987). Is there a common denominator for the antimanic effect of lithium and anticonvulsants? *Pharmacopsychiatry*, **20**, 37–47.

Willow, M., Kuenzel, E.A. and Catterall, W.A. (1984). Inhibition of voltage-sensitive sodium-channels in neuroblastoma cells and synaptosomes by the anticonvulsant drugs diphenylhydantoin and carbamazepine. *Mol. Pharmacol.*, **25**, 228–234.

Zeise, M.L., Kasparow, S. and Zieglgänsberger, W. (1991). Valproate suppresses N-methyl-D-aspartate-evoked, transient depolarizations in the rat neocortex *in vitro*. *Brain Res.*, **544**, 345–348.

Zieglgänsberger, W. and Völger, J. (1987). Zum Wirkungsmechanismus von Carbamazepin: Neurophysiologische Aspekte. In: Krämer, G. and Hopf, H.C. (Eds), *Carbamazepin in der Neurologie*, Thieme Verlag, Stuttgart, pp. 18–25.

Zona, C. and Avoli, M. (1990). Effects induced by the antiepileptic drug valproic acid upon the ionic currents recorded in rat neocortical neurons in cell culture. *Exp. Brain Res.*, **81**, 313–317.

Zona, C., Tancredi, V., Palma, E., Pirrone, G.C. and Avoli, M. (1990). Potassium currents in rat cortical neurons in culture are enhanced by the antiepileptic drug carbamazepine. *Can. J. Physiol. Pharmacol.*, **68**, 545–547.

The Temporal Lobes and the Limbic System
Edited by M.R. Trimble and T.G. Bolwig

7

In vivo Imaging of the Temporal Lobe Limbic System

JEROME ENGEL JR
Departments of Neurology and Anatomy and Cell Biology and the Brain Research Insitute, UCLA School of Medicine, Los Angeles, California, USA

INTRODUCTION

The past decade has witnessed tremendous advances in noninvasive neurodiagnostic technologies capable of producing three-dimensional images of both structure and function of the human brain. With spatial resolution now in the range of millimetres for these techniques, intersubject variations in cerebral anatomy, as well as intersubject and intrasubject variations in a variety of aspects of function within specific cerebral structures, can be identified. Consequently, modern clinicians and scientists can noninvasively define abnormalities of mesial temporal limbic structure and function associated with various neurological and psychiatric clinical conditions, and examine alterations in functions of these cerebral structures associated with normal as well as abnormal behaviours. Until recently, our understanding of the role of mesial temporal limbic structures in normal and abnormal behaviours of humans was based on inferences derived from post-mortem studies of brain structure, effects of pathological lesions, physiological experiments carried out in animal models and, in a limited extent, intracranial EEG recordings of patients with temporal lobe epilepsy. These new imaging techniques make it possible to design experiments that will more directly investigate the role of the mesial temporal limbic system in human health and disease.

STRUCTURAL IMAGING

The standard clinical diagnostic tests for imaging cerebral structure have depended on roentgenographic techniques including plain skull X-rays, cerebral angiography, pneumoencephalography, and, more recently, X-ray computed tomography (XCT). The development of magnetic resonance imaging (MRI) now provides the highest spatial resolution of all structural imaging rechniques, without the risks associated with radiation exposure. XCT and MRI have largely replaced earlier diagnostic radiographic evaluations of cerebral structure in most medical centres. MRI is usually preferred except for conditions associated with subtle intracerebral calcifications that may be better visualized on XCT, and in patients with indwelling ferrous appliances, such as pacemakers, that would be adversely affected by the strong magnetic field. MRI also is associated with a small but disturbingly real risk of death for patients who need to be sedated for the procedure and, therefore, must be left for long periods of time in the bowels of the scanner, where adequate cardiorespiratory monitoring is impossible.

Magnetic resonance imaging

MR images are constructed from complex signals emitted from tissues with differential magnetic susceptibilities that are revealed by application of high strength magnetic fields (Brant-Zawadzki and Norman, 1987). Exceptional cerebral anatomic detail can now be displayed on the T1-weighted images obtained with the latest generation 1.5 Tesla scanners. T1-weighted images are particularly helpful for identifying specific structural lesions such as tumours and vascular malformations, as well as atrophy. Of particular relevance to this book is the fact that hippocampal anatomy is readily identified with T1 images of the 1.5 Tesla MRI, particularly when coronal sections are used (Fig. 1). In patients with temporal lobe epilepsy, asymmetries of hippocampal volume can often be readily appreciated by visual analysis of these images, with the smaller hippocampus corresponding to the presence of hippocampal sclerosis (Berkovic *et al.*, 1991). Quantitative volumetric measurement techniques are now being used to identify statistically significant asymmetries (Cascino *et al.*, 1991); however, the advantage of this quantitative approach over more qualitative visual analysis remains to be demonstrated.

T2-weighted MRI images reveal a different aspect of cerebral structure with high intensity signals reflecting areas of higher water content, such as oedema or CSF. Localized zones of high intensity on the T2-weighted image that are unassociated with corresponding disturbances on the T1-weighted image have been referred to as 'unidentified bright objects' (UBOs). Mesial temporal UBOs are commonly encountered in patients with temporal lobe epilepsy (Laster *et al.*, 1985; Lattack *et al.*, 1986), but no definitive pathological substrate has yet been identified, and this finding has been considered nonspecific (Sperling *et al.*, 1986). Although it has been suggested that these abnormal signals reflect physiological, rather

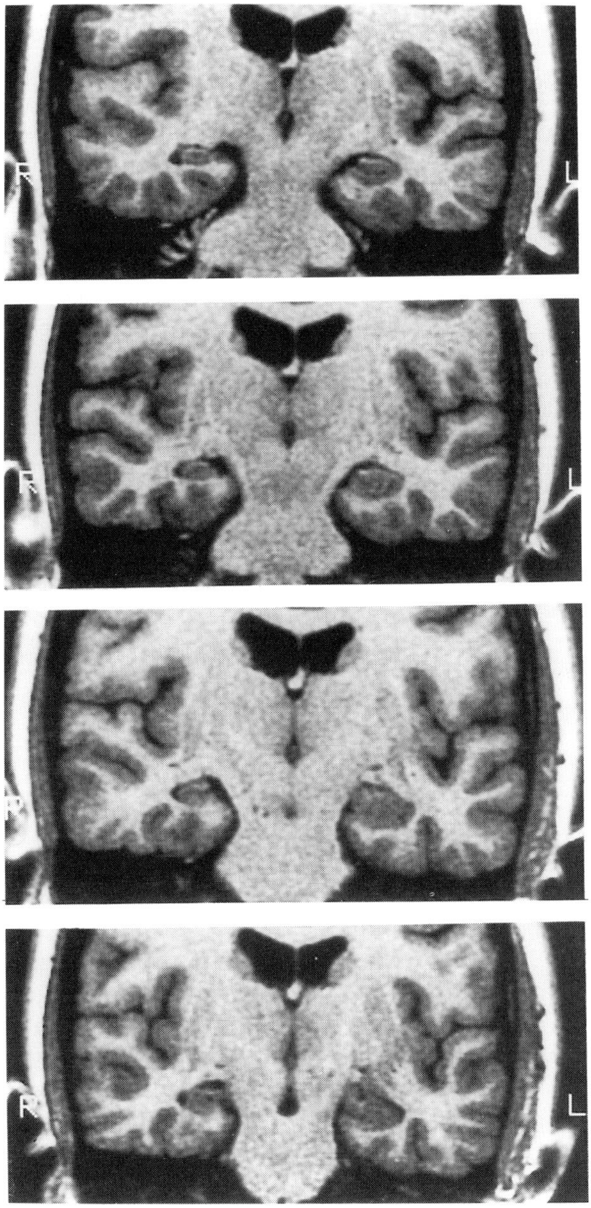

Figure 1. High resolution MRI inversion recovery image using a 1.5 Tesla GE Sigma Scanner, TR:1500, TE:20.0, TI:650. The exquisite anatomical detail that is revealed allows clear visualization of mesial temporal structures. In this patient with temporal lobe epilepsy, the hippocampal asymmetry is apparent, with the smaller hippocampus being the site of seizure onset. (Reproduced by courtesy of Dr John Bentson, UCLA Department of Radiology.)

than structural, disturbances related to epileptogenicity, there is no evidence that they change in relation to seizure occurrence (Ryvlin *et al.*, 1992a). Discrete 'hippocampal' hyperintensity on the T2-weighted image, however, often corresponds to hippocampal atrophy seen on the T1 image, and these two findings taken together appear to strongly indicate the presence of hippocampal sclerosis (Berkovic *et al.*, 1991). In this situation, the hyperintensity on the T2-weighted image most likely represents CSF within the temporal horn, which is dilated as a result of hippocampal atrophy, rather than the parenchymal hyperintensity that characterizes a UBO.

In addition to identifying specific lesions and atrophy underlying limbic system pathology, structural imaging is also useful for basic research on the normal human brain. For instance, anatomical differences between right and left hemisphere structure in the same individual can be correlated with hemispheric dominance for specific behaviours (Galaburda *et al.*, 1978). MRI-reconstructed images are also useful as anatomical templates for data obtained from tests of cerebral function. For instance, results of PET studies can be superimposed on corresponding MRI cross-sectional images (Zhang *et al.*, 1990; Pelizzari *et al.*, 1989; Mazziotta *et al.*, 1990), and the scalp distribution of event-related EEG potentials can be superimposed on MRI reconstruction of the cortical surface (Gevins *et al.*, 1990) of individual subjects, to determine more precisely which cerebral structures are involved in the functional changes under investigation.

Roentgenographic studies

Standard skull X-rays, as well as cerebral angiography and XCT, still have their place in clinical diagnosis of neurologic disorders. The last application of pneumoencephalography, localization of intracerebral structures for depth electrode implantation, has now been replaced in almost all centres by XCT, or, more recently, by MRI stereotactic techniques (Levesque *et al.*, 1990). Cerebral angiography is particularly important for precise identification of cerebrovascular abnormalities when surgery is necessary, and in defining the normal vascular supply of cerebral structures when stereotactic procedures are being planned. Stereotactic digital subtraction angiography is now commonly used for this latter purpose, and can be superimposed on stereotactically-acquired MRI images for planning depth electrode trajectories (Levesque *et al.*, 1990). Cerebral angiography is also important for defining the extent of vascular distribution of the carotid artery, and presence or absence of contralateral perfusion, in order to analyse the results of the modified intracarotid amytal test (Wada test) used to assess memory function of each hemisphere independently. Aberrant vascular distributions can result in inaccurate conclusions regarding the ability of one mesial temporal lobe to support memory (Rausch and Risinger, 1990). Because blood vessels can be visualized on MRI scans as a flow void, cerebral angiograms reconstructed from high resolution MRI scans may eventually replace invasive cerebral angiography.

FUNCTIONAL IMAGING

Positron emission tomography (PET) and single photon emission computed tomography (SPECT) are the two techniques in current use for *in vivo* functional imaging of the human brain. PET utilizes tracers labelled with positron emitting isotopes. Positron annihilation results in the release of two photons, which travel in opposite directions. Therefore, a technique known as coincidence detection can be used to reconstruct high resolution images of tracer localization within the brain (Phelps *et al.*, 1983). Positron-emitting isotopes can readily be incorporated into a wide variety of biologically active compounds, providing the opportunity to measure many different aspects of cerebral function. Because these isotopes are short-lived, they can be used for relatively dynamic studies; but it is necessary to have ready access to a medical cyclotron. SPECT, on the other hand, uses standard single photon-emitting radionuclide tracers that can be obtained commercially without the need for a cyclotron facility. Spatial resolution, however, is considerably less than for PET, and only tracers that measure cerebral perfusion non-quantitatively are currently readily available. SPECT does have one major advantage over PET for studies of epilepsy. Tracers labelled with single photon-emitting isotopes can be kept by the bedside and easily injected on call, permitting routine performance of ictal or immediate postictal SPECT scans of spontaneous seizures.

Positron emission tomography

Table 1 shows a list of cerebral functions that can be monitored by tracers used in positron emission tomography. Most clinical studies of limbic system pathophysiology carried out on patients with epilepsy have used ^{18}F-fluorodeoxyglucose (FDG), which provides images of local cerebral metabolic rate for glucose (LCMRGlc). Spatial resolution of the latest generation PET scanners, with FDG, is about 5 mm, which provides excellent visualization of cerebral structures as small as the hippocampus in the resting state. Quantitative analysis of PET scan data has been greatly enhanced by the techniques that allow superimposition of PET scans on MRI scans, in order to construct specific anatomical regions of interest that permit small structures such as the hippocampus to be distinguished from adjacent temporal cortex (Zhang *et al.*, 1990; Pelizzari *et al.*, 1989; Mazziotta *et al.*, 1990).

Table 1. Examples of tracers used in positron emission tomography of brain.

Process	*Tracer*
Blood flow	$H_2{}^{15}O$, $C^{15}O_2$, ^{85m}Kr, $CH_3{}^{18}F$, ^{11}C-alcohols
Blood volume	$C^{15}O$-RBC, ^{11}CO-RBC, ^{68}Ga-labelled EDTA
Tissue pH	^{11}C-DMO, $^{11}CO_2$
Transport and metabolism	
Oxygen	^{15}O-O_2
Glucose, glucose analogues, carbohydrates	2-deoxy-2-^{18}F-fluoro-D-glucose, 2-^{11}C-deoxy-D-glucose, ^{11}C-D-glucose, 3-O-^{11}C-methyl-D-glucose, ^{11}C-lactate, -pyruvate, -acetate, -succinate, -oxaloacetate
Amino acids: ^{13}N	L-^{13}N-glutamate, -glutamine, -alanine, -aspartate, -leucine, -valine, -isoleucine, -methionine
Amino acids: ^{11}C	L-^{11}C-aspartate, -glutamate, -valine, -leucine, -phenylalanine, -methionine; D,L-^{11}C-1-aminocyclopentane carboxylic acid, -1-aminocyclobutane carboxylic acid
Molecular diffusion	^{68}Ga-EDTA
Protein synthesis	L-1-^{11}C-leucine, -methionine, -phenylalanine, L-^{11}C-methyl-methionine
Receptor systems	
Dopaminergic	^{18}F-spiperone, ^{11}C-spiperone, ^{11}C-raclopride, ^{75}Br- and ^{76}Br-*p*-bromospiperone, ^{18}F-haloperidol, ^{11}C-pimozide, ^{11}C-methyl-, -ethylspiperone, L-^{11}C-dopa, 6-^{18}F-fluoro-L-dopa, ^{18}F-ethyl-spiperone
Cholinergic	^{11}C-imipramine, ^{11}C-QNB
Benzodiazepine	^{11}C-flunitrazepam, -diazepam, -RO15-1788, ^{18}F-fluorovalium
Opiate	^{11}C-etorphine, N-methyl-^{11}C-morphine, ^{11}C-heroin, -carfentanil
Adrenergic	^{11}C-norepinephrine, -propranolol
Anticonvulsants	^{11}C-valproate, -diphenylhydantoin

Reproduced with permission, from Engel, 1989.

Studies of epilepsy with FDG-PET have revealed zones of hypometabolism in the interictal state which include, but are usually larger than, the epileptogenic region identified electrophysiologically, and the specific structural epileptogenic lesion identified by pathological analysis of surgically resected tissue (Fig. 2) (Engel *et al.*, 1982a,b,c; Theodore *et al.*, 1984; Abou-Khalik *et al.*, 1987). Interictal hypometabolism is much more commonly encountered in patients with complex partial seizures of mesial temporal origin than in patients with epileptogenic regions involving neocortex (Henry *et al.*, 1992). Hippocampal sclerosis is usually associated with localized hypometabolism that involves lateral as well as mesial temporal cortex, and often extratemporal structures, most commonly ipsilateral thalamus, followed by ipsilateral basal ganglia and frontal lobe (Henry *et al.*, 1990). Involvement of these structures in the enduring interictal dysfunction associated with temporal lobe epilepsy suggests a role in genesis or propagation of complex partial seizures that remains to be eluci-

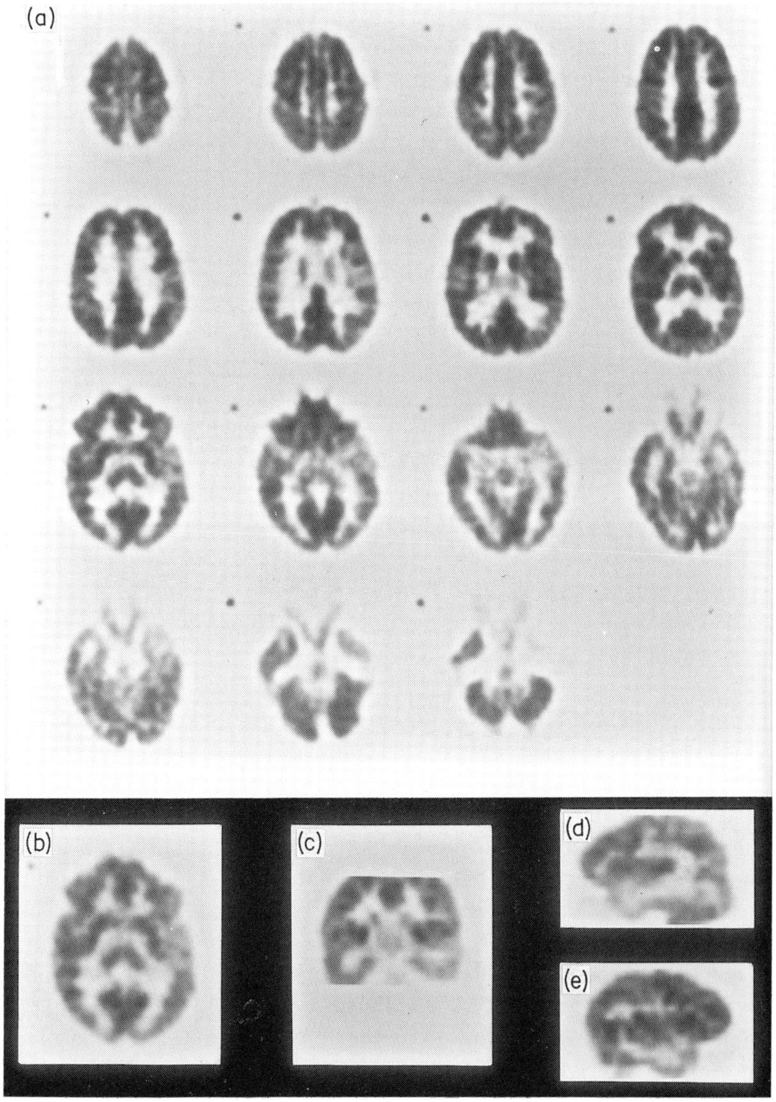

Figure 2. PET scan with FDG from a patient with complex partial seizures of left mesial temporal origin. This scan was performed on a Siemens-CTI 831 tomograph with an in plane resolution of approximately 5 mm. Fifteen horizontal planes of section are obtained simultaneously, and one or more sets of planes can then be reformatted into coronal, sagittal, or other planes as desired. The PET scan of this patient demonstrates mild left temporal hypometabolism, which can be seen on all horizontal planes of section through the temporal lobe shown in (a), and enlarged for one section in (b). The hypometabolism can also be appreciated in the coronal section (c) and in sagittal section through the left temporal lobe (d), when compared with the sagittal section through the right temporal lobe (e). (Reproduced with permission, from Engel, 1989.)

dated. Interictal hypometabolism of the epileptogenic region is presumed to reflect hypoactivity of neurons in the areas where habitual seizures originate, and either reduced input to, or primary hypoactivity in, their projection fields (Engel, 1990). This hypoactivity may be due to enhanced inhibitory tone that develops in response to epileptic seizures in order to maintain the interictal state and to prevent spread of ictal discharge. The mechanisms of naturally-occurring seizure-suppressing influences are unknown; however, it is unlikely to involve GABA-mediated inhibition, since this is associated with hyper- rather than hypometabolism (Ackermann *et al.*, 1984).

A variety of ictal metabolic patterns have been demonstrated with FDG-PET obtained during spontaneous seizures. Complex partial seizures of limbic origin are usually associated with hypermetabolism in the area of ictal onset and immediate propagation, and hypometabolism in the remainder of the brain (Engel *et al.*, 1983). The hypometabolism is believed to reflect postictal contributions to the functional image, which is averaged over 40–60 min. In some cases, limbic seizures may be associated only with localized hypometabolism, perhaps representing more restricted postictal changes. Simple partial seizures, without alteration in consciousness, can produce widespread areas of hypermetabolism without hypometabolism, presumably due to less pronounced postictal disturbances (Engel *et al.*, 1983). Petit mal absences, which have no associated postictal depression, either behaviourally or electrographically, produce profound generalized hypermetabolism on PET (Engel *et al.*, 1985), while generalized convulsions may yield diffuse hyper- or hypometabolism, depending upon the duration of postictal depression (Ackermann *et al.*, 1986). These complicated ictal metabolic patterns can be analysed in more detail by superimposing the PET scan on an MRI scan in order to identify the specific anatomical structures involved in hyper- and hypometabolic changes (Colour section, Plate 1), and by correlating these findings with ictal electrographic propagation recorded with depth electrodes (Engel *et al.*, unpublished observations). It is anticipated that comparison of data from these analyses with results of interictal PET studies will allow the use of routine interictal PET to predict the cerebral structures involved in some specific ictal events, and to determine the anatomical substrates of certain individual ictal behaviours. Such investigations could also elucidate the role of specific limbic structures in normal behaviours.

Other positron emitting isotope-labelled tracers have been used to study patients with epilepsy. PET images of cerebral blood flow and oxygen metabolism have demonstrated interictal and ictal patterns that qualitatively resemble those obtained with FDG (Kuhl *et al.*, 1980; Bernardi *et al.*, 1983; Yamamoto *et al.*, 1983). More recently, disturbances in μ opiate (Frost *et al.*, 1988; Mayberg *et al.*, 1991) and benzodiazepine (Savic *et al.*, 1988) receptor binding have been identified in temporal lobes of patients with complex partial seizures. The opiate receptor studies are of particular interest since they demonstrated enhanced receptor binding in the temporal neocortex ipsilateral to ictal onset, that correlated directly with the degree of hypometabolism seen with FDG. Endogenous opioids are known to exert an inhibitory influence on principal cortical neurons (Dingledine, 1981), to suppress epileptic seizures (Caldecott-Hazard and Engel, 1987; Rocha *et al.*, 1991), and to produce cortical hypometabolism (Chugani *et al.*, 1984); consequently, interictal seizure-suppressing mechanisms may be mediated in part by endogenous opioids, which in turn could contribute to localized hypometabolism. If this were the case, the presence and degree of hypometabolism seen on FDG-PET might be used as a measure of interictal seizure-suppressing influences.

Endogenous opioids participate in the appearance of certain postictal behaviours in experimental animal models (Caldecott-Hazard and Engel, 1987), and it has been postulated that enduring alterations in opioid mechanisms may account for certain interictal behavioural disturbances such as depression (Engel *et al.*, 1991). Therefore, PET with FDG, as well as PET with specific opioid ligand tracers, might help to elucidate the mechanisms and anatomical substrates of disabling interictal psychopathology associated with epilepsy, and perhaps provide insights into the aetiology of similar behaviours that occur spontaneously. Thus far, however, FDG-PET studies have revealed frontal, but not temporal, hypometabolic zones in major depression (Baxter, 1991).

PET has been used to image metabolic disturbances associated with a variety of other neurological and psychiatric disorders, some of which consistently involve temporal limbic structures. Mesial temporal hypofunction demonstrated with PET represents limbic disturbances that can be correlated with memory deficits seen in temporal lobe epilepsy (Rausch *et al.*, 1992), amnesic syndrome (Volpe and Hearst, 1983) and dementia (Kamo *et al.*, 1987). PET, therefore, might provide an opportunity to study anatomical substrates of human memory functions, not only when disrupted by pathological processes, but in normal subjects, using activation paradigms that involve specific memory tasks. Anxiety is associated with temporal lobe hyperperfusion on PET (Reiman *et al.*, 1989), and patients with panic disorder have decreased blood flow in related areas (Reiman *et al.*, 1984), suggesting opportunities to study human emotion with functional imaging. Limbic dysfunction is also described with PET studies of obsessive compulsive behaviour (Baxter, 1991), and mesial temporal hypermetabolism has been seen in patients who have abused cocaine (Baxter *et al.*, 1988).

Single photon emission computer tomography

Patients with partial epilepsy demonstrate interictal zones of cerebral hypoperfusion, and ictal zones of hyper- and hypoperfusion with SPECT that resemble the hypo- and hypermetabolic zones seen with FDG-PET (Magistretti *et al.*, 1983; Lee *et al.*, 1986; Rowe *et al.*, 1991). However, the yield of positive interictal studies with SPECT is considerably less than with PET (Stefan *et al.*, 1987; Ryvlin *et al.*, 1992b) and spatial resolution remains inferior. There is controversy concerning the patterns of ictal perfusion obtained with SPECT during partial seizures, with reports of varying postictal hyperperfusion lasting as long as days (Lang *et al.*, 1988). Most recently, a consistent time course has been described for changes in temporal lobe perfusion during the following complex partial seizures, consisting of initial hyperperfusion of mesial and lateral structures, followed by lateral hypoperfusion, and finally by mesial hypoperfusion (Rowe *et al.*, 1991) (Colour section, Plate 2). This characteristic time course of hyper- and hypoperfusion may accurately identify which temporal lobe is involved in a given complex partial seizure, and help to lateralize an epileptogenic region when resective surgical treatment is being considered. However, it has not been demonstrated that this pattern is unique to seizures of mesial temporal limbic onset, since ictal events that originate extratemporally, for instance in frontal lobe, and rapidly project to ipsilateral mesial temporal structures, have not yet been studied with this technique.

A variety of SPECT tracers are being used clinically, all of which reflect cerebral perfusion. As yet, however, the resultant data cannot be quantitatively analysed. In the future, it may be possible to develop SPECT tracers which can be routinely used to measure other aspects of cerebral function as well. Although SPECT is not as versatile as PET, and its spatial resolution remains inferior, it is more readily available and its increasing clinical use should yield important insights into temporal limbic dysfunction underlying neurologic and psychiatric disorders. It could also be that SPECT provides images of a different aspect of cerebral function than PET, and that these two functional imaging approaches should be viewed as complementary rather than redundant.

CONCLUSIONS

The advent of modern noninvasive neuroimaging techniques now provides opportunities to evaluate the structure and function of the human temporal lobes *in vivo* with extraordinary spatial resolution. Combined use of MRI and PET, for instance, allows quantitative measures of glucose metabolism, blood flow, oxygen metabolism, and a variety of neurotransmitter functions, in specific temporal lobe structures, such as the hippocampus. These techniques have already been used to elucidate the anatomical substrates of certain pathological behaviours, particularly complex partial seizures in patients with temporal lobe epilepsy. Such clinical studies should also provide insights into the neuronal basis of other, non-epileptic, cerebral functions as well. Experiments can be designed, using patients with disorders presumed to involve limbic mechanisms, as well as volunteer subjects, to identify anatomical substrates and fundamental mechanisms of normal limbic-mediated human behaviours. Available data already suggest that memory, affective disturbances such as depression and anxiety, and perhaps aspects of more normal emotion, could be productively explored with these techniques.

ACKNOWLEDGEMENTS

Original research reported by the author was supported in part by Grants NS-02808, NS-15654 and GM-24839, from the National Institutes of Health, and Contract DE-AC03-76-SF00012 from the Department of Energy.

REFERENCES

Abou-Khalil, B.W., Siegel, G.J., Sackellares, J.C., Gilman, S., Hichwa, R. and Marshall, R. (1987). Positron emission tomography studies of cerebral glucose metabolism in chronic partial epilepsy. *Ann. Neurol.*, **22**, 480–486.

Ackermann, R.F., Finch, D.M., Babb, T.L. and Engel Jr, J. (1984). Increased glucose metabolism during long-duration recurrent inhibition of hippocampal pyramidal cells. *J. Neurosci.*, **4**, 251–264.

Ackermann, R.F., Engel Jr, J. and Baxter, L. (1986). PET and autoradiographic studies of glucose utilization following electroconvulsive seizures in humans and rats. *Ann. N.Y. Acad. Sci.*, **462**, 263–269.

Baxter Jr, L.R. (1991). PET studies of cerebral function in major depression and obsessive-compulsive disorder: the emerging prefrontal cortex consensus. *Ann. Clin. Psychiatry*, **3**, 103–109.

Baxter Jr, L.R., Schwartz, J.M., Phelps, M.E., Mazziotta, J.C., Barrio, J., Rawson, R.A., Engel Jr, J., Ackermann, R., Guze, B.H., Selin, C. and Sumida, R. (1988). Localization of the neurochemical effects of cocaine and other stimulants in the human brain. *J. Clin. Psychiatry*, **49** (Suppl.), 2.

Berkovic, S.F., Andermann, F., Olivier, A., Ethier, R., Melanson, D., Robitaille, Y., Kuzniecky, R., Peters, T. and Feindel, W. (1991). Hippocampal sclerosis in temporal lobe epilepsy demonstrated by magnetic resonance imaging. *Ann. Neurol.*, **29**, 175–182.

Bernardi, S., Trimble, M.R., Frackowiak, R.S.J., Wise, R.J.S. and Jones, T. (1983). An interictal study of partial epilepsy using positron emission tomography and the oxygen-15 inhalation technique. *J. Neurol. Neurosurg. Psychiatry*, **46**, 473–477.

Brant-Zawadzki, M. and Norman, D. (Eds) (1987). *Magnetic Resonance Imaging of the Central Nervous System*, Raven Press, New York.

Caldecott-Hazard, S. and Engel Jr, J. (1987). Limbic postictal events: anatomical substrates and opioid receptor involvement. *Prog. Neuropsychopharmacol. Biol. Psychiatry*, **11**, 389–418.

Cascino, G.D., Jack, C.R., Parisi, J.E., Sharbrough, F.W., Hirschorn, K.A., Mayer, F.B., Marsh, W.R. and O'Brien, P. (1991). Magnetic resonance imaging-based volumetric studies in temporal lobe epilepsy: pathological correlations. *Ann. Neurol.*, **30**, 31–36.

Chugani, H.T., Ackermann, R.F., Chugani, D.C. and Engel Jr, J. (1984). Opioid-induced epileptogenic phenomena: anatomical, behavioral, and electroencephalographic features. *Ann. Neurol.*, **15**, 361–368.

Dingledine, R. (1981). Possible mechanisms of enkephalin action on hippocampal CA1 pyramidal neurons. *J. Neurosci.*, **1**, 1022–1035.

Engel Jr, J. (1989). *Seizures and Epilepsy*, F.A. Davis, Philadelphia.

Engel Jr, J. (1990). Functional explorations of the human epileptic brain and their therapeutic implications. *Electroencephalogr. Clin. Neurophysiol.*, **76**, 296–316.

Engel Jr, J., Brown, W.J., Kuhl, D.E., Phelps, M.E., Mazziotta, J.C. and Crandall, P.H. (1982a). Pathological findings underlying focal temporal lobe hypometabolism in partial epilepsy. *Ann. Neurol.*, **12**, 518–528.

Engel Jr, J., Kuhl, D.E., Phelps, M.E. and Crandall, P.H. (1982b). Comparative localization of epileptic foci in partial epilepsy by PCT and EEG. *Ann. Neurol.*, **12**, 529–537.

Engel Jr, J., Kuhl, D.E., Phelps, M.E. and Mazziotta, J.C. (1982c). Interictal cerebral glucose metabolism in partial epilepsy and its relation to EEG changes. *Ann. Neurol.*, **12**, 510–517.

Engel Jr, J., Kuhl, D.E., Phelps, M.E., Rausch, R. and Nuwer, M. (1983). Local cerebral metabolism during partial seizures. *Neurology*, **33**, 400–413.

Engel Jr, J., Lubens, P., Kuhl, D.E. and Phelps, M. (1985). Local cerebral metabolic rate for glucose during petit mal absences. *Ann. Neurol.*, **17**, 121–128.

Engel Jr, J., Bandler, R., Griffith, N.C. and Caldecott-Hazard, S. (1991). Neurobiological evidence for epilepsy-induced interictal disturbances. In: Smith, D., Treiman, D. and Trimble, M. (Eds), *Advances in Neurology, Vol. 55*, Raven Press, New York, pp. 97–111.

Frost, J.J., Mayberg, H.S., Fisher, R.S., Douglass, K.H., Dannals, R.F., Links, J.M., Wilson, A.A., Ravert, H.T., Rosenbaum, A.E., Snyder, S.H. and Wagner, H.N. (1988). Mu-opiate receptors measured by positron emission tomography are increased in temporal lobe epilepsy. *Ann. Neurol.*, **23**, 231–237.

Galaburda, A.M., LeMay, M., Kemper, T.L. and Geschwind, N. (1978). Right-left asymmetries in the brain. Structural differences between the hemispheres may underlie cerebral dominance. *Science*, **199**, 852–856.

Gevins, A., Brickett, P., Costales, B., Le, J. and Reutter, B. (1990). Beyond topographic mapping: towards functional-anatomical imaging with 124-channel EEGs and 3D MRIs. *Brain Topography*, **3**, 53–64.

Henry, T.R., Mazziotta, J.C., Engel Jr, J., Christenson, P.D., Zhang, J.-X., Phelps, M.E. and Kuhl, D.E. (1990). Quantifying interictal metabolic activity in human temporal lobe epilepsy. *J. Cerebral Blood Flow Metab.*, **10**, 748–757.

Henry, T.R., Sutherling, W.W., Engel Jr, J., Risinger, M.W., Levesque, M.F., Mazziotta, J.C. and Phelps, M.E. (1992). Interictal cerebral metabolism in partial epilepsies of neocortical origin. *Epilepsy Res.*, in press.

Kamo, H., McGeer, P.L., Harrop, R. *et al.* (1987). Positron emission tomography and histopathology in Pick's disease. *Neurology*, **37**, 439–445.

Kuhl, D.E., Engle Jr, J., Phelps, M.E. and Selin, C. (1980). Epileptic patterns of local cerebral metabolism and perfusion in humans determined by emission computed tomography of ^{18}FDG and $^{13}NH_3$. *Ann. Neurol.*, **8**, 348–360.

Lang, W., Podreka, I., Suess, E., Müller, C., Zeitlhofer, J. and Deecke, L. (1988). Single photon emission computerized tomography during and between seizures. *J. Neurol.*, **235**, 277–284.

Laster, D.W., Penry, J.K., Moody, D.M., Ball, M.R., Witcofski, R.L. and Riela, A.R. (1985). Chronic seizure disorders: contributions of MR imaging when CT is normal. *Am. J. Neuroradiol.*, **6**, 177–180.

Latack, J.T., Abou-Khalil, B.W., Segal, G.J., Sackellares, J.C., Gabrielsen, T.O. and Aisen, A.M. (1986). Patients with partial seizures: evaluation by MR, CT and PET imaging. *Radiology*, **159**, 159–163.

Lee, B.I., Markand, O.N., Siddiqui, A.R., Park, H.M., Mock, B., Wellman, H.H., Worth, R.M. and Edwards, M.K. (1986). Single photon emission computed tomography (SPECT) brain imaging using N,N,N′-trimethyl-N′-(2 hydroxy-3-methyl-5-^{123}I-iodobenzyl)-1,3-propanediamine 2 HC1 (HIPDM): intractable complex partial seizures. *Neurology*, **36**, 1471–1477.

Levesque, M.F., Zhang, J.-X., Wilson, C.L., Behnke, E.J., Harper, R.M., Lufkin, R.B., Engel Jr, J. and Crandall, P.H. (1990). Stereotactic investigation of limbic epilepsy using a multimodal image analysis system. *J. Neurosurg.*, **73**, 792–797.

Magistretti, P.L., Uren, R.F., Royal, H.D., Parker, A.J., Front, D. and Kolodny, G.M. (1983). *n*-isopropyl-^{123} I-*p*-iodoamphetamine imaging in epilepsy. In: Magistretti, P. (Ed.), *Functional Radionuclide Imaging of the Brain*, Raven Press, New York.

Mayberg, H.S., Sadzot, B., Meltzer, C.C., Fisher, R.S., Lesser, R.P., Dannals, R.F., Lever, J.R., Wilson, A.A., Ravert, H.T., Wagner Jr, H.N., Bryan, R.N., Cromwell, C.C. and Frost, J.J. (1991). Quantification of mu and non-mu opiate receptors in temporal lobe epilepsy using positron emission tomography. *Ann. Neurol.*, **30**, 3–11.

Mazziotta, J.C., Valentino, D., Pelizzari, C.A., Chen, G.T. and Bookstein, F. (1990). Structure–function correlation of the living human brain with MRI and PET: a means of anatomical and functional localization. *Clin. Neuropharmacol.*, **13** (Suppl. 2), 460–461.

Pelizzari, C.A., Chen, G.T.Y., Spelbring, D.R., Weichselbaum, R.R. and Chen, C.T. (1989). Accurate three-dimensional registration of CT, PET and/or MR images of the brain. *J. Comput. Assist. Tomogr.*, **13**, 20–26.

Phelps, M.E., Schelbert, H.R. and Mazziotta, J.C. (1983). Positron computed tomography for studies of myocardial and cerebral function. *Ann. Intern. Med.*, **98**, 339–359.

Rausch, R. and Risinger, M. (1990). Intracarotid sodium amobarbital procedure. In: Boulton, A.A., Baker, G.B. and Hiscock, M. (Eds), *Neuromethods, Vol. 17: Neuropsychology*, Humana Press, Clifton, New Jersey, pp. 127–146.

Rausch, R., Henry, T.R., Ary, C.M., Engel Jr, J. and Mazziotta, J. (1992). Relation of asymmetric interictal glucose hypometabolism to cognitive performance in patients with unilateral mesial temporal lobe epilepsy. *Arch. Neurol.*, in press.

Reiman, E.M., Raichle, M.E., Butler, F.K., Herscovitch, P. and Robins, E. (1984). A focal brain abnormality in panic disorder, a severe form of anxiety, *Nature*, **310**, 683.

Reiman, E.M., Fusselman, M.J., Fox, P.T. and Raichle, M.E. (1989). Neuroanatomical correlates of anticipatory anxiety. *Science*, **243**, 1071–1074.

Rocha, L., Engel Jr, J. and Ackermann, R.F. (1991). Effects of chronic naloxone pretreatment on amygdaloid kindling in rats. *Epilepsy Res.*, **10**, 103–110.

Rowe, C.C., Berkovic, S.F., Austin, M.C., McKay, W.J. and Bladin, P.F. (1991). Patterns of postictal cerebral flow in temporal lobe epilepsy: qualitative and quantitative analysis. *Neurology*, **41**, 1096–1103.

Ryvlin, P., Froment, J.C., Turjman, F., Fischer, C., Revol, M. and Mauguière, F. (1992a). Test-retest stability of MRI hyperintense T_2 signals in temporal lobe epilepsy. In press

Ryvlin, P., Philippon, B., Linotti, L., Froment, J.C., Lebars, D. and Mauguière, F. (1992b). Functional neuro-imaging strategy in temporal lobe epilepsy: a comparative study of ^{18}FDG-PET and ^{99m}Tc-HMPAO. In press.

Savic, I., Persson, A., Roland, P., Pauli, S., Sedvall, G. and Widen, L. (1988). *In vivo* demonstration of reduced benzodiazepine receptor binding in human epileptic foci. *Lancet* **ii**, 863–866.

Sperling, M.R., Wilson, G., Engel Jr, J., Babb, T.L., Phelps, M.E. and Bradley, W. (1986). Magnetic resonance imaging in intractable partial epilepsies: correlative studies. *Ann. Neurol.*, **20**, 57–62.

Stefan, H., Pawlik, G., Böcher-Schwarz, H.G., Biersack, H.J., Burr, W., Penin, H. and Heiss, W.-D. (1987). Functional and morphological abnormalities in temporal lobe epilepsy: a comparison of interictal and ictal EEG, CT, MRI, SPECT and PET. *J. Neurol.*, **234**, 377–384.

Theodore, W.H., Newmark, M.E., Sato, S., De LaPaz, R., DiChiro, G., Brooks, R., Patronas, N., Kessler, R.M., Manning, R., Margolin, R. Channing, M. and Porter, R.J. (1984). ^{18}F-fluorodeoxyglucose positron emission tomography in refractory complex partial seizures. *Ann. Neurol.*, **14**, 429–437.

Volpe, B.T. and Hearst, W. (1983). Characterization of an amnesic syndrome following hypoxic ischemic injury. *Arch. Neurol.*, **40**, 436–440.

Yamamoto, Y.L., Ochs, R., Gloor, P., Ammann, W., Meyer, E., Evans, A.C., Cooke, B., Sako, K., Gotman, J., Feindel, W.H., Diksic, M., Thompson, C.J. and Robitaille, Y. (1983). Patterns of rCBF and focal energy metabolic changes in relation to electroencephalographic abnormality in the interictal phase of partial epilepsy. In: Baldy-Moulinier, M., Ingvar, D.-H. and Meldrum, B.S. (Eds), *Current Problems in Epilepsy: 1. Cerebral Blood Flow, Metabolism and Epilepsy*, John Libbey, London, pp. 51–62.

Zhang, J.-X., Levesque, M.F., Wilson, C.L., Harper, R.M., Engel Jr, J. and Behnke, E. (1990). Multimodality imaging of brain structures for stereotactic surgery. *Radiology*, **175**, 435–441.

The Temporal Lobes and the Limbic System
Edited by M.R. Trimble and T.G. Bolwig

8

Localization Related Epileptic Syndromes

MOGENS DAM
University Clinic of Neurology, Hvidovre Hospital, Denmark

INTRODUCTION

Complex partial seizures are epileptic seizures characterized by impairment but without total loss of consciousness. The EEG during seizures has unilateral or often bilateral discharges, diffuse or focal in temporal or frontotemporal regions. The interictal expression is unilateral or bilateral, generally an asynchronous focus, usually in the temporal regions.

The onset may be as a simple partial seizure, an aura with simple partial features, followed by impairment of consciousness. They may however start with impairment of consciousness and only involve this symptom, or be followed by an automatism. Both simple partial seizures and complex partial seizures may then evolve to secondary generalized tonic–clonic seizures. The fundamental distinction between simple partial seizures and complex partial seizures is the presence of or the impairment of the fully conscious state. Consciousness has been defined as 'the integrating activity by which man grasps the totality of his phenomenal field and incorporates it into his experience'. It corresponds to 'Bewusstsein' in German and is thus much more than 'vigilance', for were it only vigilance (which is a degree of clarity) then only confusional states would be representative of disordered consciousness.

Operationally, in the context of classification, consciousness refers to the degree of awareness or responsiveness of the patient to externally applied stimuli. *Responsiveness* refers to the ability of the patient to carry out simple commands or willed movements, and *awareness* refers to the patient's contact with events during the period in question. A person aware and unresponsive will be able to recount the events that occurred during an attack and his inability to respond by movement or speech. In this context, unresponsiveness is other than the result of paralysis, aphasia or apraxia.

PHENOMENOLOGY

Implicit in the discussion of complex partial seizures are three assumptions (Gloor, 1987):

1. Complex partial seizures are the result of some form of brain pathology, a lesion therefore always exists.
2. If a brain lesion can be demonstrated in a patient with seizures, the likelihood that the seizures are in some way the consequence of this lesion is high.
3. The area from which seizures originate is likely to lie within the confines or at least in the vicinity of the demonstrated brain lesion, but its precise anatomical site and extent are not necessarily coextensive with that lesion.

Given the numerous inadequacies inherent in any of our structural or functional investigations used to delineate the site of seizure onset, the most secure evidence in favour of having identified it with as much certainty as is possible is the fact that the topographic information derived from a number of mutually independent structural and functional tests converges on one and the same site. There does not seem to be any characteristic ictal expression which will unequivocally and reliably identify the temporal lobe site of origin of a clinical seizure. This is the reason for the fact that presurgical selection must be multifactorial, looking for convergence among neuroanatomical, neurophysiological, and neurobehavioural information.

PARTIAL SEIZURES

1. With motor signs

Any portion of the body may be involved in partial seizure activity, depending on the site of origin of the attack along the motor strip. Partial motor seizures may remain strictly focal, or they may spread to contiguous cortical areas and produce a sequential involvement of body parts in an epileptic 'march', which is then known as a Jacksonian seizure. Consciousness may be preserved in the initial phase; however, the discharge may spread to structures whose participation is likely to result in impaired consciousness and then perhaps to loss of consciousness and generalized convulsions. Other partial motor attacks may be versive, with the head turning to one side, usually the side contralateral to the discharge. If speech is involved, this is often speech arrest or aphasia, or vocalization. Occasionally, a partial dysphasia is seen in the form of epileptic palilalia with involuntary repetition of a syllable or phrase. Often the pronunciation is affected with a more or less pronounced dysarthria.

Following partial seizure activity there may be a localized paralysis in the previously involved region. This is known as Todd's paralysis and may last from minutes to hours, or even days. When partial motor seizure activity is continuous, it is known as a simple partial status epilepticus, previously called epilepsia partialis continua (Kojevnikow's syndrome).

2. With somatosensory or special sensory symptoms

Somatosensory seizures arise from those areas of cortex subserving sensory function. They belong to the simple partial seizures, which also may 'march' and may spread at any time to become a complex partial seizure. The sensation accompanying these seizures is usually described as pins and needles or a feeling of numbness. Special sensory seizures include visual seizures that may vary in elaborateness (depending on whether the primary or association areas are involved) from flashing lights to structured visual hallucinatory phenomena, including persons and scenes.

Case history

One patient experienced each time a swimming pool area where people were sitting between waving palm trees drinking cocktails. In most instances this simple partial seizure would develop into a secondary generalized convulsion.

Like visual seizures, auditory seizures may also run the gamut from crude auditory sensations to such highly integrated functions as discussions between people with whom the patient is familiar, or even music.

Case history

A lady, in her sixties, suffered from simple partial seizures during which she felt that she was hearing a discussion between her bridge friends. They talked about her, but she could not exactly identify the content of their discussion. As the seizures increased in frequency she felt persecuted or paranoid, feeling that they talked about her behind her back. She suffered from an inoperable tumour and the seizures could only be controlled by antiepileptic drugs for a restricted period of time. When they increased in frequency she finally could not clearly distinguish between her real experiences and the experiences she had during her simple partial seizures.

Olfactory sensations, usually in the form of unpleasant odours, may occur.

Case history

A girl, in her twenties, working as a laboratory technician had simple partial seizures during which she smelled smoke. She ran around in the laboratory in order to find the fire, a little astonished by the fact that nobody else could smell burning. As this often recurred she realized that it must be a seizure, which was verified at the epilepsy clinic.

Gustatory sensations may be pleasant but are usually odious taste hallucinations.

Vertiginous symptoms include sensations of falling in space, floating, as well as rotatory vertigo in a horizontal or vertical plane.

3. With autonomic symptoms

Pallor, flushing, vomiting, sweating, piloerection, pupil dilatation, borborygmia, and incontinence may occur as part of complex partial seizures.

4. With psychic symptoms (disturbance of higher cerebral function)

These symptoms usually occur as complex partial seizures.

(a) Dysmnesic symptoms

These symptoms include a distorted memory experience such as a distortion of the time sense, a dreamy state, a flashback, or a sensation as if a naïve experience had been experienced before (known as déjà vécu) or as if a previously experienced sensation had not been experienced (known as jamais vécu). Occasionally, as a form of forced thinking, the patient may experience a rapid recollection of episodes from his past life, known as panoramic vision.

(b) Cognitive disturbances

These include dreamy states, distortions of time sense, sensations of unreality, detachment, or depersonalization.

Case history

A young fellow, about 18 years of age, suffered from seizures with distortion of time sense consisting of a feeling that everything was happening at an increased speed. He therefore had to rush in order to keep pace with his surroundings. This resulted in accidents as he rushed out of the house into the street or even rode on his bike faster and faster, trying to reach the same speed he felt everything else had.

(c) Affective symptoms

A sensation of extreme pleasure or displeasure, as well as fear and intense depression with feelings of unworthiness and rejection, may be experienced with seizures. Unlike the symptoms of psychiatrically induced depression, these symptoms tend to come in attacks lasting only a few minutes, but they may be long lasting, sometimes one or two days. Anger and rage is occasionally experienced. Epileptic anger is apparently unprovoked and abates rapidly.

Case history

A 22 year-old man had epilepsy from childhood with infrequent seizures. His temperament was said to be excitable. He became angry for no apparent reason and would throw around everything within reach. With the help of the local authority he was trained as a potter. This gave certain problems when he had a temper tantrum. He would break everything he had made, including the moulds and tools. One evening he was being driven home from a party by his fiancée. He did not drive and had no driving licence. Suddenly, on the highway, he demanded to drive the car. His fiancée could see that he was becoming angry and, as he is a powerful man, she did not dare refuse to let him take the wheel. He drove for about one kilometre, then slowly came to himself and, somewhat confused, gave her the wheel. He repeated many times, 'what am I doing?'. As they changed seats, a police patrol drove up. They had noticed the changing of driver and demanded to see their driving licences. The result was that he was fined 600 DKr and his girlfriend 250 DKr for having handed the wheel over to him. This, the patient felt, was unjust as he had no recollection of what had happened. He applied to the local epilepsy association and was referred to our epilepsy clinic. At first we suspected he was just trying to dodge the fine, but when we looked more closely at the cause of the incident and his fiancée confirmed all that had happened, we were sure that the events were related to epilepsy. This not only had led to the infrequent convulsive seizures but also to complex partial seizures with affective symptoms. He was treated with carbamazepine and since then there have only been isolated incidents of temper, and no seizures. The patient and his fiancée had their fines rescinded.

Fear or terror are the most frequent symptoms; they are sudden in onset, usually unprovoked, and may lead to running away.

In gelastic seizures, the laughter should not be classified under affective symptoms because it is usually without an associated affect and without true mirth.

Case history

A 24 year-old girl had suffered from epilepsy for 2 years, presumably after an encephalitis. Among her seizures she had gelastic fits which gave her some trouble. She cleaned in a factory and she had great difficulties in explaining to her colleagues why she suddenly would laugh or chuckle for half an hour to an hour. She herself could find no reason for her laughing and felt no true mirth. As her seizures could not be controlled by antiepileptic drugs she had an amygdalohippocampectomy. Since then she has been seizure-free.

(d) Illusions

These symptoms take the form of distorted perceptions in which objects may appear deformed. Monocular diplopia, distortions of size, macropsia, or micropsia, may occur. Similarly, distortions of sound, including microacusis or macroacusis are reported. Depersonalization, as if the person were unreal, or sometimes outside his body, may occur as may derealisation, the experience of the surrounding world as flat, affectless and unreal. Altered perception of size and weight of a limb may be noted.

(e) Structured hallucinations

Hallucinations may occur as manifestations or perceptions without a corresponding external stimulus and may affect somatosensory, visual, auditory, olfactory, or gustatory senses. If the seizure arises from the primary receptive area, the hallucination would tend to be rather primitive. In the case of vision, flashing lights may be seen; in the case of auditory perception, rushing noises may occur. With more elaborate seizures involving visual or auditory association areas with participation of mobilized memory traces, formed hallucinations occur; these may take the form of scenery, persons, spoken sentences, or music. The character of these perceptions may be normal or distorted.

(f) Automatisms

Gastaut (1973) describes automatisms in the following way: they are more or less coordinated, adapted, involuntary motor activities occurring during the state of clouding of consciousness either in the course of or after an epileptic seizure, and usually followed by amnesia for the event. The automatism may be simply a continuation of an activity that was going on when the seizure occurred.

Case history

A 34 year-old man, a refugee from Lebanon with epilepsy after an encephalitis in his childhood, went into a store in order to buy some videos. Exactly at the moment when he took down the videos from the shelf he had an automatism. He went out of the store with the videos without paying. He was immediately arrested and could not react to what was going on as he was in the postictal confusional state. When he regained consciousness he told the police that he suffered from epilepsy, but was not believed. The next day he therefore came to the epilepsy clinic and described the event. He was full of shame. Showing some photocopies of the relevant pages from the book Epilepsy—Prejudice and Fact (Dam and Gram, 1985) to the police solved the matter, and the police felt that they had learned something about epilepsy.

Automatisms may also be characterized by new activity developed in association with the ictal impairment of consciousness. Usually, the actions are commonplace in nature, often provoked by the subject's environment, or by his sensations during the seizure; exceptionally, fragmentary, primitive, or infantile behaviour is seen.

Case history

Dr E. Sindrup has a charming video recording of a shy 16 year-old boy, who during a seizure went up to the EEG technician and gave her a kiss. He went back to the chair still in his seizure and then the automatism stopped. The technician asked him what he had done; he could not, however, recall the event. It was evident that this shy boy would never have done this if it was not during a seizure. He had presumably realized that the EEG technician was a very attractive girl, and because of the seizure his inhibitions had disappeared.

Antisocial behaviour is only rarely described. From a symptomatological point of view the following are distinguished: (i) eating automatisms (chewing, swallowing); (ii) automatisms of mimicry, expressing the subject's emotional state (usually of fear) during the seizure; (iii) gestural automatisms, crude or elaborate, directed toward either the subject or his environment; (iv) ambulatory automatisms; (v) verbal automatisms.

Ictal epileptic automatisms usually represent the release of automatic behaviour under the influence of clouding of consciousness. There seems to be little doubt that automatisms are a common feature of different types of epilepsy. Although they do not lend themselves to simple anatomical interpretation, they appear to have in common a discharge involving various areas of the limbic system bilaterally. Crude and elaborate automatisms do occur in patients with absences as well as complex partial seizures. The precise descriptive history of the seizures, the age of the patient, and the presence or absence of confusion are of great clinical significance. The EEG is of cardinal localizational importance here.

ANATOMICAL–CLINICAL CORRELATIONS

Temporal lobe seizures

The majority of complex partial seizures originate in the temporal lobes. Reports from the UCLA and Yale programmes suggest that 70–85% of complex partial seizures originate in the temporal lobes (Cahan *et al.*, 1984; Williamson, 1986). Temporal lobe seizures are those clinical electrical events that are the consequence of localized epileptic discharges from neurons within the temporal lobe. There are two approaches to defining these phenomena: (a) the consequences of external stimulation of the temporal lobe in humans; (b) the behaviour as a consequence of apparent localized spontaneous epileptiform discharges within the temporal lobe.

Several authors have attempted to clarify this issue by observing the response to stimulation of the temporal lobe in humans under varying circumstances (Gloor, 1982; Penfield and Perot, 1963; VanBuren, 1958). While this provides useful information, the interpretation of the data is subject to limitations. One can summarize the data by saying that stimulating *the anterior temporal gyrus of Heschl* produces unformed auditory sensations such as a buzz or a whistle; stimulating *the superior temporal convolution* produces formed auditory hallucinations or illusions; stimulating *the posterior temporal cortex*, especially on the non-dominant side, tends to produce formed visual hallucinations or illusions; and that stimulating *other parts of the neocortex* tends to produce experiences of déjà vécu, reproduction of memory and experiences, and changes in mood.

Stimulation of *the insula* is associated with visceral sensations; stimulation of *the amygdaloid and periamygdaloid area* is associated with vague emotional sensations of anxiety or fear, decreased awareness, and a wide variety of behaviours of a non-directed sort such as chewing movements, vocalizations, arrest of motor activity, contraversive deviation of the head, and elaborate functional behaviour including learned acts. Stimulation of *the hippocampus* is associated with memory disturbances, fear, grooming, and sexual and pleasurable sensations.

Primary signs of involvement of *posterior neocortical structures* are disturbances in speech or elementary or complex auditory hallucinations. However, vestibular sensations, complex illusions, hallucinations, dreamy states, fear, and epigastric discomfort and other vegetative sensations all can appear when neocortical areas are stimulated.

Seizures arising in the limbic system tend to come either from the hippocampus or amygdala. Associations described include olfactory hallucinations, visceral motor and signs of oroalimentary activity (e.g. salivation and swallowing), apnoea, cardiovascular and gastrointestinal disturbances, mimic gesticulatory and verbal automatisms, memory troubles, transient and retrograde amnesia and occasionally some tonic motor behaviour.

Among the anatomical–clinical correlations that have been suggested by a number of authors are that olfactory sensations arise from the uncus and amygdala; that gustatory sensations usually are combined with olfactory sensations and stem from various parts of the limbic system; and that oroalimentary manifestations originate from the amygdala (Penfield and Jasper, 1954; Bancaud *et al.*, 1965). The Penfield and the Bancaud schools disagree about many particulars. One could argue that there really is no single anatomical correlation of vocalization, adversive movements of the head and eyes, pupillary changes, flushing and palpitation, and the abdominal and thoracic sensations (rising aura). All of these sensations and behaviours can arise from different parts of the temporal lobe and from different parts of the brain.

Wieser (1983) proposed a classification of five typical spontaneous seizure types for psychomotor epilepsy from an anatomical point of view. He takes into account the projections which exist from parts of the brain to other parts of the brain. His classification ignores the historical anatomical separation of temporal, parietal, occipital, and frontal lobes to focus on the more functional inter-relationships.

Four of the Wieser seizure types were allegedly of temporal lobe origin: temporobasal-limbic, temporal polar, opercular and posterior temporal neocortical. There was a significant degree of overlap among the seizure types, but there were some salient features that served to distinguish between the groups.

The temporobasal-limbic syndrome

Auras were most common in the temporobasal-limbic syndrome and included epigastric sensations, déjà vécu, as well as more complex memory flashbacks. A motionless stare was often a feature of these seizures but was not by itself reliable. Oroalimentary automatisms were uncommon.

The temporal polar syndrome

The seizures had prominent early autonomic changes and very early oroalimentary automatisms.

The opercular syndrome

The seizures with suggestive origin near Heschl's gyrus, had prominent auditory hallucinations, face and upper extremity motor features, and focal sensory symptoms. Aphasia apparently was not a reliable dominant versus non-dominant lateralizing clinical expression.

The posterior temporal neocortical syndrome

The seizure had complex visual hallucinations and vestibular features.

These results are, however, not easy to interpret, as the study was based on a small number of patients. After a mean follow-up of 6 years, only 57% were seizure free, and 14% unchanged. 29% had a marked or moderate reduction of seizure frequency. As a result of surgical treatment of drug resistant epilepsy these results are acceptable. However, the purity of the ictal localization is, at best, suspect.

In a retrospective study of medical records of patients whose interictal scalp EEGs suggested a site of seizure origin within the temporal lobe, 83% of the patients reported auras with over half describing more than one type of event. Visceral phenomena and fear, strangeness, and déjà vécu were the most frequent events described. 80% of the patients also had focal tonic and clonic motor activity (King and Ajmone-Marsan, 1977).

Delgado-Escueta and Walsh analysed video-taped complex partial seizures and defined two types of events (Delgado-Escueta, 1979; Walsh, 1984; Delgado-Escueta and Walsh, 1985): *Type I* were most common and began with an arrest reaction and a motionless stare. After the stare there were stereotypic automatisms with oroalimentary behaviour as the most prominent feature. *Type II* seizures exhibited neither arrest reactions nor the automatisms but had some associated semi-purposeful motor activity. Based upon results of surgery and intracranial recording, they concluded that the Type I seizures originated in the medial temporal lobe and Type II were of extratemporal origin.

Along with certain portions of the frontal lobe, the temporal lobe is the easiest structure to excite into epileptic activity. This is due to the low seizure threshold or 'hyperexcitability' of the hippocampus. Numerous attempts have been made to draw circuits indicating the linkage of neocortical to rhinencephalic structures in the temporal lobe and from those structures to the rest of the brain. While many of these interconnections can be experimentally confirmed, there is no way to know which, if any, are involved in the provocation of any individual seizure or for any class of seizure. A bland onset with arrest or simple stereotyped automatisms including vocalization can occur with seizures of extratemporal origin. Consequently, the utility of the clinical expression of a seizure for localizing its site of origin would appear to be suspect (Williamson *et al.*, 1987).

Most simplistically it can be said that the temporal lobes have tracts which connect them to every other area of the brain. Therefore, depending upon what circuits are relatively activated in a given patient at a given time, with variable factors such as medication reduction, fatigue, or other factors affecting the modification of the seizure threshold, a variable clinical expression will result.

Therefore, we can conclude that there is no characteristic ictal expression which will unequivocally and reliably identify the temporal lobe site of origin of a clinical seizure (Gates and Gumnit, 1991).

Frontal lobe seizures

Although most complex partial seizures originate in the temporal lobes, about 10% are thought to originate from the frontal lobes (Williamson and Spencer, 1986). It has been suggested that frontal lobe seizures comprise most of the complex partial seizures of extratemporal origin (Swartz and Delgado-Escueta, 1987). The typical symptoms of these seizures are initial prominent motor activity involving the axial regions, often symmetric. Resulting behaviours are disorganized thrashing, frequent postural change, bimanual or bipedal activity, spitting, or eccentric breathing. Often verbal automatisms are observed with shouting, cursing or other material with significant affective components. The automatism may differ from one seizure to the next depending on the setting. Postictal confusion is often absent or slight. The seizures are short, in the range of 10–30 s and there may be no reorientation phase. The seizure frequency will in general be higher than in temporal lobe epilepsy and many of the seizures will be nocturnal, occurring in clusters. The tendency to cluster may fuse with the occurrence of complex partial status epilepticus. Spontaneous remissions lasting for years may occur.

It is common for seizures that begin in the temporal region to develop features of frontal lobe involvement as they evolve (Waterman *et al.*, 1987). This anterior propagation may be very fast and the patient's subjective aura may be overlooked or masked by amnesia. Ictal recordings are extremely important in solving this problem.

EPIDEMIOLOGY

There are few reliable studies on the incidence and prevalence of different seizure types in the community, as hospital investigation is often necessary to classify seizures accurately. Complex partial seizures seem to be the most prevalent of any single seizure type. According to Juul-Jensen and Foldspang (1983) the incidence of complex partial seizures with or without secondary generalization is about 50%. Some evidence for an increasing prevalence of these seizures was found by Hauser and Kurland (1975) in their longitudinal study of a population in Rochester. Zielinski (1974) and Gastaut *et al.* (1975)

also found a high prevalence of complex partial seizures, although the percentage of temporal lobe epilepsy was a great deal higher in the Polish and French studies than in those from Rochester and Tonbridge. When complex partial seizures occur, they are by far the most frequent seizure type in the individual patient.

CONCLUSION

It is concluded that there is no characteristic ictal expression which will unequivocally and reliably identify the temporal lobe site of origin of a clinical seizure. If this is the case, we cannot expect to be able to identify the individual syndromes reflecting temporal lobe disturbance, if they exist, with the knowledge and the technical armamentarium we have today.

REFERENCES

Bancaud, J., Talairach, J., Bonis, A., Schaub, A., Szikala, G., Morel, P. and Bordas-Ferrer, M. (1965). *La Stereo-electroencephalographie dans l'Epilepsie*, Masson, Paris.

Cahan, L.D., Sutherling, W., McCullough, M.A., Rausch, R., Engel, J. and Crandall, P.H. (1984). Review of the 20-year UCLA experience with surgery for epilepsy. *Cleveland Clin. Q.*, **51**, 313–318.

Dam, M. and Gram, L. (1985). *Epilepsy—Prejudice and Fact*, Munksgaard, Copenhagen.

Delgado-Escueta, A.V. (1979). Epileptogenic paroxysms: modern approaches and clinical correlations. *Neurology*, **29**, 1014–1022.

Delgado-Escueta, A.V. and Walsh, G.O. (1985). Type I complex partial seizures of hippocampal origin: excellent results of anterior temporal lobectomy. *Neurology*, **35**, 143–154.

Gastaut, H. (1973). Definitions. In: *Dictionary of Epilepsy, Part I*, World Health Organization, Geneva.

Gastaut, H., Gastaut, J.L., Goncalves e Silva, G.E. and Fernandez Sanohez, G.R. (1975). Relative frequency of different types of epilepsy: a study employing the classification of the International League Against Epilepsy. *Epilepsia*, **16**, 457–461.

Gates, J.R. and Gumnit, R.J. (1991). Partial seizures of temporal lobe origin. In: Dam, M. and Gram, L. (Eds), *Comprehensive Epileptology*, Raven Press, New York, pp. 187–195.

Gloor, P. (1982). The role of limbic system and experiental phenomena of temporal lobe epilepsy. *Ann. Neurol.*, **12**, 129–144.

Gloor, P. (1987). Commentary: approaches to localization of the epileptogenic lesion. In: Engel, J. (Ed.), *Surgical Treatment of the Epilepsies*, Raven Press, New York, pp. 97–100.

Hauser, W.A. and Kurland, L.T. (1975). The epidemiology of epilepsy in Rochester, Minnesota, 1935 through 1967. *Epilepsia*, **16**, 1–66.

Juul-Jensen, P. and Foldspang, A. (1983). Natural history of epileptic seizures. *Epilepsia*, **24**, 297–312.

King, D.W. and Ajmone-Marsan, C. (1977). Clinical features and ictal patterns in epileptic patients with EEG temporal lobe foci. *Ann. Neurol.*, **2**, 138–147.

Penfield, W. and Jasper, H. (1954). *Epilepsy and the Functional Anatomy of the Human Brain*, Little, Brown, Boston.

Penfield, W. and Perot, P. (1963). The brain's record of auditory and visual experience: a final summary and discussion. *Brain*, **86**, 595–696.

Swartz, B.E. and Delgado-Escueta, A.V. (1987). Complex partial seizures of extratemporal origin: 'The Evidence for'. In: Wieser, H.G., Speckmann, E.J. and Engel, J. (Eds), *Current Problems in Epilepsy*, John Libbey, London, pp. 137–174.

VanBuren, J.M. (1958). Some autonomic concomitants of interictal automatisms: a study of temporal lobe attacks. *Brain*, **81**, 505.

Walsh, G.O. and Delgado-Escueta, A.V. (1984). Type II complex partial seizures: poor results of anterior temporal lobectomy. *Neurology*, **34**, 1–13.

Waterman, K., Purves, S., Kosaka, B., Strauss, E. and Wada, J. (1987). An epileptic syndrome caused by mesial frontal lobe foci. *Neurology*, **37**, 577–582.

Wieser, H.G. (1983). *Electroclinical Features of the Psychomotor Seizure*, Gustav Fischer, New York.

Williamson, P.D. (1986). Intensive monitoring for complex partial seizures. In: Gumnit, R. (Ed.), *Advances in Neurology*, Raven Press, New York, pp. 69–84.

Williamson, P.D. and Spencer, S.S. (1986). Clinical and EEG features of complex partial seizures of extratemporal origin. *Epilepsia*, **27** (Suppl. 2), S46–S63.

Williamson, P.D., Wieser, H.G. and Delgado-Escueta, A.V. (1987). Clinical characteristics of partial seizures. In: Engel, J. (Ed.), *Surgical Treatment of the Epilepsies*, Raven Press, New York, pp. 101–120.

Zielinski, J.J. (1974). *Epidemiology and Medical-Social Problems of Epilepsy in Warsaw*, Psychoneurological Institute, Warsaw.

The Temporal Lobes and the Limbic System
Edited by M.R. Trimble and T.G. Bolwig

9

The Aetiology of Mesial Temporal Sclerosis

AGNETE MOURITZEN DAM
Virum, Denmark

INTRODUCTION

Pathological studies of the temporal lobes have played an outstanding role in epilepsy research. This work was initiated primarily by neuropathologists and later involved neurophysiologists and other neuroscientists, as experimental research on seizure mechanisms and neurotransmitters increased in order to explore the aetiologies of epilepsy.

With improved technical devices the gross pathology of uncal atrophy, as described in the early nineteenth century by Bouchet and Cazauviehlh (1825), has been studied in more refined detail in human brains post-mortem and, after surgical intervention was introduced, on resected temporal lobes (Mouritzen Dam, 1979; Babb *et al.*, 1984). Experimental studies have added further information on the effects of the application to the brain of well defined noxious stimuli able to simulate the pathology of epilepsy. Although loss of neurons has been the focus of attention in mesial temporal sclerosis, which is synonymous with neuron loss in the centro-medial part of the temporal lobe, other pathoanatomical aspects have been studied. Changes in the dendritic tree were described in specimens of resected temporal lobes (Scheibel and Scheibel, 1973) and interest in microdysgenesis has recently been revived in research.

DEFINITIONS OF MESIAL TEMPORAL SCLEROSIS AND OTHER TYPES OF PATHOLOGY IN THE TEMPORAL LOBES

The hippocampus has been the focus of the investigations ever since Sommer (1880) described restricted neuron loss on one side as a remarkable feature

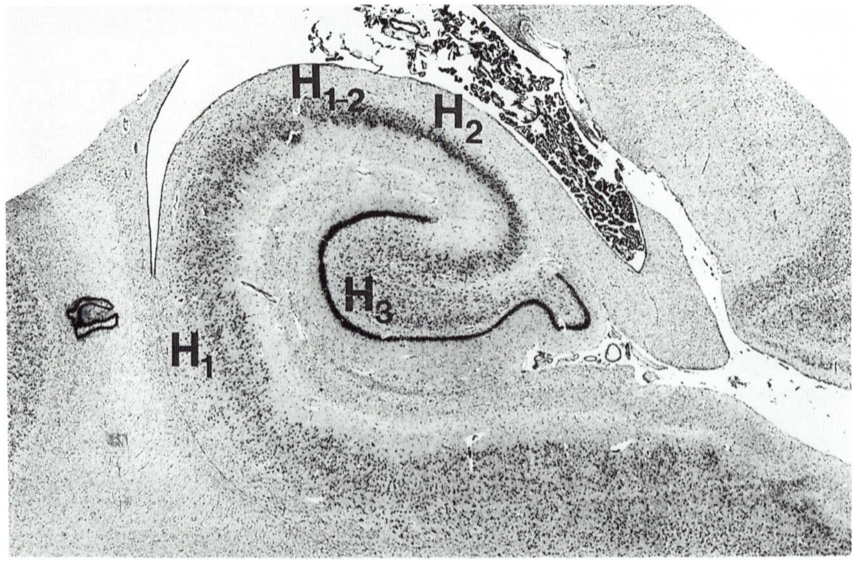

Figure 1. The human hippocampus with subdivisions of the pyramidal cells.

in some brains from patients with epilepsy. The area has since borne his name. His contemporaries (Meynert, 1868; Bratz, 1899) agreed with the unilateral occurrence, and Meynert also described the 'patchy pattern' due to the varying degree of neuron loss throughout the hippocampus. Later studies discovered not only that Sommer's sector was involved, but also that the neuron loss was different in the different areas.

Scholz (1959) subdivided the hippocampal pyramidal band and described fields H_1, H_2 and H_3. Field H_1 is analogous with Sommer's sector (Fig. 1). Fields H_1 and H_3 were both affected but field H_2 seemed resistant. Also granule cells in the fascia dentata were damaged. In 1966, Corsellis described two types of pathology in brains from patients with epilepsy (Margerison and Corsellis, 1966). One he named the classical type and it was closest to Sommer's description. The other type he called mesial temporal sclerosis, which covered more wide-spread damage not unilateral and extending out of the hippocampus to include the amygdalae, uncus and the parahippocampal gyrus. Mesial temporal sclerosis was the most common lesion in resected temporal lobes.

After the meticulous work of Corsellis, in which he stressed the importance of the loss of neurons with gliosis, quantification was introduced in studies of the hippocampus from post-mortem brains (Mouritzen Dam, 1979) as well as studies on surgical specimens (Babb *et al.*, 1984).

The pyramidal cells and the granule cells of the fascia dentata were counted because of the unique pattern and the frequent occurrence of

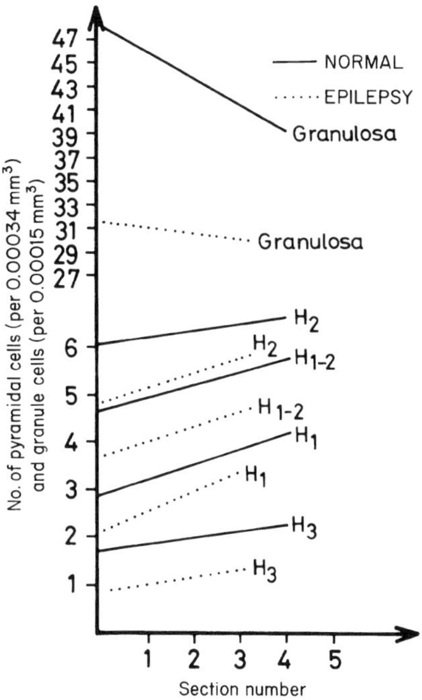

Figure 2. Neuron densities in the different H fields and the granule cells (*y*-axis) related to the anterior–posterior direction of the hippocampus (*x*-axis), from the study on post-mortem brains (Mouritzen Dam, 1979).

neuron loss seen in that particular part of the temporal lobes in epilepsy. Hippocampal sclerosis was described.

In the post-mortem study of Mouritzen Dam (1979), quantification was performed in each pyramidal field, H_1, H_2 and H_3 and on the granule cells, and in different blocks from the anterior to the posterior end of the hippocampal structure and in both right and left side. Control groups were included for the first time in the history of pathology in the hippocampus in relation to epilepsy. The neuronal numbers were given as volume densities, and related to different clinical parameters of the epilepsy.

It was found that no region was spared. Neuron loss occurred in all subfields of pyramidal cells and granule cells. In the post-mortem study this was particularly marked in fields H_3 and H_1 and in the granule cells and less in field H_2. The neuron loss of H_1 was related to early onset of the seizures. There was no systematic side difference.

In resected temporal lobes, the loss of granule cells was less. The neuron loss was shown particularly in the anterior part in both studies (Fig. 2), and in the surgical group there was a better outcome if the loss was mainly in the anterior part than in cases with patchy neuron loss throughout the structure. Other types of pathology in the temporal lobes include the recently described reorganization of mossy fibres in deafferented hippocampal tissue with secondary sprouting (Babb *et al.*, 1991) and changes in the dendritic tree with loss of spines described by Scheibel and Scheibel (1973) in temporal lobe specimens. Their role is uncertain, they may be non-specific changes and seem to be reversible under some conditions.

Heterotopia, which is localized clustering of neurons and cortical dysplasia or dystopia, is often found in the cerebrum and cerebellum in patients with epilepsy. It may be due to a developmental anomaly. It was first described in cortex in relation to temporal lobe epilepsy and in cerebellum in relation to symptomatic epilepsy with hippocampal neuron loss (Taylor *et al.*, 1971). Its role in symptomatic epilepsy is not known and the recent descriptions of a similar phenomenon called microdysgenesis in idiopathic epilepsies (Meencke and Janz, 1984) have revived interest in the phenomenon.

Dual pathology with the co-existence of extrahippocampal lesions including tumours combined with hippocampal sclerosis is found in 8–25% of brains in epilepsy (Armstrong and Bruton, 1987). It is difficult to say which is the epileptogenic focus.

Supporting cells such as glia have also been studied, but no conclusion can be drawn. Such studies are difficult as differentiation is not easy and is time-consuming. Better delineation will possibly be the result of refined substructure identification and will, together with the new and faster stereological method of quantification (Gundersen and Jensen, 1987), make such studies worth considering.

THE AETIOLOGIES OF MESIAL TEMPORAL SCLEROSIS AND OTHER TYPES OF PATHOLOGY IN HIPPOCAMPUS

Sommer and his contemporaries believed that the loss of neurons in the hippocampus had occurred before delivery, during pregnancy. However, hypoxic damage as the cause of neuron loss has long been the most defended aetiology and is still controversial. The German school with Spielmeyer (1927) and Scholz (1959) as its spokesmen, put forward the theory at the beginning of this century. The demonstration of similar occurrences of neuron loss in relation to status epilepticus has supported these ideas (Norman, 1964). More specific mechanisms were hypothesized after surgical intervention was introduced. Damage due to temporal herniation during birth was the theory of Earle *et al.* (1953), and febrile convulsions have been held responsible in the studies by Falconer and Taylor (1968).

The quantitative study of post-mortem brains found a relationship between long duration of the epilepsy and many generalized convulsions. In the quantitative study of temporal resections on the other hand, neuron loss was found to be of early occurrence and not progressive. The hypothesis of Penfield and Jasper (1954) of 'ripening' of the focus was not confirmed by these investigations. The apparent discrepancy in the two last-mentioned studies may be explained by the fact that they studied two different types of patients with epilepsy. The temporal resections were performed on younger patients with few generalized convulsions and relatively short duration of the epilepsy compared with the study of post-mortem brains.

The possible role of seizure-like activity in the brain, also acting perhaps interictally, is a matter of dispute today. Experimental studies have shown that neurons disappear in relation to seizures elicited by mechanisms which possibly influence the excitatory/inhibitory balance in hippocampus and is seen if the animals have a genetic trait to seizures (Mouritzen Dam *et al.*, 1981). Seizures elicited by external stimuli which possibly do not influence these factors do not destroy the neurons even if applied in high numbers although not as status epilepticus (Mouritzen Dam, 1982; Berthram *et al.*, 1990).

One observation of interest is that the neuron loss in field H_1 is selective without gliosis and delayed in occurrence (Kirino, 1982). This is interesting in relation to the classical type of hippocampal sclerosis in particular and may suggest that there is a different aetiology for neuron loss in that field. The role kindling may play in these processes is not yet clear in man, but deserves further consideration.

The recently described mossy fibre reactive synaptogenesis observed by ultrastructural and histochemical studies in human fascia dentata in resected temporal lobes (Babb *et al.*, 1991) has given rise to the hypothesis that this may result in enhanced excitation and contribute to seizure development.

CONCLUSIONS

Characteristic pathology has been described and studied in the temporal lobes or in the hippocampus proper in patients with epilepsy for over a century. The pathology is probably always associated with changes elsewhere in the brain, but apart from loss of Purkinje cells in the cerebellum (Dam, 1972; Dam *et al.*, 1984), these other pathological lesions are not specifically related to epilepsy. Every attempt has been made to correlate the loss of neurons in the hippocampus with the epilepsy.

The main causes of neuron loss are probably hypoxia, in particular around the time of birth, and the seizure activity itself. The importance of effective and early treatment in order to stop epileptic seizures and seizure activity has been emphasized. The resection of the temporal lobe in cases of medical intractability has had a revival over the last 10 years with improved presurgical evaluation.

The relation between neuron loss and the clinical manifestations of the epilepsy is not well established. Epileptic seizures express the properties of the brain region where they are elicited. Hughlings Jackson and Stewart (1899) were the first clinicians to propose a close relationship between the temporal lobes and epileptic seizures with psychosensory events including smell, taste and fear; and stimulation of the hippocampus is associated with memory disturbances, fear, sex and pleasure sensations, which to some degree supports Hughlings Jackson's idea.

Such seizure components as olfactory hallucinations, oromandibular activity, cardiovascular and gastrointestinal disturbances are, however, according to Gloor (1982), related to the amygdala-hippocampal complex and not of pure hippocampal origin. In patients with intractable temporal lobe epilepsy bound for surgical intervention, motor arrest and stereotypic automatisms with oromandibular movements were the most prominent signs of the seizures on the EEG- and video-monitoring before operation (Delgado-Escueta and Walsh, 1985).

The speed at which seizures spread in the temporal lobes makes it difficult to localize the exact site of origin (Williamson *et al.*, 1987), and Gates and Gumnit (1991) concluded that there is no characteristic ictal expression which will unequivocally and reliably identify the site of origin in the hippocampus of a clinical seizure. Hippocampal sclerosis defined as a specific pattern of neuron loss in the hippocampus pyramidal band cannot actually be more specifically related to either the clinical expressions of motor phenomena of the epileptic seizures or the concomitant psychological/psychiatric manifestations.

REFERENCES

Armstrong, D.D. and Bruton, C.L. (1987). What terminology is appropriate for tissue pathology? How does it predict outcome? In: Engel Jr, J. (Ed.), *Surgical Treatment of the Epilepsies*, Raven Press, New York.

Babb, T.L., Jann Brown, W., Pretorius, J., Davenport, C., Lieb, J. and Crandall, P.H. (1984). Temporal lobe volumetric cell densities in temporal lobe epilepsy. *Epilepsia*, **25**, 729–740.

Babb, T.L., Kupper, W.R., Pretorius, J.K., Crandall, P.H. and Levesque, M.F. (1991). Synaptic reorganization by mossy fibres in human epileptic fascia dentata. *Neurosci.*, **42**, 351–363.

Berthram, E.H., Lothman, E.W. and Lenn, N.J. (1990). The hippocampus in experimental chronic epilepsy: a morphometric analysis. *Ann. Neurol.*, **27**, 42–48.

Bouchet and Cazauviehlh (1825). Epilepsie et l'alienation mentale. *Arch. Gen. Med.*, **9**, 510–542.

Bratz, F. (1899). Ammonshorn Befunde der Epileptischen. *Arch. Psychiatr. Nervenkr.*, **31**, 820–936.

Dam, M. (1972). The density and ultrasturcture of Purkinje cells following diphenylhydantoin treatment in animals and man. *Acta. Neurol. Scand.*, (Suppl.) 1–65.

Dam, M., Bolwig, T., Hertz, M., Bajorek, J., Lomax, P. and Mouritzen Dam, A. (1984). Does seizure activity produce Purkinje cell loss? *Epilepsia*, **25**, 747–751.

Delgado-Escueta, A.V. and Walsh, G.O. (1985). Type I complex partial seizures of hippocampal origin: excellent results of anterior temporal lobectomy. *Neurology*, **35**, 143–154.

Earle, K.M., Baldwin, M. and Penfield, W. (1953). Incisural sclerosis and temporal lobe seizures produced by hippocampal herniation at birth. *Arch. Neurol. Psychiatry*, **69**, 27–42.

Falconer, M.A. and Taylor, D.C. (1968). Surgical treatment of drug-resistant epilepsy due to mesial temporal sclerosis. *Arch. Neurol.*, **19**, 353–361.

Gates, J.R. and Gumnit, R.J. (1991). Partial seizures of temporal lobe origin. In: Dam, M. and Gram, L. (Eds), *Comprehensive Epileptology*, Raven Press, New York, pp. 187–195.

Gloor, P. (1982). The role of the limbic system and experimental phenomena of temporal lobe epilepsy. *Ann. Neurol.*, **12**, 129–144.

Gundersen, H.J.G. and Jensen, E.B. (1987). The efficiency of systematic sampling in stereology and its prediction. *J. Microsc.*, **147**, 229–263.

Hughlings Jackson, J. and Stewart, P. (1899). Epileptic attacks with a warning of a crude sensation of smell and with the intellectual aura and symptoms of disorder in the right tempero-sphenoidal lobe. *Brain*, **22**, 534–549.

Kirino, T. (1982). Delayed neuronal death in the gerbil hippocampus following ischemia. *Brain Res.*, **239**, 57–69.

Margerison, J.H. and Corsellis, J.A.N. (1966). Epilepsy and the temporal lobes. *Brain*, **89**, 499–530.

Meencke, H.J. and Janz, D. (1984). Neuropathological findings in primary generalized epilepsy: a study of 8 cases. *Epilepsia*, **25**, 8–21.

Meynert, T. (1868). Studien über das pathologisch-anatomische Material der Wiener Irren-Anstalt. *Vierteljahrzeitschr. Psychiatr.*, **3**, 381–402.

Mouritzen Dam, A. (1979). The densities of neurons in the human hippocampus. *Neuropathol. Appl. Neurobiol.*, **5**, 249–264.

Mouritzen Dam, A. (1982). Hippocampal neuron loss in epilepsy and after experimental seizures. *Acta Neurol. Scand.*, **66**, 601–642.

Mouritzen Dam, A., Bajorek, J. and Lomax, P. (1981). Hippocampal neuron densities and seizures in the mongolian gerbils. *Epilepsia*, **22**, 667–674.

Norman, R.M. (1964). The neuropathology of status epilepticus. *Med. Sci. Law*, **4**, 46–51.

Penfield, W. and Jasper, H. (1954). *Epilepsy and the Functional Anatomy of the Human Brain*, Little, Brown, Boston.

Scheibel, M. and Scheibel, A. (1973). Hippocampal pathology in temporal lobe epilepsy. A Golgi survey. *Forum Med. Sci. Univ. Calif.*, **17**, 311–337.

Scholz, W. (1959). The contribution of pathoanatomy to the problem of epilepsy. *Epilepsia*, **1**, 36–55.

Sommer, W. (1880). Erkrankung des Ammonshorns als ätiologisches Moment der Epilepsie. *Arch. Erkrank. Nervenheilk.*, **10**, 631–675.

Spielmeyer, W. (1927). Die pathogenese des epileptischen krampfes. *Z. Dtsch. Gesamte. Neurol. Psychiatr.*, **109**, 501–520.

Taylor, D.C., Falconer, M.A., Bruton, C.J. and Corsellis, J.A.N. (1971). Focal dysplasia of the cerebral cortex in epilepsy. *J. Neurol. Neurosurg. Psychiatry*, **34**, 369–387.
Williamson, P.D., Wieser, H.G. and Delgado-Escueta, A.V. (1987). Clinical characteristics of partial seizures. In: Engel, J. (Ed.), *Surgical Treatment of the Epilepsies*, Raven Press, New York, pp. 101–120.

The Temporal Lobes and the Limbic System
Edited by M.R. Trimble and T.G. Bolwig

10

The Gastaut–Geschwind Syndrome

MICHAEL R. TRIMBLE
The Institute of Neurology, Queen Square, London, UK

INTRODUCTION

The relationship between epilepsy and personality disorders has had a long history and only in recent years has it become so controversial. The title of this chapter acknowledges the recrudescence of interest in the clinical aspects of this problem, which largely stems from the work of Gastaut in France and Geschwind in the United States of America. However, pride of place in crystallizing the concept of personality changes associated with epilepsy must surely reside with the French and German authors of the mid-nineteenth century.

THE CONTRIBUTIONS OF MOREL AND FALRET

Morel (1860) noted, '*Il est dans la nature des maladies nerveuses, d'imprimer à l'idiosyncrasie physique et morale des malades un cachet tout à fait particulier*'. (It is in the nature of these nervous diseases to impart a very specific aspect to the mental and physical idiosyncracies of patients.) Included were anger, irritability and fury, and from these ideas the concept of larval or masked epilepsy developed. Morel recognized that paroxysmal behavioural disturbances could coincide with the ictus, or be independent of it. It was therefore only a short step to suggesting the concept of epilepsy without seizures, masked and identified by behavioural changes only. The changes of character listed by Morel included marked instability, increased motor activity, polymorphic delusions, sudden explosive behaviour, episodic repetition of stereotyped insanity and sudden shouting.

Such ideas received support from the writing of Falret. He recognized peri-ictal disorders, those associated in time with the seizure, inter-paroxysmal disorders, and patients who entered a prolonged delirium, folie épileptique or epileptic insanity proper (Falret, 1860; 1861). He also noted cases in which slight epileptic paroxysms were unrecognized or developed late in the illness. He stated that in some cases, '*Le delire épileptique se substitue en quelque sorte aux convulsions épileptiques*'. (Epileptic delirium in some ways replaces epileptic convulsions.)

THE GERMAN CONTRIBUTION

Similar ideas were being discussed in Germany at the same time. Griesinger (1867) suggested that psychical disturbances could occur before epilepsy became manifest and in established cases could alternate with epileptic attacks. The term epileptic equivalent seems first to have been used by Hoffman in 1862. He noted in a short paper that, 'Eventually epileptic seizures may be missed completely, but the mental disease can reveal through its particular symptoms and signs that it is an equivalent of epilepsy, especially of convulsions and coma'.

Samt (1875, 1876), a psychiatrist from Berlin elaborated on the concept of epileptic insanity, and recognized two major forms, namely psychic equivalents and post-epileptic insanity. Psychic equivalents were recognized by their clinical form which included episodes of violence, religious ecstasy, anxious delirium and stupor. Kraepelin (1904) also noted the religious hallucinations and delusions of patients with epilepsy and discussed the acute mood changes. The latter were taken up by Aschaffenberg (1906) and Gaupp (1903). It was but a short step to the concepts of such authors as Bratz and Leubuscher (1907) of affect epilepsy, attacks precipitated by psychological factors which consisted of loss of consciousness, dizziness, hallucinations and rage.

THE MODERN ERA

The introduction of the EEG into clinical studies permitted a clear delineation of temporal lobe epilepsy and gave credence to the idea of a clinical association of behaviour disturbances with that form of epilepsy. Gibbs and Stamps (1953) commented that: 'The patient's emotional reactions to his seizures, to his family and to his social situation are less important determinants of psychiatric disorder than the site and type of the epileptic discharge'. Gibbs (1951) noted that 32% of patients with anterior temporal discharges had severe personality disorders, and suggested that pathological and physiological involvement of temporal lobe structures were therefore related to their presentation.

In France, Gastaut and his group clearly documented the underlying neuropathological changes of psychomotor seizures, re-emphasizing the importance of Ammon's horn sclerosis. They identified the association between behavioural disorders and seizures arising from such medial temporal structures. In one of the earliest controlled studies of personality in epilepsy, they compared 43 patients with psychomotor epilepsy with 21 with generalized epilepsy and a smaller group with symptomatic epilepsy and neocortical surface lesions. Only patients with lesions involving limbic structures, the majority of whom presented with psychomotor seizures and temporal lobe EEG abnormalities, showed personality disorders.

Gastaut (1956) commented further on the temporal lobe personality in his critical study of the artist Van Gogh, summing up his views as follows:

> *Nous croyons avoir demontré, en effet, que Van Gogh a presenté des crises épileptiques de type psychomotor secondaires à une lesion irritative temporale et declenchées par des excés alcooliques agissant sur un terrain neurolabile congenital. Nous croyons avoir demontré, egalement, que les troubles psychiques survenus à sa majorité et continuées dans l'intervalle de ses crises ne different pas des troubles characteriels intercritiques habituellement rencontrés chez les épileptiques psychomoteurs et dont l'aspect est souvant schizomorph.*
>
> (We believe we have demonstrated that Van Gogh had epileptic attacks of a psychomotor type secondary to an irritative temporal lesion and triggered by alcoholic excess acting on a congenital neurolabile disposition. We believe we have also demonstrated that the psychic problems he developed as he matured and which continued between attacks were the same as the personality problems usually found in the psychomotor epileptic when the pattern is often schizomorphic.)

RATING SCALE STUDIES

The more scientific studies of the concept of the epileptic personality began in the 1960s. Tizard (1962) critically reviewed the concept, and pointed out that the studies done up to that time had major methodological difficulties which included selection bias, assessment reliability, validity, and inadequate techniques, heavily relying on the Rorchach test, notorious for the subjective nature of its interpretation. However, since that time a plethora of studies have been carried out, and these can be divided into two main groups. Those that have used the Minnesota Multiphasic Personality Inventory, and those that have used other scales. These are briefly reviewed here.

Table 1. Personality and epilepsy – adult MMPI studies since 1962.

Authors[a]	*n*	*Result*
Guerrant *et al.*, 1962	32 TLE 26 Primary generalized 26 Chronic medical illness	All three groups similar: med illness more N; gen. more personality disturbance; TLE more P
Small *et al.*, 1962	25 Psychomotor 25 Centrencephalic or extratemporal foci	No differences – high scores both groups
Kløve and Dorhring, 1962	20 Epilepsy, unknown aetiology 20 Symptomatic epilepsy 20 Brain damage, no epilepsy 20 Affective disturbances 20 Controls	Epilepsy of unknown aetiology highest on scores
Meier and French, 1965	53 TLE	Bilateral > unilateral esp. F, D, Pa, Sc, Ca. Independent > dependent
Matthews and Kløve, 1968	51 Non-neurological controls 48 Brain damage, no epilepsy 65 Epilepsy, known aetiology (23 major motor, 22 psychomotor; 20 mixed) 69 Unknown aetiology (29 major motor, 22 psychomotor, 18 mixed)	No differences depression most frequently elevated in epileptic patients; most abnormalities in non-neuro controls
Mignone *et al.*, 1970	98 Psychomotor 53 Non-psychomotor	No differences between psychomotor and non-psychomotor; schizophrenia increase in those psychomotor with generalized seizures; % deviant responses, dominant > non-dominant
Stevens *et al.*, 1972	29 Psychomotor 14 Generalized 6 Local	No differences; schizophrenia scale high scores for psychomotor and generalized
Rodin *et al.*, 1976	78 TLE 78 Controls	TLE higher on depression and paranoia
Lachar *et al.*, 1979	37 TLE 28 non-TLE	No differences
Hermann *et al.*, 1980	47 TLE	Adolescent onset associated with increased Pd, Pt, Sc, Pa compared with child and adult onset
Hermann *et al.*, 1982a	TLE – ictal fear 11 other aura 14 generalized 14	Ictal fear higher than others on Pd, Pa, Pt, Sc, Si; Goldberg's system GE, normal: TLE, other aura, abnormal neurotic: TLE, fear, abnormal psychotic

Hermann *et al.*, 1982b	33 CPS 34 CPS with secondary generalized	CPS with 2 generally score higher
Dikmen *et al.*, 1983	37 CPS, 25 secondary generalized 34 CPS with generalization 48 Primary generalized	CPS with 2 generally higher D

[a]Full details of all references may be found in Trimble (1991).
Abbreviations: Ca, caudality; CPS, complex partial seizure; D, depression, F, validity; N, neurosis; P, psychosis; Pa, paranoia; Sc, schizophrenia; Si, social introversion.

MMPI Studies

Table 1 gives an overview of the MMPI studies. Several conclusions emerge. First, the earlier studies fail to show significant differences between temporal lobe epilepsy or its variants and other forms of seizures. Some of the studies however are complicated in that non-epileptic control groups also score high on psychopathology (Guerrant *et al.*, 1962; Matthews and Kløve, 1968), or alternative psychological tests suggest that the 'centrencephalic' or generalized seizure group have more cerebral damage than one would suspect from patients with a primary generalized seizure disorder. Secondly, some differences do emerge, especially in subcategories of patients with temporal lobe disorder. Bilateral findings appear to lead to more disturbances of personality than unilateral lesions while those with multiple seizure types or secondary generalized seizures also have more deviant profiles (Meier and French, 1965; Mignone *et al.*, 1970; Rodin *et al.*, 1976; Hermann *et al.*, 1982).

Rodin *et al.* (1976) explored this in most detail, comparing patients with temporal lobe seizures and one seizure type with those of more than one seizure type, and then comparing control patients who have one seizure type with those who have more than one seizure type. The first analysis revealed higher evaluation of MMPI scores in patients with more than one seizure type, while the second evaluation did not. In other words, behavioural abnormalities did not increase solely as the result of having more than one seizure type and were over represented in a temporal lobe population.

Thirdly, the scales which tend to be reported abnormal most frequently are the depression scale (D), the paranoia scale (Pa), the schizophrenia scale (Sc) and the psychaesthenia scale (Pt). These cover such personality attributes as suspiciousness, oversensitivity, ideas of reference, phobias and obsessive compulsive behaviour.

There have been many criticisms of these MMPI studies; one of the most important being that many of the negative studies may have arisen because the MMPI was not designed to assess psychopathology in epilepsy and a more sensitive instrument is required. It was in part to overcome such difficulties that Bear and Fedio (1977) developed their rating scale (BFI) which

Table 2. Non-MMPI studies of personality and epilepsy.

Authors[a]	*Scale*	*n*	*Result*
Standage and Fenton, 1975	Present state Examine, non-psychotic: EPI	27 Epilepsy 27 Medical controls	No difference; both groups high scores; TLE v. non-TLE no difference
Bech *et al.*, 1977	Marke–Nyman Inventory	30 JME 29 Psychomotor 30 Grand Mal 22 Controls (menières)	Low validity in JME
Trimble and Perez, 1990	Middlesex Hosp. Questionnaire	281 51% generalized 36% TLE and generalized 8% TLE alone	No major difference
Kogeorgos *et al.*, 1982	General Health Questionnaire Crown–Crisp Experimental Index	66 Epilepsy 50 Neurological controls	No major difference
Sorensen *et al.*, 1988	EPI Bellak Interview	28 TLE 15 Psoriasis 15 Primary generalized 15 Controls	Ego functioning poorer in those with more than one seizure type. No R/L differences
Bear and Fedio, 1977	BFI MMPI	27 TLE 15R 12L 12 Normal 9 Neuromuscular disorders	MMPI no differences; BFI many differences between TLE and others; R v. L esp. paranoia, elation, dependence, anger
Hermann and Riel, 1981	BFI	14 Generalized 14 CPS	TLE significantly greater on personal destiny, dependence; paranoia, philosophical interest
Nielsen and Kristensen, 1981	BFI	Lateral focus 14L 11R Mediobasal focus 9L 8R	Mediobasal focus > lateral; guilt and paranoia; L/R differences noted
Bear *et al.*, 1982	BFI	TLE10 10 Other seizures 10 Affectives 10 Schizophrenia 10 Aggresiveness	TLE and other seizures, TLE greater on religiosity, philosophical interests, sadness, emotionally and overall mean
Mungas, 1982	BFI	14 TLE 14 Neurological and behaviour disorders 14 Psychiatric	No differences
Rodin and Schmaltz, 1984	BFI	148 Epilepsy – 16 RTLE – 16 LTLE 18 Pain patients 15 Psychiatric 40 Controls	TLE scored higher on 13 categories, hypergraphia esp.; no R/L differences; relationship to anti-convulsant drugs;

Master *et al.*, 1984	BFI	55 TLE 16 Primary generalized 27 Psychiatric 40 Controls	no differences between patient groups; no R/L differences
Brandt *et al.*, 1985	BFI	28 LTLE 19 RTLE 10 Primary generalized 14 Controls	LTLE and generalized patients most different from controls, esp. circumstantiality, humourlessness, sadness, viscosity, dependence, obsessionality and paranoia
Stark-Adamec *et al.*, 1985	BFI	70 Seizure pts CPS, gen, CPS+ Gen 92 Psychiatric 28 Dialysis 447 Non patients	Seizure patients do not differ from each other; links of psychopathology in epilepsy to auras

[a]Full details of all references may be found in Trimble (1991).
Abbreviations: BFI, Bear–Fedio inventory; CPS, complex partial seizures; EPI, Eysenck personality inventory; JME, juvenile myoclonic epilepsy; MMPI, Minnesota multiphasic inventory; TLE, temporal lobe epilepsy.

was derived from prior reports of descriptions of personality in patients with epilepsy. Their data are shown in Table 2, which includes other studies of personality in epilepsy which have not used the MMPI.

Non-MMPI studies

As with the MMPI the results of these investigations, including those with the BFI are somewhat mixed. In their original report, Bear and Fedio compared patients with unilateral temporal lobe epilepsy with normal subjects and with a group having neuromuscular disorders. They noted that epileptic patients reported a different profile of responses to non-epileptic subjects and controls, noting such personality features as humourlessness, dependence, circumstantiality, increased sense of personal destiny and others as being distinctive. There were differences between self-reported behaviour profiles and independent profiles from a close family member or friend. Laterality differences were noted: patients with left temporal epilepsy described more anger, paranoia and dependence, while those with right temporal foci reported more elation.

Subsequent investigations have tended either to confirm or refute their findings. Authors of the latter studies suggest that the scale does no more than assess non-specific psychopathology (Mungas, 1982; Rodin and Schmaltz, 1984; Master *et al.*, 1984). This is largely based on comparisons between patients hospitalized for psychiatric illness and patients with temporal lobe epilepsy, few or no differences being noted between these populations. While not supportive for a profile of psychopathology distinctive for temporal lobe epilepsy, these critics miss the point that there is a cerebral basis to psychopathology in the absence of epilepsy and that patients with conditions other than epilepsy may have disturbed function within their temporal lobe.

Of more interest are the positive findings. Several studies report an increase in paranoia in temporal lobe groups, (Bear and Fedio, 1977; Hermann and Riel, 1981; Nielsen and Kristensen, 1981; Brandt *et al.*, 1985). Another trait which is distinguishing in several studies is that of hypergraphia (Bear and Fedio, 1977; Nielsen and Kristensen, 1981; Rodin and Schmaltz, 1984).

One criticism of the BFI studies is that they have failed to confirm that all patients with temporal lobe epilepsy suffer from a distinctive personality profile which can be detected by the scale. While Bear and Fedio (1977) do refer to a consistent profile of changes noted in patients, they did not suggest that it would be seen in all patients at all times, an unrealistic expectation.

Adamec (1989) has discussed the complexity of these studies, and added contributions of his own. He gave a modified BFI to 114 patients with epilepsy of varying diagnoses, to 91 psychiatric patients, to 43 patients with chronic illness other than epilepsy, and to 100 normal controls. Three classifications of seizure patients emerged from an item cluster analysis followed by discriminate function analysis; namely, correctly classified seizure patients, those classified as psychiatric patients, and those classified as non-patients. The 25% classified as psychiatric patients were distinguished from other seizure patients on depression, mood and metaphysical (religious) clusters. In addition, they had five of 33 aura experiences intensely and frequently. Adamec referred to these as limbic auras.

This is one of several studies which use some marker of limbic system function to identify patients with mediolimbic seizures where an association between the latter seizure type and psychopathology has been demonstrated. Another is that of Wieser (1983), who used depth electrode recordings to verify the site of origin of seizures in patients with temporal lobe epilepsy. He noted that patients with a medial focus scored higher on a number of BFI subscales when compared with patients with either temporal neocortical involvement or extratemporal foci.

CLINICAL STUDIES

The view that there is an interictal behaviour syndrome associated with temporal lobe epilepsy has been most strongly supported from the clinical point of view by Geschwind and colleagues (Waxman and Geschwind, 1975). In their report they highlighted, with striking examples, changes in sexual behaviour, hypergraphia and religiosity. They also highlighted stickiness or viscosity, patients showing a marked preoccupation with detail and concerns over moral and ethical issues.

Religiosity in association with epilepsy has been noted on many occasions. It is commented on in the early writings of the French and German authors, for example in Morel. The English psychiatrist Maudsley specifically mentioned the development of exaggerated sentiment as part of the character change in epilepsy, and quoted Swedenborg as an example (Maudsley, 1874, 1879).

Such religiosity was the subject of a special study by Howden (1873). He thought it was not uncommon and recognized strong devotional feelings in patients which could manifest either as simple piety, or as religious delusions. He gave several case histories, emphasizing different shades of religiosity which could arise, and suggested that, 'Many religious fanatics were epileptics'. He included amongst these Mohammed, Ann-Lee (the mother of the Shakers) and Swedenborg. Others who have written on this subject include Echeverria (1873), Clouston (1896) and Clark and Lesko (1939). The latter authors described four patients with a chronic schizophrenia-like illness in epilepsy, three of whom had religious delusions or hallucinations. Slater and Beard (1963) commented that mystical illusions were remarkably common in their series, occurring in 38% of cases, and Bruens (1971) noted that 'Religious contents were fairly common' to all hallucinations in his patients.

Dewhurst and Beard (1970) reviewed the literature and described six cases of their own all of whom had temporal lobe epilepsy and who underwent religious conversions, not having been particularly religious prior to the conversion. Hyper-religiosity was one of the 18 traits selected by Bear and Fedio for their rating scale, although no clear conclusions about the association of epilepsy and religiosity can be obtained from the studies using the scale.

It is most likely that personality traits such as religiosity and hypergraphia seen in patients with epilepsy represent an all-or-none phenomenon and are seen in a minority of patients. It is not a graded characteristic, for example like obsessionality, and therefore does not emerge as a prominent factor in questionnaire studies unless a sufficiently large number of patients are evaluated.

CONCLUSIONS

The association of epilepsy with personality and character change is one which goes back to the writings of ancient times. The French and German authors of the last century re-emphasized this connection, and two different ideas emerged: first, that of a chronic organic brain change secondary to a lesion in the brain, most notably in the medial temporal lobes, which was responsible both for the epilepsy and the personality change. Sommer was an early exponent of this view which has become crystallized through the writings of authors such as Gibbs, Gastaut and Geschwind. The other line of literature related to the development of personality changes in the absence of seizures, or some kind of alternating phenomenon whereby seizures are replaced by behaviour changes. This has been subject to much less investigation and has been an area of controversy ever since the ideas were introduced over a century ago.

It is not suggested that all patients with temporal lobe epilepsy will automatically succumb to adverse personality changes and many of the traits noted need not be seen in a majority. Indeed, a full blown syndrome is seen quite rarely, hence part of the controversy. Rodin *et al.* (1984) in their MMPI study removed subjects with high and low scores on certain EPI derived items and then performed a cluster analysis. The cluster which corresponded to the complete features of the epileptic personality was present in association with a temporal lobe seizure disorder in 7% of patients.

REFERENCES

Adamec, R.E. (1989). Kindling, anxiety and personality. In: Bolwig, T.G. and Trimble, M.R. (Eds), *The Clinical Relevance of Kindling*, Wiley, Chichester, pp. 117–135.

Aschaffenberg, G. (1906). *Uber die Stimmungs-Schwankungen der Epileptiker*, Marhold, Halle.

Bear, D.M. and Fedio, P. (1977). Quantitative analysis of interictal behaviour in temporal lobe epilepsy. *Arch. Neurol.*, **34**, 454–467.

Brandt, B.J., Seidman, L.J. and Kohl, D. (1985). Personality characteristics of epileptic patients. *J. Clin. Exp. Neuro. Psychol.*, **7**, 25–28.

Bratz, H. and Leubuscher, H. (1907). Die affect-epilepsie. *Dtsch. Med. Wschr.*, **33**, 592–593.

Bruens, J.H. (1971). Psychosis in epilepsy. *Psychiatr. Neurol. Neurochir.*, **74**, 174–192.

Clark, R.A. and Lesko, J.M. (1939). Psychoses associated with epilepsy. *Am. J. Psychiatry*, **96**, 595–607.

Clouston, T.S. (1896). *Clinical Lectures on Mental Diseases. 4th edn*, Churchill, London.

Dewhurst, K. and Beard, A.W. (1970). Sudden religious conversions in temporal lobe epilepsy. *Br. J. Psychiatry*, **117**, 497–507.

Echeverria, M.G. (1873). On epileptic insanity. *Am. J. Insanity*, 301–351.

Falret, J. (1860, 1861). D'l'état mental des épileptiques. *Arch. Gen. Med.*, **16**, 661–699; **17**, 461–491; **18**, 423–443.

Gastaut, H. (1956). Etude électroclinique des épisodes psychotiques survenant en dehors des crises cliniques. Chez les épileptiques. *Rev. Neurol.*, **94**, 587–594.

Gaupp, H. (1903). Zür Frage der Kombinierten psychosen. *Zentralbl. Nervenheilk. Psychiatrie*, **26**, 766–775.

Gibbs, F.A. (1951). Ictal and non-ictal psychiatric disorders in temporal lobe epilepsy. *J. Nerv. Ment. Dis.*, **113**, 522–528.

Gibbs, F.A. and Stamps, F.W. (1953). *Epilepsy Handbook*, Thomas, Springfield, IL.
Griesinger, W. (1967). *Mental Pathology and Therapeutics*, New Sydenham Society, London.
Guerrant, J., Anderson, W.W., Fischer, A., Weinstein, M.R., Jaros, R.M. and Deskins, A. (1962). *Personality in Epilepsy*, Charles C. Thomas, Springfield.
Hermann, B.P. and Riel, P. (1981). Interictal personality and behaviour traits in temporal lobe and generalised epilepsy. *Cortex*, **17**, 125–128.
Hermann, B.P., Schwartz, M.S., Karnes, W.E. and Valdat, P. (1980). Psychopathology in epilepsy: relationship of seizure type to age of onset. *Epilepsia*, **21**, 15–23.
Hermann, B.P., Dikmen, S. and Wilensky, A. (1982). Incidence of psychopathology associated with multiple seizure types. Fact or artifact? *Epilepsia*, **23**, 587–598.
Hoffman, H. (1862). *see* Aschaffenberg, 1906.
Howden, J.C. (1873). The religious sentiments of epileptics. *J. Ment. Sci.*, **18**, 491–497.
Kraepelin, E. (1904). *Lectures on Clinical Psychiatry*, William Wood, New York.
Master, D.R., Toone, B.K., and Scott, D.F. (1984). Interictal behaviour in temporal lobe epilepsy. In: Porter, R. (Ed.), *Advances in Epileptology: 15th Epilepsy International Symposium*, Raven Press, New York, pp. 557–565.
Matthews, C.H.G. and Kløve, H. (1968). MMPI performance in major motor, psychomotor and mixed seizure classifications of known and unknown aetiology. *Epilepsia*, **9**, 43–53.
Maudsley, H. (1874). *Responsibility in Mental Disease*, Henry King, London.
Maudsley, H. (1879). *Body and Mind*, Appleton, New York.
Meier, M. and French, L.A. (1965). Some personality correlates of unilateral and bilateral EEG abnormalities in psychomotor epileptics. *J. Clin. Psychopathol.*, **21**, 3–9.
Mignone, R.J., Donnelly, E.F. and Sadowsky, D. (1970). Psychological and neurological comparisons of psychomotor and non-psychomotor epileptic patients. *Epilepsia*, **11**, 345–349.
Morel, B.A. (1860). *Traité des Maladies Mentales*, Masson, Paris.
Mungas, D. (1982). Interictal behaviour abnormality in temporal lobe epilepsy. *Arch. Gen. Psychiatry*, **39**, 108–111.
Nielsen, H. and Kristensen, O. (1981). Personality correlates of sphenoidal EEG foci in temporal lobe epilepsy. *Acta Neurol. Scand.*, **64**, 289–300.
Rodin, E. and Schmaltz, S. (1984). The Bear–Fedio personality inventory. *Neurology*, **34**, 591–596.
Rodin, E., Katz, M. and Lennox, D. (1976). Differences between patients with temporal lobe seizures and those with other forms of epileptic attacks. *Epilepsia*, **17**, 313–320.
Rodin, E., Schmaltz, S. and Twitty, G. (1984). What does the Bear–Fedio inventory measure? *Epilepsy International Symposium*, Raven Press, New York, pp. 551–555.
Samt, P. (1875, 1876). Epileptische Irreseins Formen. *Arch. Psychiatr. Nervenkr.*, **5**, 393–444; **6**, 110–216.
Slater, E. and Beard, A.W. (1963). The schizophrenia-like psychoses of epilepsy V. Discussion and conclusions. *Br. J. Psychiatry*, **109**, 95–150.
Tizard, B. (1962). The personality of epileptics: a discussion of the evidence. *Psychol. Bull.*, **59**, 196–210.
Trimble, M.R. (1991). *The Psychoses of Epilepsy*, Raven Press, New York, pp. 112–118
Waxman, S.G. and Geschwind, N. (1975). The interictal behaviour syndromes of temporal lobe epilepsy. *Arch. Gen. Psychiatry*, **32**, 1580–1586.
Wieser, H.G. (1983). Depth recorded limbic seizures and psychopathology. *Neurosci. Behav. Rev.*, **7**, 427–440.

The Temporal Lobes and the Limbic System
Edited by M.R. Trimble and T.G. Bolwig

11

Psychosis and Epilepsy: The Link to the Temporal Lobe

BETTINA SCHMITZ
Institute of Neurology, Department of Neurology, Queen Square, London, UK and Department of Neurology, Rudolf Virchow Clinic, Berlin, Germany

INTRODUCTION

Wilhelm Sommer

One of the first authors to explore the relationship between temporal lobe pathology and psychosis was Wilhelm Sommer while working as a psychiatrist in the lunatic asylum of Allenberg in Germany. He wrote two extensive papers on these topics. In the first of these (1880), Sommer analysed neuropathological findings in the Ammon's horn of 90 epilepsy patients. This material represented all previously published cases supplemented by five of Sommer's own patients from Allenberg. For each of the 90 patients Sommer specified seizure symptomatology, psychopathology and neuropathological findings, thus allowing us to do statistical analyses in retrospect (Table 1).

Sommer described a characteristic cell loss in the CA1 region of his cases ('Sommer sector'). In his opinion pathological changes in the hippocampus, which he thought was a major sensory centre, were of significant aetiological importance for the development of epilepsy and substantiated this by emphasizing the frequency of sensory impairments and hallucinations in epilepsy patients.

One year later, in 1881, Sommer published an article on 'Postepileptisches Irresein' (postepileptic insanity) in which he developed an extensive classification of the various subforms of epileptic insanity, including also aetiology and prognosis. He based his hypotheses on quantitative analyses of large series of well-described patients. This approach was different to most of Sommer's contemporary epileptologists whose concepts were based mainly on single case studies.

Table 1. Relationship between history of psychosis and lateralization of hippocampus pathology in 90 patients with epilepsy (after Sommer, 1880).

Lateralization		*Non-affective psychosis*[a] *n = 10*	*Affective psychosis*[b] *n = 3*	*No psychosis*[c] *n = 77*
Left	*n* = 31	5	2	24
Right	*n* = 14	2	1	11
Bilateral	*n* = 39	3	–	36
Unknown	*n* = 6	–	–	6

These figures derive from a retrospective analysis of Sommer's original data. Sommer's descriptions of the psychiatric states of his patients were classified by a psychiatrist who was blinded to the lateralization of hippocampus pathology.
[a]Hallucinations, delusions, ideas of persecution, religious excitation, insanity, delirium.
[b]Depression, mania.
[c]Normal (*n* = 2) and unknown mental state (*n* = 9), dysphoria, irritability, raving madness, irascibility, malevolence, excitation, mental weakness, idiocy, stupidity, dementia.

Sommer distinguished postepileptic stupidity and episodic postepileptic insanity (after Samt, 1875). Postepileptic stupidity was the final consequence of a dementing process which was initiated by recurrent postictal twilight states and consecutively followed by progressive forgetfulness, circumstantiality, word finding difficulties, impairment of perception and changes in character with religiosity, hypocrisy, irascibility and irritability.

With respect to episodic insanity, in 63 patients Sommer distinguished psychoses which occur pre-ictally (*n* = 5), postictally (*n* = 47) or instead of seizures (epileptic equivalents, *n* = 11). In Sommer's opinion these episodes were directly related to epileptic activity, in contrast to the rare cases of combinations of epilepsy with true madness (schizophrenia), melancholy or paralysis. In these cases he believed that the insanity was not caused by the epilepsy but that both were related to the same underlying pathology. Sommer not only characterized in detail the psychopathology of epileptic psychoses but also investigated 'risk factors' and emphasized that insanity was much more frequent in patients with 'petit mal' epilepsies (absence seizures and complex focal seizures) compared with patients with grand mal epilepsies—only one of many findings subsequently confirmed in the modern literature (Schmitz, 1988).

Modern literature

After a period of neglect, psychoses in epilepsy were 'rediscovered' in the 1950s and 1960s (Landolt, 1953; Tellenbach, 1965). English and American authors (Gibbs, 1951; Pond, 1962; Slater and Beard, 1963) emphasized again the link to temporal lobe epilepsy (TLE). However, in contrast to psychiatrists in the early twentieth century who, like Sommer, saw episodic psychoses in epilepsy as quite separate from schizophrenia and others who assumed an antagonism between epilepsy and schizophrenia, they stressed the similarity between psychosis in epilepsy and schizophrenia and therefore favoured a positive relationship between both disorders. Since then the growing international interest in links between psychosis and epilepsy has generated a multitude of studies. Research has been very much concentrated on the identification of biological risk factors.

The role of the temporal lobe in the development of psychoses in epilepsy has been a matter of considerable disagreement in the literature. The pathophysiological basis of a possible relationship is still not well explained. This paper will discuss specific methodological problems and concentrate on findings deriving from clinical studies concerning the temporal lobe hypothesis.

CLASSIFICATION

Classification of psychoses in epilepsy

A classification system for psychoses in epilepsy should ideally consider psychopathology, duration and course of psychosis, type of epilepsy, relation to seizure activity, drug treatment, EEG findings and psycho-social factors. Unfortunately, these criteria are not strictly intercorrelated (Table 2). 'Atypical' combinations are not unusual, such as ictal and postictal psychoses in clear consciousness (Wolf, 1973). Variations in phenomenology and precipitation can also be seen intra-individually in patients who experience recurrent psychotic episodes (Sherwin, 1984; Bash and Mahnig, 1984). In addition to this there is also some evidence for an aetiological overlap between syndromes (Wolf, 1991). The usefulness for both clinical application and research purposes of previously proposed syndromatic classification systems (Bruens, 1974; Helmchen, 1975; Köhler, 1980; Fenton, 1981) is therefore limited.

For the time being a comprehensive description considering each of the above-mentioned criteria separately is recommended. Epileptic syndromes and seizures should be classified according to the proposals of the ILAE (Commission on Classification and Terminology of the ILAE, 1981, 1989). Psychoses should also be classified following international systems such as the ICD 9 (World Health Organization, 1980) and the DSM IIIR (American Psychiatric Association, 1987). However, when applied in psychosis in epilepsy, these classifications have some problems which necessitate adaptations. In the DSM IIIR the existence of epilepsy automatically leads to a diagnosis of 'organic mental syndromes and disorders' and does not allow the diagnosis of 'functional' psychoses such as schizophrenia, even if all required criteria are met (Trimble, 1991).

Table 2. Relationship between impairment of consciousness and relationship to seizures, duration of episodes and course of psychoses in 28 consecutive epilepsy patients with mixed psychoses (Schmitz, 1988).

	Consciousness impaired *n = 15*	*Consciousness not impaired* *n = 13*
Relation to seizures		
Periictal	12	4
Alternative	1	2
No relation	2	7
Not significant		
Duration of episodes[a]		
Days	9	1
Weeks	4	4
Months	1	6
$p < 0.05$		
Course		
Single episode	5	3
Recurrent episodes	10	5
Chronicity (> 6 months)	0	5
$p < 0.05$, χ^2 test		

[a]Unknown in three cases.

Having emphasized the limitations of syndromatic classifications, Table 3(a)–(e) is an amalgam from a range of authors of the descriptions of the psychotic syndromes seen grouped according to their relation to seizures. Pre-ictal syndromes are not considered because they very rarely manifest as psychosis (Wolf, 1976).

Classification of temporal lobe epilepsy

Because temporal lobe epilepsy (TLE) is frequent and often drug-resistant (Wieser, 1991), epileptologists have spent much effort in studying the phenomenological variety of seizures arising from this particular part of the brain. The terminology which has been developed and applied to describe temporal lobe epilepsies and seizures in the last century is, unfortunately very confusing (Table 4). Even the recent Proposal for Classification of the ILAE is more discouraging than helpful for clinical needs. It suggests that reliable classification requires sophisticated, often invasive EEG methods because clinical seizure symptomatology is not specific and can therefore be misleading, as can the routine scalp EEG. This classification seems to have been unduly influenced by the needs of epilepsy surgeons since it is strictly localization-related and does not consider functional anatomy. Limbic epilepsy for example, which arises from a recognized functional system (Trimble, 1991), has no place in the classification because it crosses anatomical boundaries.

Table 3(a). Ictal psychoses.

Literature	Lennox, 1945; Ballenger *et al.*, 1983
Subtypes and synonyms	Absence-status, spike-wave-stupor, non-convulsive status, status psychomotoricus, status of complex focal seizures, aura continua, ictal twilight states
Type of epilepsy	Localization-related (temporal lobe and frontal lobe epilepsy) and generalized epilepsies (Lennox–Gastaut syndrome, pyknolepsy, juvenile absence epilepsy)
Seizure types	Complex focal seizures, absence seizures
Clinical characteristics	Impaired consciousness, subtle epileptic motor phenomena such as oral automatisms and lid myoklonias
Duration	Hours to days, rarely longer (if unrecognized)
Termination	Intravenous antiepileptic drugs, spontaneous generalized tonic–clonic seizures
EEG	Focal or generalized status epilepticus
Precipitation	Non-compliance, withdrawal of antiepileptic drugs
Risk factors	Severe epilepsies
Prognosis	Recurrence risk dependent on seizure management, recurrent non-convulsive status in children is correlated with dementia
Prophylaxis	Seizure control

Table 3(b). Postictal psychoses.

Literature	Logsdail and Toone, 1988, Savard *et al.*, 1991
Subtypes and synonyms	–
Type of epilepsy	Localization-related and generalized epilepsies
Seizure types	Primary or secondary generalized tonic–clonic seizures, complex focal seizures
Clinical characteristics	Lucid interval between seizures and psychosis 1 to 2 days, phenomenological polymorphism
Duration	Days
Termination	Antiepileptic drugs, neuroleptic drugs rarely necessary
EEG	Increased epileptic activity and slowing
Precipitation	Non-compliance, withdrawal of antiepileptic drugs, series or status epilepticus
Risk factors	Severe epilepsies
Prognosis	Recurrence risk dependent on seizure control
Prophylaxis	Seizure control, early interruption of series and status epilepticus

Table 3(c). Parictal psychoses.

Literature	Wolf, 1976
Subtypes and synonyms	–
Type of epilepsy	Localization-related and generalized epilepsies
Seizure types	Primary or secondary generalized tonic–clonic seizures, complex focal seizures
Clinical characteristics	Gradual development, disturbance of consciousness and confusion more often than in postictal psychoses
Duration	Days, weeks
Termination	Antiepileptic drugs, neuroleptic drugs rarely necessary
EEG	Increased epileptic activity and slowing
Precipitation	Increase of seizure frequency, not necessarily due to noncompliance or reduction of antiepileptic drugs in the presurgical assessment
Risk factors	Severe epilepsies
Prognosis	Recurrence risk dependent on seizure control
Prophylaxis	Seizure control, monitoring of psychiatric symptoms in the presurgical assessment

Table 3(d). Interictal psychoses.

Literature	Slater and Beard, 1963; Trimble, 1991
Subtypes and synonyms	Schizophrenia-like, schizomorph, endoform, paranoid–hallucinatory psychoses
Type of epilepsy	Localization-related epilepsies (temporal lobe epilepsy, frontal lobe epilepsy?) more often than generalized epilepsies?
Seizure types	Complex focal seizures, absence seizures
Clinical characteristics	Schizophrenia-like with hallucinations and delusions, no affective flattening, catatonia and thought disorders
Duration	Weeks to months
Termination	Neuroleptic drugs
EEG	Unchanged
Precipitation	–
Risk factors	Severe, longstanding epilepsy, social disintegration
Prognosis	High recurrence risk, long-term prognosis better than in schizophrenia, residual symptoms and personality deterioration less frequent
Prophylaxis	Optimal epilepsy management including medical treatment and psychosocial care

Table 3(e). Alternative psychoses.

Literature	Landolt, 1953; Tellenbach, 1965; Wolf, 1991
Subtypes and synonyms	Forced normalization, paradoxical normalization
Type of epilepsy	Generalized more frequent than localization-related epilepsies
Seizure types	Pyknoleptic absences, complex focal seizures
Clinical characteristics	Prodromal phase with insomnia, anxiety and social withdrawal (prepsychotic dysphoria), delusional-hallucinatory symptomatic less frequent than non-psychotic syndromes (such as depressive, hypochondriacal and hysterical states)
Duration	Days to weeks
Termination	Sleep regulation, epileptic seizures, spontaneous
EEG	'Normalized' (no epileptic activity, less well organized alpha-rhythm, lower amplitude, more interspersed slow activity)
Precipitation	Effective antiepileptic treatment, especially with ethosuximide, vigabatrin?
Risk factors	Absence seizures in adults
Prognosis	Generally good, recurrence risk dependent on seizure management, very rarely chronic course with alternating of psychotic symptoms and epileptic seizures
Prophylaxis	Recognition and therapy of prodromal symptoms, careful medical treatment of absences in adults

Differences in definition of TLE, either based on seizure symptomatology ('psychomotor epilepsy'), involvement of specific functional systems ('limbic epilepsy') or on anatomical localization as detected by depth EEG or neuroimaging ('amygdalo-hippocampal epilepsy') have considerable impact on the interpretation of the literature on epilepsy and psychosis with respect to the nature of a possible link to temporal lobe epilepsy. In many studies frontal and temporal lobe epilepsies are not sufficiently differentiated. An observed link to psychosis in such studies is thus not necessarily evidence for localization.

THE LINK BETWEEN EPILEPSY AND PSYCHOSIS IN GENERAL AND BETWEEN TLE AND PSYCHOSIS IN PARTICULAR

Epidemiological studies

The majority of authors who write on psychosis in epilepsy come to the conclusion that psychoses are frequent complications of epilepsy. This

Table 4. Synonyms for temporal lobe epilepsy and temporal lobe seizures.

Synonyms	*Authors*	*Year*
Fugues épileptiques	Morel	1860
Petit mal intellectuel	Falret	1861
Epileptoide Zustände	Griesinger	1868
Psychomotorische Zustände	Griesinger	1868
Automatismes ambulatoires	Charcot	1874
Epilepsie de l'intelligence	Legrand du Saulle	1877
Epileptische rudimente	Sommer	1880
Dreamy states	Jackson	1888
Uncinate group of epileptic fits	Jackson	1889
Epilepsie psychique pure	Laroussinie	1895
Psychomotorism	Turner	1907
Psychomotorische äquivalente	Förster	1926
Psychic variant	Wilson	1935
Psychomotor epilepsy	Gibbs *et al.*	1938
Dämmerattacken	Meyer-Mickeleit	1950
Limbic epilepsy	Fulton	1953
Rhinenephalic epilepsy	Fulton	1953
Automatisms and psychical seizures	Penfield and Jasper	1954
Oral-petit mal	Hallen	1954
Complex focal seizures	ILAE	1981
Frontal lobe complex partial seizures	Williamson et al.	1983
Type I, Type II seizures	Delgado-Escueta and Walsh	1985
Mesiobasal limbic epilepsy	Wieser and Yasargil	1982
Amygdalo-hippocampal seizures	ILAE	1989
Lateral temporal epilepsies	ILAE	1989

Modified from Janz (1969).

opinion, however, is mainly based on selected case series and is not in keeping with findings from epidemiological studies (Zielinski, 1986).

There are only two population-based studies on the frequency of mixed psychoses in epilepsy. Zielinski found in a field study of the Warsaw population prevalence rates for psychoses in epilepsy of 2–3% (Zielinski, 1974). Gudmundsson in a study on the frequency of mixed psychoses in epilepsy in the population of Iceland found prevalence rates for males of 6% and for females of 9% (Gudmundsson, 1966). These figures can be compared with findings of an earlier study by Helgason, who looked at the risk of psychosis in the general population of Iceland using the same diagnostic criteria as Gudmundsson. Helgason found prevalence rates of 7% for males and 5% for females. The comparison of Helgason's and Gudmundsson's studies suggests a similar risk for psychosis in people with and without epilepsy, being only slightly higher in females with epilepsy but slightly lower in males with epilepsy.

There are two possible explanations for the discrepancies between clinical observations and epidemiological findings.

1. Epidemiological studies underestimate the rate of psychosis in epilepsy, or
2. Uncontrolled clinical studies overestimate the rate of psychosis.

Explanation 1

Gudmundsson's and Helgason's data taken together do not support the conclusion that the frequency of mixed psychoses in patients with epilepsy in large case series or epidemiological studies is underestimated. With respect to schizophrenia, however, there is a possible reason for a bias towards underestimation of prevalence rates in epilepsy patients. Several authors have pointed out, that the so-called schizophrenia-like psychoses in epilepsy are different from true schizophrenia in terms of a much better prognosis without deterioration of personality and other residual symptoms (Slater and Beard, 1963; Sherwin, 1984). Although not confirmed by all authors (Helmchen, 1975; Toone *et al.*, 1982; Oyebode and Davison, 1989), such a difference in prognosis would favour an underestimation of these psychoses compared with functional schizophrenia. This could for example account for the low figures of patients with epilepsy and schizophrenia in clinical series of psychiatric institutions in the old literature. The data by Ganter (1925), who found one patient with epilepsy and schizophrenia among 487 psychiatric patients (0.2%), and Wyrsch (1933), who found 16 patients with epilepsy and schizophrenia among 10 000 psychiatric patients (0.2%), were interpreted as an indication for an antagonism between epilepsy and schizophrenia. Whether psychoses in epilepsy are 'schizophrenia-like' or not depends critically on the definition of schizophrenia used, which is internationally different and may be based for example either on Schneiderian first rank symptoms (positive symptoms) or Bleulerian fundamental symptoms (negative symptoms).

Explanation 2

Looking at the prevalence rates for psychosis in epilepsy as a function of the source of patients (Table 5) it becomes obvious that psychoses are considerably overrepresentated in more specialized centres. Zielinski (1974) could demonstrate that the rate of psychoses in epilepsy patients is higher when these are known to medical services as compared with people with epilepsy who never sought medical treatment for their epilepsy (3% versus 2%). Zielinski could also show that the probability for a patient to be seen in a specialized centre was higher when he or she suffered from more than one medical problem. The high prevalence rate of schizophrenia in epilepsy in case series from Third World countries (Gureje, 1991; Matuja, 1990) could be explained by a similar mechanism. In a retrospective study of 697 outpatients

Table 5. Frequency of mixed psychoses in epilepsy (Europe, Japan, USA).

Source of patients	*Authors*	*Year*	*Prevalence*
Field study	Gudmundsson	1966	7%
	Zielinski	1974	2%
General practices	Edeh and Toone	1987	5%
Neurological departments	Roger *et al.*	1956	9%
	Standage and Fenton	1975	8%
Epileptological departments	Bruens	1973	6%
	Sengoku *et al.*	1983	6%
	Schmitz	1988	4%
Psychiatric departments	Roger *et al.*	1956	41%
	Betts	1974	21%
	Bash and Mahnig	1984	60%

with epilepsy, consecutively referred to an epilepsy clinic, it could be shown that patients with psychoses were followed up significantly longer and significantly rarely referred to other facilities compared with patients without psychoses (Schmitz, 1988). This necessarily leads to a progressive accumulation of patients with psychosis and could explain the relative higher prevalence rate of psychosis in studies not considering consecutively referred patients but patients registered at a fixed time or having appointments in a defined interval.

Controlled studies on the relationship of psychosis to different forms of epilepsy

It is widely accepted in clinical epileptology that psychoses are positively linked to temporal lobe epilepsy. However, this hypothesis was introduced on the basis of uncontrolled case series (Gibbs, 1951; Slater and Beard, 1963) and has not yet been confirmed unequivocally by controlled studies (Stevens, 1991).

There is a general consensus that psychoses are very rare in patients with neocortical extratemporal epilepsies (Gibbs, 1951; Dongier, 1959; Stevens, 1966; Bruens, 1974; Onuma, 1983; Sengoku *et al.*, 1983; Schmitz, 1988). The findings are less unequivocal regarding TLE and generalized epilepsies. Most controlled studies have shown that psychoses are no less frequent in generalized epilepsies than in temporal lobe epilepsies (Gastaut, 1956; Small *et al.*, 1962; Stevens, 1966; Mignone *et al.*, 1970; Bruens, 1971; Standage and Fenton, 1975; Sengoku *et al.*, 1983; Schmitz, 1988). There are three studies which can be quoted to show an elevated risk for psychoses in TLE compared with generalized epilepsies. Shukla *et al.* (1979) investigated psychiatric symptoms in 62 patients with TLE and 80 demographically similar patients with grand mal epilepsy. Eleven (18%) of the patients with temporal lobe epilepsy were found to have psychoses in contrast to only three (3%) of those with grand mal epilepsy. Grand mal epilepsy however is not identical to generalized epilepsy and carried in fact a well recognized low risk for psychoses (Gibbs, 1951). Sengoku *et al.* (1983) found a significantly higher prevalence of paranoid symptoms in patients with temporal lobe epilepsies compared with patients with generalized epilepsy (9% versus 3%). Paranoid symptoms however are not necessarily indicative of psychoses with epilepsy and might also occur in personality disorders, which have also been linked to TLE. In the third study, Gureje (1991) investigated interictal psychopathology in patients (not consecutive referrals) in a neuropsychiatric clinic in Nigeria. Psychoses were three times more common in patients with TLE than in patients with generalized epilepsies. Since medical services in Nigeria are presumably very different from those of industrial countries, Gureje's data cannot easily be compared and might be biased by different referral systems. In summary, there is no strong evidence that mixed psychoses are more common in TLE than in generalized epilepsy.

There are however several studies showing that psychoses in generalized epilepsies differ from psychoses in TLE (Trimble, 1991). The former are more likely to be short lasting and confusional (Dongier, 1959; Stevens, 1966; Bruens, 1971; Dörr-Zegers and Rauh, 1980). Alternative syndromes (Table 3) with paradoxical normalization of the EEG, which are especially common in generalized epilepsies are mostly relatively mild and often remit before reaching the extent of paranoid-hallucinatory psychoses (Wolf, 1991). Schneiderian first rank symptoms are less frequent in patients with generalized epilepsy compared with temporal lobe epilepsy (Trimble and Perez, 1982). In a retrospective analysis of 28 patients with mixed psychoses (Schmitz, 1988) there was no relationship between short-lasting confusional psychoses and generalized epilepsy or between paranoid-hallucinatory psychoses and TLE. However, it was found that five of six chronic psychoses (defined by a duration of longer than 6 months) occurred in patients with TLE. Although this relation was not significant, possibly due to small numbers, it also suggests that psychoses in TLE tend to be more 'severe' than those in generalized epilepsy.

In summary, published studies to date suggest that: (i) psychoses are rare complications in the whole group of people suffering from epilepsy; (ii) that patients with epilepsy and psychoses are over-representated in special centres, and (iii) that there is a link between more 'severe' and more 'Schneiderian' psychoses and TLE as compared with generalized epilepsy. The low overall prevalence of psychosis in epilepsy does not mean the problem of psychosis with epilepsy can be in any way neglected. Even if these patients represent a minority in terms of epidemiology, the need for more frequent attendances and inpatient treatments means that patients with psychosis and epilepsy represent a significant clinical management problem especially in specialized units and referral centres.

RISK FACTORS FOR PSYCHOSIS

The literature on risk factors for psychoses in epilepsy is highly controversial. Since the task of this chapter is to explore the relationship to the temporal lobe, in the following possible risk factors will be grouped according to the degree of their relationship to TLE.

Risk factors directly related to TLE

Seizure symptomatology

Complex hallucinations and delusions have been described as frequent aura symptoms of psychotic patients by Jensen and Larsen (1979). Hermann and Chabria (1981) noted a relationship between ictal fear and high scores on paranoia and schizophrenia scales of the Minnesota Multiphasic Personality Inventory (MMPI). Kristensen and Sindrup (1978a) found an excess of dysmnesic and epigastric auras in their psychotic group and emphasized the localizing significance with respect to periamygdalar dysfunction. However, Schmitz (1988) could not find a relationship between psychosis and simple seizure symptomatology when classified as 'limbic' or 'extra-limbic' in a retrospective controlled study. There was however a significant relationship with the presence of both complex focal seizures and absence seizures. This was interpreted as an indication of widespread dysfunction and as being of more significance than a localizable pathology since simple seizure symptomatology is more reliable in terms of localization than complex focal seizure symptomatology (Commission on Classification and Terminology of the ILAE, 1981). Kristensen and Sindrup found a higher rate of ictal amnesia among their psychotic patients which again might indicate that ictal impairment of consciousness plays a role in the development of psychoses. This finding has not however been universal (Flor-Henry, 1969; Sengoku *et al.*, 1983).

EEG findings

Looking at EEG studies, Kristensen and Sindrup (1978b) investigated psychotic and non-psychotic TLE patients with scalp and sphenoidal electrodes and found an excess of sphenoidal spikes in the psychotic group, which like the seizure symptomatology they interpreted as an indication for temporobasal dysfunction. Schmitz (1988) could not find significant differences between the scalp EEGs of psychotic and non-psychotic patients with epilepsy in terms of focus localization. There was however a trend (p <10%, χ^2 test) towards a higher frequency of generalized slowing and foci characterized by both epileptic discharges and slowing in the psychotic group as compared with other types of foci.

Neuropathology

Neuropathological studies of resected temporal lobes from patients with TLE have suggested a link between psychosis and the presence of cerebral malformations such as hamartomas and gangliogliomas as compared with mesial temporal sclerosis (Taylor, 1971). These findings have been seen as consistent with recent findings of structural abnormalities found in the brains of schizophrenic patients without epilepsy which arise during fetal brain development (Roberts *et al.*, 1990).

Epilepsy surgery

The role of epilepsy surgery in TLE for the development of psychosis is controversial (Falconer, 1973). The incidence of psychosis following surgery is high, ranging from 7–37%, (Ferguson and Rayport, 1965; Jensen and Larsen, 1979; Horowitz and Cohen, 1968; Taylor, 1972; Rausch *et al.*, 1977). There remains some doubt whether this really reflects the *de novo* onset of psychosis following surgery rather than recurrence of pre-existing psychosis, which is crucial when considering whether to exclude patients with a history of psychosis from surgery or not. However, there remains little reason to assume that surgery itself can improve the psychiatric prognosis for psychoses other than those clearly related to seizures.

Laterality

Left lateralization of temporal lobe dysfunction or temporal lobe pathology as a risk factor for schizophreniform psychosis was suggested originally by Flor-Henry in 1969. The literature has recently been summarized by Trimble (1991). In a synopsis of 14 studies with 341 psychotic patients, Trimble described the following distribution: 43% of patients had left, 23% right, and 34% bilateral abnormalities. He concluded that there was a clear bias towards left laterality. Although this asymmetry is striking, it is not convincing without control data. The need for controls is important, since in unselected patients with TLE, left sided foci are more frequent than right sided foci. In some series Currie *et al.* (1971) reported left sided EEG foci occurred in 42% compared with right sided foci in 29%, figures which are comparable to Trimble's data. Sommer's original data are similar when re-examined in the same way (Table 1).

Risk factors for psychosis in epilepsy interlinked with TLE

Antiepileptic drug treatment is one of the factors which link epileptic psychosis and temporal lobe epilepsy. Phenytoin, carbamazepine and

Table 6. Risk factors for psychoses in epilepsy: intercorrelation with the occurrence of complex focal seizures.

Factors correlated with psychoses	*Correlation with complex focal seizures*
Immigration status	+
Low vocational status	−
Low professional qualification following good school results	−
Long duration of follow-up in the outpatient clinic	+
Multiple seizure types	+
Poor tonic–clonic seizure control	+
Non-compliance	+
EEG foci with both epileptic discharges and slowing	+
Generalized slowing in the EEG	+

Twenty-eight patients with psychosis were compared with 669 non-psychotic patients (Schmitz, 1988).

vigabatrin are associated with psychosis (Sander *et al.*, 1991; Wolf, 1977; McDamal and Bolman, 1975; Franks and Richter, 1979). These drugs are also more often used in TLE than in generalized epilepsies.

The literature on brain damage and epileptic psychosis is very controversial. Some authors could not find an association with psychosis (Flor-Henry, 1969; Schmitz, 1988), others have suggested a higher rate of pathological neurological examinations, diffuse slowing in the EEG and mental retardation in those epileptic patients with psychosis (Commission on Classification and Terminology of the ILAE, 1981). If brain damage is a risk factor for psychosis in epilepsy this could also explain an association with TLE since brain damage is seen more frequently in this group.

The strongest risk factors for psychosis in epilepsy are those factors which indicate severity of epilepsy. These are long duration of epilepsy (Slater and Beard, 1963), multiple seizure types (Schmitz, 1988; Ounsted, 1969; Commission on Classification and Terminology of the ILAE, 1981; Bruens, 1974; Sengoku *et al.*, 1983; Rodin *et al.*, 1976; Hermann *et al.*, 1982; Lindsay *et al.*, 1979), and poor response to drug treatment (Lindsay *et al.*, 1979; Schmitz, 1988). Again, most of these factors are also related to TLE, which has a relatively poor prognosis among epileptic syndromes (Wieser, 1991).

In the retrospective study by Schmitz (1988) all biological factors associated with psychoses were also correlated with the occurence of complex focal seizures (Table 6). In contrast, social factors were not intercorrelated. These findings raise the question of whether severity of epilepsy may be the main risk factor for the development of psychosis.

Risk factors unrelated to TLE

There are in fact only very few risk factors left which are not related to TLE. A history of status epilepticus is not closely related to TLE, and there is an isolated study showing an elevated risk for mixed psychoses in patients with a history of status epilepticus (Schmitz, 1989). Many authors with few exceptions (Sengoku *et al.*, 1983, Schmitz, 1988) described a lower seizure frequency in psychotic patients compared with non-psychotic patients (Standage, 1973; Slater, 1969; Flor-Henry, 1969; Sengoku *et al.*, 1983). Low seizure frequency is definitely not linked to TLE but is difficult to assess retrospectively and one presumes that some authors only studied the seizure frequency during the psychosis and not before the onset of psychosis. This is not always clarified.

SUMMARY AND CONCLUSIONS

It has been shown that psychoses are infrequent complications of epilepsy if the whole population of patients with epilepsy is considered. Because of the problems with respect to the diagnosis of schizophrenia in epilepsy the question of whether the two disorders may be antagonistic or agonistic cannot be answered conclusively. Patients with epilepsy and psychoses are over-representated in specialized units. This group of patients which represents only a minority of the wider population with epilepsy is also more likely to suffer from severe epilepsies. They thus require more intensive and multidisciplinary care than do other epilepsy patients.

The nature of the link between TLE and psychosis remains unclear. The links to other risk factors for psychosis in epilepsy especially those factors indicating severity of epilepsy are remarkable but require further confirmation and specification. Thus, we are left with the following important question. Is psychosis in epilepsy related to temporal lobe pathology, severity of epilepsy or a combination of both factors? Future research must recognize the methodological difficulties involved in differentiating these related aspects in its attempt to clarify these issues.

ACKNOWLEDGEMENTS

The author is grateful to the Deutsche Forschungsgemeinschaft (DFG) for financial support (Grant 864/1-2) and to Dr Michael Trimble and the Raymond Way Neuropsychiatry Research Group for advice and support.

REFERENCES

American Psychiatric Association. (1987). *Diagnostic and statistical manual of mental disorders. Third edition—Revised*, American Psychiatric Association, Washington, DC.

Ballenger, C.E., King, D.W. and Gallagher, B.B. (1983). Partial complex status epilepticus. *Neurology*, **33**, 1545–1552.
Bash, K.W. and Mahnig, P. (1984). Epileptiker in der psychiatrischen Klinik. Von der Dämmerattacke zur Psychose. *Eur. Arch. Psychiatr. Neurol. Sci.*, **234**, 237–249.
Betts, T.A. (1974). A follow-up study of a cohort of patients with epilepsy admitted to psychiatric care in an English city. In: Harris, P. and Maudsley, C. (Eds), *Proceedings of the Hans Berger Symposium*, Churchill Livingstone, Edinburgh, pp. 326–336.
Bruens, J.H. (1971). Psychoses in epilepsy. *Psychiatr. Neurol. Neurochir.*, **74**, 174–192.
Bruens, J.H. (1973). Zur Frage der kausalen Beziehung zwischen Psychose und Epilepsie. In: Penin, H. (Ed.), *Psychische Störungen bei Epilepsie*, Schattauer, Stuttgart, pp. 67–74.
Bruens, J.H. (1974). Psychoses in epilepsy. In: Vinken, P.J. and Bruyn, G.W. (Eds), *Handbook of Clinical Neurology, Vol. 15*, North Holland, Amsterdam, pp. 593–610.
Commission on Classification and Terminology of the ILAE (1981). Proposal for revised clinical and electroencephalographic classification of epileptic seizures. *Epilepsia*, **22**, 489–501.
Commission on Classification and Terminology of the ILAE (1989). Proposal for revised classification of epilepsies and epileptic syndromes. *Epilepsia*, **30**, 389–399.
Currie, S., Heathfield, K.W.G., Henson, R.A. and Scott, D.F. (1971). Clinical course and prognosis of temporal lobe epilepsy: a survey of 666 patients. *Brain*, **94**, 173–190.
Delgado-Escueta, A.V. and Walsh, G.O. (1985). Type I complex partial seizures of hippocampal origin: excellent results of anterior temporal lobectomy. *Neurology*, **35**, 143–154.
Dongier, S. (1959). Statistical study of clinical and electroencephalographic manifestations of 536 psychotic episodes occurring in 516 epileptics between clinical seizures. *Epilepsia*, **1**, 117–142.
Dörr-Zegers, O. and Rauh, J. (1980). Different kinds of psychoses as related to different kinds of epilepsy. Presented at study group of psychoses of epilepsy. 12th International Epilepsy Congress, Copenhagen (unpublished).
Edeh, J. and Toone, B. (1987). Relationship between interictal psychopathology and the type of epilepsy. *Br. J. Psychiatry*, **151**, 95–101.
Falconer, M.A. (1973). Pathological substrates in temporal lobe epilepsy with psychoses. In: Laitinen, L.V. and Livingston, K.E. (Eds), *Surgical Approaches in Psychiatry*, MTP, Lancaster, pp. 121–124.
Fenton, G.W. (1981). Psychiatric disorders in epilepsy: classification and phenomenology. In: Reynolds, E.H. and Trimble, M.R. (Eds), *Epilepsy and Psychiatry*, Churchill Livingstone, pp. 12–26.
Ferguson, S.M. and Rayport, M. (1965). The adjustment to living without epilepsy. *J. Nerv. Ment. Dis.*, **140**, 26–37.
Flor-Henry, P. (1969). Psychosis and temporal lobe epilepsy: a controlled investigation. *Epilepsia*, **10**, 363–395.
Franks, R.D. and Richter, A.J. (1979). Schizophrenia-like psychosis associated with anticonvulsant toxicity. *Am. J. Psychiatry*, **136**, 973–974.
Ganter, R. (1925). Ein mit Schizophrenie kombinierter Fall von Epilepsie. *Arch. Psychiatr. Nervenkr.*, **74**, 829–837.
Gastaut, H. (1956). Etude électronique des episodes psychotiques surviennent chez les épileptiques en dehors des crises cliniques. *Rev. Neurol.*, **95**, 587–616.

Gibbs, F.A. (1951). Ictal and non-ictal psychiatric disorders in temporal lobe epilepsy. *J. Nerv. Ment. Dis.*, **113**, 522–528.

Griesinger, W. (1868). Über einige epileptoide Zustände. *Arch. Psychiatr. Nervenkr.*, **1**, 320–333.

Gudmundsson, G. (1966). Epilepsy in Iceland: a clinical and epidemiological investigation. *Acta Neurol. Scand.*, **43** (Suppl. 25), 1–123.

Gureje, O. (1991). Interictal psychopathology in epilepsy—prevalence and pattern in a Nigerian clinic. *Br. J. Psychiatry*, **158**, 700–705.

Helmchen, H. (1975). Zerebrale Bedingungskonstellationen psychopathologischer Syndrome bei Epileptikern. In: Helmchen, H. and Hippius, H. (Eds), *Entwicklungstendenzen biologischer Psychiatrie*, Thieme, Stuttgart, pp. 125–148.

Hermann, B.P. and Chabria, S. (1980). Interictal psychopathology in patients with ictal fear. *Arch. Neurol.*, **37**, 667–668.

Hermann, B.P., Dikmen, S., Schwartz, M.S. and Karnes, W.E. (1982). Psychopathology in TLE patients with ictal fear: a quantitative investigation. *Neurology*, **32**, 7–11.

Horowitz, M.J. and Cohen, F.M. (1968). Temporal lobe epilepsy: effect of lobectomy on psychosocial functioning. *Epilepsia*, **9**, 23–41.

Janz, D. (1969). *Die Epilepsien*, Thieme, Stuttgart.

Jensen, I. and Larsen, J.K. (1979). Mental aspects of temporal lobe epilepsy: follow-up of 74 patients after resection of a temporal lobe. *J. Neurol. Neurosurg. Psychiatry*, **42**, 256–265.

Köhler, G.K. (1980). Zur Einteilung der Psychosen bei Epilepsie. Zum Begriff Psychosen bei Epilepsie bzw epileptische Psychosen. In: Wolf, P. and Koehler, G.K. (Eds), *Psychopathologische und pathogenetische Probleme psychotischer Syndrome bei Epilepsie*, Huber, Bern, pp. 11–18.

Kristensen, O. and Sindrup, E.H. (1978a). Psychomotor epilepsy and psychosis. I. Physical aspects. *Acta Neurol. Scand.*, **57**, 361–369.

Kristensen, O. and Sindrup, E.H. (1978b). Psychomotor epilepsy and psychosis. II. Electroencephalographic findings. *Acta Neurol. Scand*, **59**, 1–9.

Landolt, H. (1953). Serial electroencephalographic investigations during psychotic episodes in epileptic patients and during schizophrenic attacks. In: Lorentz de Haas, A.M. (Ed.), *Lectures on Epilepsy*, Elsevier, Amsterdam, pp. 91–133.

Lennox, W.G. (1945). The treatment of epilepsy. *Med. Clin. North Am.*, **29**, 1114–1128.

Lindsay, J., Ounsted, C. and Richards, P. (1979). Long-term outcome in children with temporal lobe seizures. III. Psychiatric aspects in childhood and adult life. *Devel. Med. Child Neurol.*, **21**, 630–636.

Logsdail, S.J. and Toone, B.K. (1988). Postictal psychoses. A clinical and phenomenological description. *Br. J. Psychiatry*, **152**, 246–252.

McDamal, C. and Bolman, W. (1975). Delayed idiosyncratic psychosis with diphenylhydantoin. *J. Am. Med. Assoc.*, **231**, 1063.

Matuja, W.B. (1990). Psychological disturbance in African Tanzanian epileptics. *Trop. Geogr. Med.*, **42**, 359–364.

Mignone, R.J., Donnelly, E.F. and Sadowsky, D. (1970). Psychological and neurological comparisons of psychomotor and non-psychomotor epileptic patients. *Epilepsia*, **11**, 345–359.

Onuma, T. (1983). Limbic lobe epilepsy with paranoid symptoms: analysis of clinical features and psychological tests. *Folia Psychiatr. Neurol. Jpn*, **37**, 239–244.

Ounsted, C. (1969). Aggression and epilepsy. Rage in children with temporal lobe epilepsy. *J. Psychosom. Res.*, **13**, 237–242.

Oyebode, F. and Davison, K. (1989). Epileptic schizophrenia: clinical features and outcome. *Acta Psychiatr. Scand.*, **79**, 327–331.

Pond, D.A. (1962). Discussion remark. *Proc. R. Soc. Med.*, **55**, 316.

Rausch, R., McCreary, C. and Crandall, P.H. (1977). Psychosocial functioning following successful surgical relief from seizures: evidence of prediction from preoperative personality characteristics. *J. Psychosom. Res.*, **21**, 141–146.

Roberts, G.W., Done, D.J., Bruton, C. and Crow, T.J. (1990). A mock up of schizophrenia: temporal lobe epilepsy and schizophrenia-like psychosis. *Biol. Psychiatry*, **28**, 127–143.

Rodin, E.A., Katz, M. and Lennox, K. (1976). Differences between patients with temporal lobe seizures and those with other forms of attacks. *Epilepsia*, **17**, 313–320.

Roger, J., Collomb, H. and Pache, D. (1956). Etude étiologique. In: Gastaut, H: Etude electronique des episodes psychotiques survenant en dehors des crises cliniques chez les épileptiques. *Rev. Neurol.*, **95**, 589–591.

Samt, P. (1875). Epileptische Irreseinsformen. *Arch. Psychiatr. Nervenkr.*, **5**, 393–444.

Sander, J.W.A.S., Hart, Y.M., Trimble, M.R. and Shorvon, S.D. (1991). Vigabatrin and psychosis. *J. Neurol. Neurosurg. Psychiatry*, **54**, 435–439.

Savard, G., Andermann, F., Olivier, A. and Remillard, G.M. (1991). Postictal psychosis after partial complex seizures: a multiple case study. *Epilepsia*, **32**, 225–231.

Schmitz, B. (1988). *Psychosen bei Epilepsie*, Thesis, Freie Universität, Berlin.

Sengoku, A., Yagi, K., Seino, M. and Wada, T. (1983). Risks of occurrence of psychoses in relation to the types of epilepsies and epileptic seizures. *Folia. Psychiatr. Neurol. Jpn*, **37**, 221–226.

Sherwin, I. (1984). Differential psychiatric features in epilepsy; relationship to lesion laterality. *Acta Psychiatr. Scand.*, **69** (Suppl. 313), 92–103.

Shukla, G.D., Srivastava, O.N., Katiyar, B.C. and Joshi, V. (1979). Psychiatric manifestations in TLE: a controlled study. *Br. J. Psychiatry*, **93**, 473–484.

Slater, E. (1969). The schizophrenia-like illnesses of epilepsy. In: Herrington, R.N. (Ed.), *Current Problems in Neuropsychiatry; Schizophrenia, Epilepsy, the Temporal Lobe*, Headley, Ashford, pp. 77–81.

Slater, E. and Beard, A.W. (1963). The schizophrenia-like psychoses of epilepsy. *Br. J. Psychiatry*, **109**, 950–1150.

Small, J.G., Milstein, V. and Stevens, J.R. (1962). Are psychomotor epileptics different? *Arch. Neurol.*, **7**, 187–194.

Sommer, W. (1880). Erkrankung des Ammonshorns als aetiologisches Moment der Epilepsie. *Arch. Psychiatr. Nervenkr.*, **10**, 631–675.

Sommer, W. (1881). Postepileptisches irresein. *Arch. Psychiatr. Nervenkr.*, **11**, 550–612.

Standage, K.F. (1973). Schizophreniform psychosis among epileptics in a mental hospital. *Br. J. Psychiatry*, **123**, 231–232.

Standage, K.F. and Fenton, G.W. (1975). Psychiatric symptom profiles of patients with epilepsy: a controlled investigation. *Psychol. Med.*, **5**, 152–160.

Stevens, J.R. (1966). Psychiatric implications of psychomotor epilepsy. *Arch. Gen. Psychiatry*, **14**, 461–471.

Stevens, J.R. (1991). Psychosis and the temporal lobe. In: Smith, D.B., Treiman, D.M. and Trimble, M.R. (Eds), *Advances in Neurology, Vol. 55, Neurobehavioral Problems in Epilepsy*, Raven Press, New York, pp. 79–96.

Taylor, D.C. (1971). Ontogenesis of chronic epileptic psychoses: a reanalysis. *Psychol. Med.*, **1**, 247–253.

Taylor, D.C. (1972). Mental state and temporal lobe epilepsy. A correlation account of 100 patients treated surgically. *Epilepsia*, **13**, 727–765.

Tellenbach, H. (1965). Epilepsie als anfallsleiden und psychose: ueber alternative psychosen paranoider praegung bei 'forcierter normalisierung' (Landolt) des elektroenzephalogramms epileptischer. *Nervenarzt*, **36**, 190–202.

Toone, B.K., Garralda, M.E. and Ron, M.A. (1982). The psychoses of epilepsy and the functional psychoses: a clinical and phenomenological comparison. *Br. J. Psychiatry*, **141**, 256–261.

Trimble, M.R. (1991). *The Psychoses of Epilepsy*, Raven Press, New York, pp. 145–149.

Trimble, M.R. and Perez, M.M. (1982). The phenomenology of the chronic psychoses of epilepsy. In: Koella, W.P. and Trimble, M.R. (Eds), *Temporal Lobe Epilepsy, Mania and Schizophrenia and the Limbic System*, Karger, Basel, pp. 98–102.

Wieser, H.G. (1991). Ictal manifestations of temporal lobe seizures. In: Smith, D.B., Treiman, D.M. and Trimble, M.R. (Eds), *Advances in Neurology. Vol. 55, Neurobehavioral Problems in Epilepsy*, Raven Press, New York, pp. 301–316.

Wieser, H.G. and Yasargil, M.G. (1982). Selective amygdalo-hippocampectomy as a surgical treatment of mediobasal limbic epilepsy. *Surg. Neurol.*, **17**, 445–457.

Wolf, P. (1973). Zur Psychopathologie epileptischer Psychosen. In: Penin, H. (Ed.), *Psychische Störungen bei Epilepsie*, Schattauer, Stuttgart, pp. 51–65.

Wolf, P. (1976). *Psychosen bei Epilepsie. Ihre Bedingungen und Wechselbeziehungen zu Anfällen*, Thesis, Freie Universität, Berlin.

Wolf, P. (1977). The role of antiepileptic drugs in epileptic psychoses. In: Majkowski, J. (Ed.), *Posttraumatic Epilepsy—Pharmacological Prophylaxis*, Polish chapter of the ILAE, Warzsawa, pp. 248–255.

Wolf, P. (1991). Acute behavioral symptomatology at disappearance of epileptiform EEG abnormality. Paradoxical or 'forced' normalization. In: Smith, D.B., Treiman, D.M. and Trimble, M.R. (Eds), *Advances in Neurology, Vol. 55, Neurobehavioral Problems in Epilepsy*, Raven Press, New York, pp. 127–142.

World Health Organization (1980). *International Classification of Impairments, Disabilities and Handicaps*, WHO, Geneva.

Wyrsch, J. (1933). Über schizophrenie bei Epileptikern. *Schweiz. Arch. Neurol. Psychiatr.*, **31**, 113.

Zielinski, J.J. (1974). *Epidemiology and Medical-Social Problems of Epilepsy in Warsaw*, Final report on research program No. 19-P-58325-F-01. DHEW, Social and Rehabilitation Services, US Government Printing Office, Washington, DC.

Zielinski, J.J. (1986). Selected psychiatric and psychosocial aspects of epilepsy as seen by an epidemiologist. In: Whitman, S. and Hermann, B.P. (Eds), *Psychopathology in Epilepsy, Social Dimensions*, Oxford University Press, New York, Oxford, pp. 38–66.

The Temporal Lobes and the Limbic System
Edited by M.R. Trimble and T.G. Bolwig

12

Behavioural Consequences of Temporal Lobe Resections

HEINZ GREGOR WIESER
Department of Neurology, University Hospital, Zürich, Switzerland

INTRODUCTION

Numerous studies have documented cognitive deficits in patients with temporal lobe epilepsy (TLE), including impaired memory functioning, reduced attention capacity, abstract reasoning difficulties, and reduced information-processing efficiency. In addition, a wide variety of psychopathology has been reported in patients suffering from complex partial seizures (CPS) ranking from brief episodes of psychical aberrations, i.e. 'psychical seizures' to peculiarities of personality and to frank psychosis.

This chapter summarizes the pre-/postoperative neuropsychological, EEG, PET, and behavioural data from our Zürich series of 364 operated patients with TLE. After a detailed presurgical evaluation including telemetric long-term monitoring of simultaneously observed behaviour and EEG from scalp and intracranial electrodes (stereo-EEG, *n*=139; foramen ovale electrodes, *n*=104), the following operations have been performed: selective amygdalahippocampectomy (AHE, *n*=279), selective temporal lobe (TL) resections outside the amygdala and hippocampus (*n*=14), anterior TL resection (*n*=66), and stereotactic lesioning of the amygdala and/or hippocampus (*n*=5).

From a pre-/postoperative comparison of neuropsychological and behavioural data, factors emerge which account for behavioural deterioration or improvement. Postoperative behavioural improvement is associated with: (i) a short duration of seizure illness; (ii) a well defined focal onset of seizures; (iii) a selective resection; (iv) complete postoperative seizure control; (v) discontinuation of anticonvulsant drugs; (vi) an improvement of social and vocational status; and (vii) 'good family support'. These variables are interrelated, and are discussed in this chapter.

PRE-/POSTOPERATIVE NEUROPSYCHOLOGICAL PERFORMANCES

Learning and memory

Patients with TLE often claim to have impaired memory functions. As a rule, memory and learning are more impaired in patients with bitemporal spike foci than in those with unilateral TL spike foci. Furthermore, they are more impaired in patients with left (dominant) compared to right (non-dominant) TL spike foci. Neuropsychological studies have confirmed a preoperative material-specific learning and memory deficit in a large percentage of candidates for surgical epilepsy therapy (Milner, 1975).

In general, the observed pre-/postoperative changes of neuropsychological performances are relatively consistent. They are related to the preoperative performance level, the postoperative outcome of the epilepsy, the site and side of the operation (dominant versus non-dominant hemisphere), the removed volume, and the pre-/postoperative EEG changes.

With regard to the preoperative performance level, we found that patients with a preoperatively existing deficit did not, as a rule, worsen postoperatively, if the seizures were completely controlled by the operation. If, however, no neuropsychological deficit was demonstrable prior to operation, learning and memory performance decreased for material specific for the operated hemisphere. This deficit was slight in cases of postoperative seizure control, but could be marked if the operation did not substantially improve the patient's seizure tendency.

With regard to the outcome of the epilepsy, patients who were seizure-free after selective AHE (Wieser and Yasargil, 1982; Yasargil and Wieser, 1987) did much better than those with persisting seizures. Moreover, we could show that the performance of the non-operated hemisphere improves more than the operated one (Wieser, 1986). This phenomenon was explained as the cessation of the pathological interference from the contralateral side after the operation. At least in some AHE cases we had the impression that a more radical removal of the parahippocampal gyrus resulted in slightly more pronounced neuropsychological deficits. This, however, is counterbalanced by the fact that a more radical removal of the parahippocampal gyrus resulted in better epileptological outcome of AHE (Siegel *et al.*, 1990). To demonstrate this relationship convincingly, unsuccessfully operated patients with differing removal of the parahippocampal gyrus during AHE must be studied.

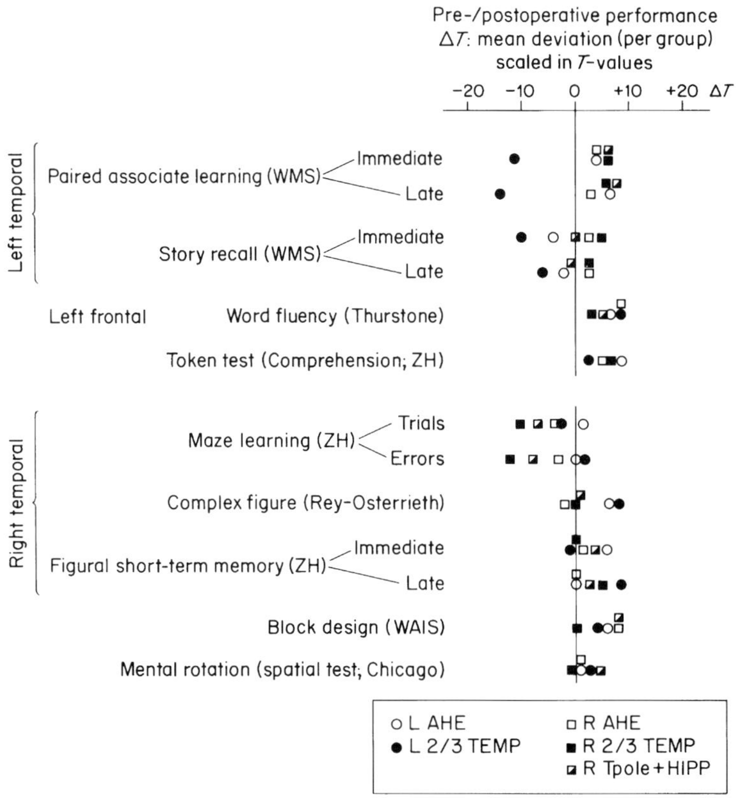

Figure 1. Comparison of pre-/postoperative performance in patients with different types of temporal lobe resections for treatment of medically refractory complex partial seizures: selective amygdalohippocampectomy (AHE; left n=3, right n=3), removal of right temporal polar area, amygdala and hippocampal formation (R Tpole + HIPP; n=3), and 'classical' two-thirds temporal lobe resection (2/3 TEMP; left n=2; right n=3). (Modified from Birri *et al.*, 1982.)

With regard to the neuropsychological outcome after anterior TL resection, as opposed to AHE, Birri *et al.* (1982) and Gonser *et al.* (1986) reported that postoperative neuropsychological performance was better in patients with selective AHE compared with patients with a classical anterior two-thirds TL resection (Fig. 1).

Figure 2 shows the up-dated results based on 70 AHE patients with pre-/postoperative changes in performance on Nadig's learning and memory test (Nadig *et al.*, 1985).

The learning performance was examined with Nadig's test consisting of three series of 15 items each drawn or written in black ink on white cards

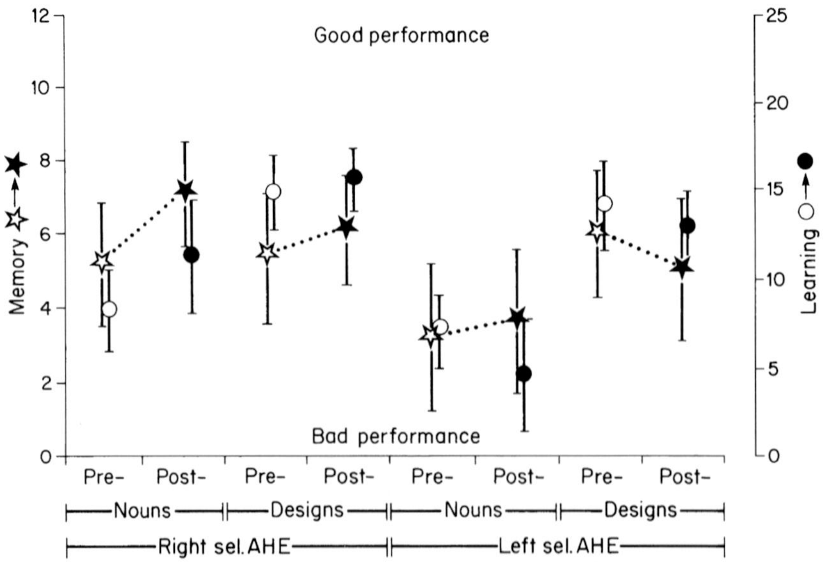

Figure 2. Pre- and postoperative performance changes in Nadig's learning and memory test battery in 35 patients with right and 35 patients with left selective amygdalohippocampectomy. Stars refer to memory, circles to learning. Open symbols indicate preoperative results, full symbols are postoperative. Symbols represent means and standard deviations. The learning performance is based on the number of trials necessary to achieve the correct reproduction of at least 12 of 15 items (see text). The performance values of the learning scale (0–25) have the following meanings: 4 = 5 trials, 8 = 4 trials, 12 = 3 trials, 16 = 2 trials. If at the fifth trial the patient is still unable to reproduce 12/15 items, the number of the correctly reproduced items is taken into account. The memory scale (0–12, left) indicates the number of items that could be reproduced after a distraction interval of 30 min.

(15 × 10 cm). The items of the first series were nonsense designs. The second consisted of drawings of common objects and the third of concrete nouns. The items were presented until the patient was able to reproduce at least 12 items, but for a maximum of five trials. The reproduction of as many items as possible of each series (designs, drawings, nouns) after a distraction interval of 30 min made up the memory performance. In order to avoid memory savings from pre- to postoperative testing, two similar but not identical parallel versions (A/B) of this test were used. Half of the patients were tested preoperatively with version A and postoperatively with version B and vice versa.

We have recently examined the effects of TL lesions on memorizing auditory nonverbal material (pure tones). Patients treated with selective AHE were included in this study. Controls and patients with mesiobasal TL

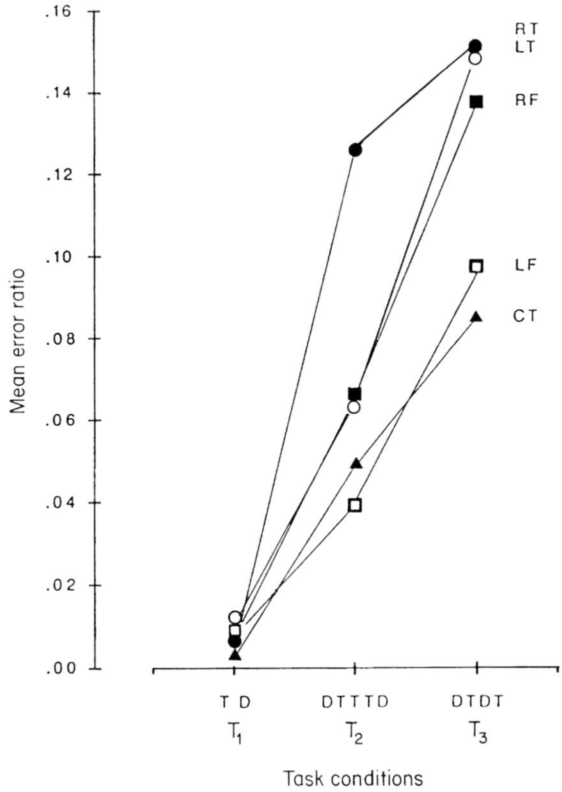

Figure 3. Mean error ratios of different groups in tone discrimination tasks (T target tone, D distractor tone). T_1, T_2 and T_3 represent different levels of task dificulty, with T_3 being the most difficult. CT, controls (*n*=20); LT, left temporal (*n*=11); RT, right temporal (*n*=13); LF left frontal (*n*=10); RF, right frontal (*n*=9) patient group. (Reproduced with permission, from Wittlieb-Verpoort and Wieser, 1992.)

or frontal lesions had to identify target tones in series consisting of target and distractor tones randomly presented. Three levels of difficulty were defined in this task. Patients with right TL lesions showed markedly reduced task performances at the most difficult task level, i.e. when more than three different target tones had to be identified (Fig. 3). The decrement in performance of these patients was attributed to: (i) poor structuring of the stimuli to reduce the memory load and (ii) inability to find an appropriate strategy. This study (Wittlieb-Verpoort and Wieser, 1992) confirms the results presented by the Montreal group analysing data from patients with varying extents of unilateral hippocampal excisions (summarized in Jones-Gotman, 1987). Our findings support the idea that the hippocampus plays a role in some, but not all, memory tasks depending on the kind of stimuli and complexity of the task. Even small differences in the experimental protocol may be sufficient to lower the performance on a task that normally is not sensitive to hippocampal dysfunction. Therefore, both the timing and sensitivity of psychometric tasks, as well as the availability of a preoperative baseline, are all important factors in determining the reliability of memory assessment following TL surgery.

More detailed neuropsychological studies of the effects of AHE remain to be done. One way to better assess the preoperative risks of selective AHE on higher cognitive functions, such as learning and memory, is selective TL-Amytal procedures. We have developed (Wieser *et al.*, 1989a,b) the following three techniques for the temporary inactivation of mesiobasal TL structures within the Amytal test, and regularly use one of the three during preoperative neuropsychological evaluation: (i) temporary balloon-occlusion distal to the anterior choroidal artery (a.ch.a) with subsequent Amytal injection into the a.ch.a., the communicans posterior and the ophthalmic artery; (ii) selective catheterization of the a.ch.a.; and (iii) the selective catheterization of the P2 segment of the posterior cerebral artery. These modifications of the 'Wada test' (Wada, 1949) have proved to be better predictors of neuropsychological outcome for selective AHE patients than the intracarotid Amytal test (Wieser *et al.*, 1989c), although the variability of the vascular supply to the hippocampus remains a problem. In the comparison of the performance before and during the selective Amytal procedure, we found memory decrements for verbal and for figural material in all patients, but the relative loss differed markedly in relation to the side of injection, the pre-injection performance level, and the technique used. The selective injection of the P2 segment of the posterior cerebral artery yielded the largest effect. Consistent with the pre-/postoperative learning and memory findings obtained with Nadig's tests, we found that the material-specific decrease following selective TL Amytal inactivation was the more pronounced the better was the performance prior to injection. Comparison with the postoperative outcome showed better results than predicted from selective Amytal procedures in patients whose postoperative course was uncomplicated (Schiess *et al.*, 1990).

Emotional decisions before and after selective AHE

No significant common personality traits among the patients who underwent AHE could be defined. In the left AHE group, however, we preoperatively observed more pedantic and matter-of-fact behaviour as well as an unexpected, heightened flow of verbal associations, whereas in the right AHE group we preoperatively observed more restlessness and dysphoria. Based on the report of several patients that they tolerate stressful situations postoperatively, much better than preoperatively, and the objectively documented fact that patients often dramatically improved after AHE in their decision-making ability, we designed a task to examine this phenomenon.

The patients' emotional behaviour was assessed by examining their spontaneous affective preferences which do not rely on higher cognitive-perceptual skills. Twenty-eight patients who underwent selective AHE (right n=15, left n=13) and 20 controls have been studied so far with a combination of preference and classification tests (Aeberli, 1990).

Subjects were instructed to spontaneously classify several stimuli which easily elicit emotional responses (14 Holtzman inkblots, 14 colour patches, and 14 piano sounds (consonant and dissonant musical chords) according to seven highly emotional German nouns (fear, anger, disgust, sadness, surprise, joy, eroticism) and to seven faces expressing the same seven emotions. In a second part of the experiment, subjects were required to create their individual preference hierarchy among the 14 stimuli of each stimulus class. They always had to choose the preferred stimulus from a pairwise stimulus presentation. Based on this forced-choice preference order and the classification, differing levels of cognitive-emotional organization of emotional behaviour were found in the three groups.

The main results were:

1. Overall, there were relatively stable preference orders within the groups (comparing pre- and postoperative results in patients, and first and second assessments in controls). The average amount of changes in all three groups was 22%.
2. In contrast to the relatively stable overall preference order, the three stimulus classes and the three groups compared within the stimulus classes differed. Differences were most pronounced in piano sounds. The smallest difference was found in the right AHE patients and the largest was in controls. The differences between the three stimulus classes (F=20.76; df=2, p=0.001), and differences between three subject groups were significant (Kruskal–Wallis 1-way-Anova, p=0.031; Wilkoxon–Rank-Sum-W-Test, control - right AHE, p=0.015; right AHE - left AHE, p=0.040.
3. Classification to emotional faces and nouns varied pre- and postoperatively mostly according to the stimulus class. Controls were more stable than the patients. The smallest differences for all groups occurred in the classifications of colour and piano sounds to emotional nouns. The following trends were found: right AHE patients showed a decrease of 'joy' and an increase of 'disgust' for faces, and an increase of 'anger' for nouns. Left AHE patients showed a decrease of 'fear' for faces.

In summary, this study showed that patients after AHE, and in particular when operated on the right side, show slight changes in their emotional preferences. The nature of the changes is consistent with the observation of many patients, close relatives, and employers that patients following AHE are more successful in their vocational and private lives because of less hesitation and more direct decision-making abilities.

Specific impairment by unilateral mesiobasal TL seizure discharges

In order to discuss pre-/postoperative changes in patients with TL epilepsy, it is important to note that postoperatively most patients were rendered seizure-free or substantially improved. It is logical to assume that seizure control *per se* has a beneficial influence on higher cognitive functions, as well as on motivation, drive and mood.

Long-lasting restricted unilateral limbic epileptic discharges constitute an ideal natural model for testing the functional implications of a localized epileptic dysfunction and at the same time the interactions between the two cerebral hemispheres. Over the years we have studied several patients with primarily limbic unilateral TL seizure discharges in order to answer the following questions:

1. Is memory impaired by the discharges?
2. Is this impairment specific to certain stimulus qualities?
3. Can the impairment be associated with functions of the discharging hemisphere?

In general our results have confirmed the strong interference of focal seizure discharges with the specific function of the neuronal substrate involved. We have recently shown during a prolonged non-convulsive unilateral left limbic status epilepticus, recorded on SEEG, that high-frequency discharges restricted to the left hippocampus abolished the capacity of the left, but not of the right hemisphere to detect function words in a tachistoscopic experiment identical to that described in Figs 4 and 5. Moreover, we demonstrated a high correlation between the performance in the sensitive lexical decision task and the locally restricted left hippocampal epileptiform EEG pattern (Wieser *et al.*, 1985). There was also a trend for the performance of the contralateral right hemisphere to improve during the breakdown of the left hemispheric function (lexical performance dropping to chance level). This finding is important since it clearly demonstrates that compensatory mechanisms have been mobilized in order to maintain the best possible performance.

Figure 4 illustrates a similar phenomenon in a 31 year-old right-handed patient in whom a spontaneous seizure restricted to the left hemisphere occurred while being tested for reading dominance. The pre-ictal normal left hemisphere dominance for lexical decision shifted to a right hemisphere dominance during the period of postictal stereo-EEG slowing and aphasia

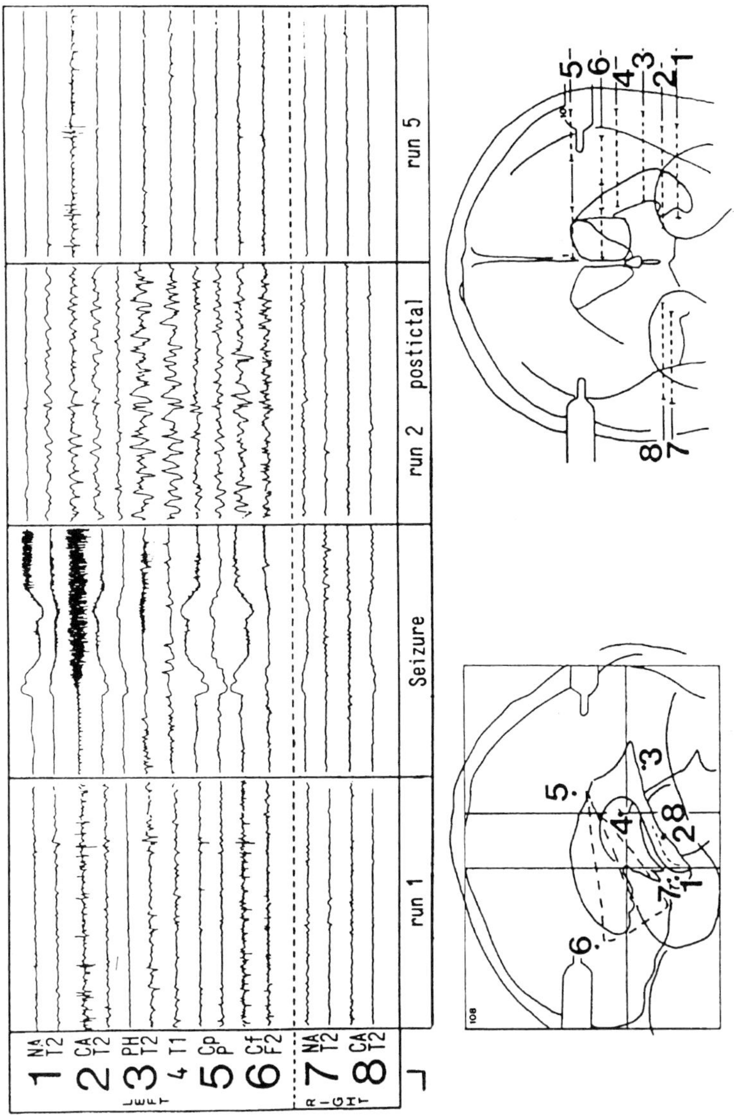

Figure 4. Seizure induced shift in hemispheric reading dominance. Example of stereo-EEG recordings, during which a tachistoscopic lexical decision task (five experimental runs) was carried out. Recording sites are indicated by numbers referring to the depth electrodes in the brain maps below. Abbreviations: NA, amygdala; CA, hippocampus; PH parahippocampal gyrus; Cp, parietal cingulate gyrus; Cf, frontal cingulate gyrus; T1, first temporal gyrus; T2, second temporal gyrus; P, parietal; F2, second frontal gyrus. The section 'Run 1' illustrates the pre-ictal, the section 'Seizure' the beginning of the spontaneous seizure discharge in the left hippocampus, and the sections 'Run 2 postictal' and 'Run 5' the early and late postictal recordings. (Reproduced with permission, from Stodieck *et al.*, 1986.)

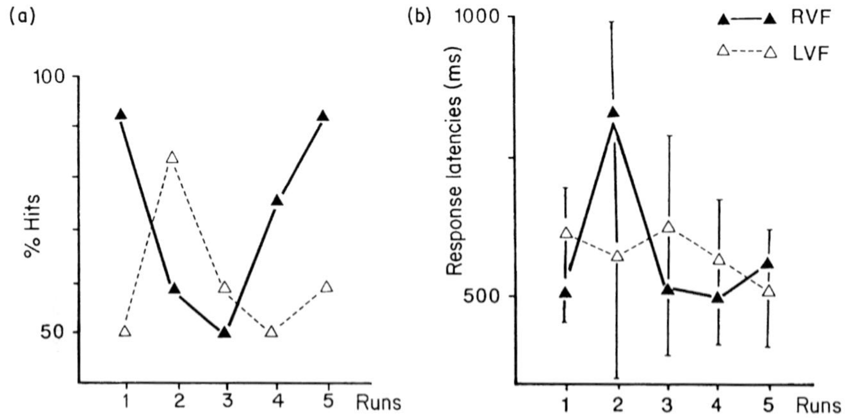

Figure 5. Seizure induced shift in hemispheric reading dominance (see also Fig. 4). (a) Diagram depicting the percentage correct responses with respect to the five tachistoscopic experimental runs. During the first run (pre-ictal phase) there is a right visual field (RVF) advantage (RVF 92%, LVF 50% hits). During the second run (immediate postical run), there is a shift to a LVF advantage (RVF 58%, LVF 83% hits). During the third to fifth run, there is a gradual restoration of the performance to the level of the first run. (b) Mean response latencies with confidence interval of 0.95 for the detection of words presented to the RVF (solid line) and LVF (dashed line) during each of the five tachistoscopic experimental runs. The slowing of response latencies for stimuli presented to the RVF in the second run (immediately postictal) is significant. (Reproduced with permission, from Stodieck *et al.*, 1986.)

with a progressive return to the previous left hemisphere dominance with normalization of the clinical and electroencephalographic state (Stodieck *et al.*, 1986).

Such observations, in particular those with long-lasting epileptic status-like discharges in certain limbic regions, have important implications for the so-called 'interictal personality and behavioural changes' observed in some, but not all patients with TL epilepsy. In the light of our findings, one is tempted to assume that the spike focus *per se* might be the primary pathogenetic mechanism in certain behavioural abnormalities seen more frequently in TL epilepsy than in other non-epileptic pathological conditions of the TL. Repetitive discharges or even isolated spikes may alter the reactivity of hodologically linked ganglionic structures leading to some kind of experimental kindling, although use of this term to describe human psychopathological conditions (Stevens and Livermore, 1978) is undesirable, given the current lack of knowledge concerning mechanisms. Similar objections might also be raised against the terms 'sensory-limbic hyperconnection' (Bear, 1979) or 'limbic dyscontrol syndrome' (Girgis and Kiloh, 1980) which might illustrate, but do not explain, the pathophysiology of the observed behavioural changes.

PSYCHOPATHOLOGY IN PATIENTS WITH TL EPILEPSY

A large variety of psychopathology in patients with TL epilepsy has been reported (Flor-Henry, 1972; Bear and Fedio, 1977; Trimble and Reynolds, 1988) (see also Chapters 10 and 11). It ranges from brief episodes of psychical aberrations (such as 'psychical' seizures—Penfield and Jasper, 1954; Gloor *et al.*, 1982; Wieser, 1979) to twilight states (such as prolonged psychomotor status—Wieser, 1980) to the above-mentioned peculiarities of personality (such as the so-called 'interictal behavioural syndrome of TLE' of Waxman and Geschwind, 1975; Geschwind, 1979), to frank psychosis (such as the so-called 'schizophrenia-like' paranoid psychosis—Slater *et al.*, 1965). Whereas the first two conditions are clearly of ictal nature, the second two are believed to be interictal phenomena, insofar as—at least at the level of scalp EEG—no underlying epileptic discharges are found. Sometimes, however, the surface EEG shows changes in the direction of a so-called 'forced normalization' (Landolt, 1960). Elsewhere (Wieser, 1983a,b; Wieser and Landis, 1983) we have presented case reports illustrating these phenomena. We found that the behavioural alterations for at least some patients

Table 1. Emotional and psychological effects of lateralized brain damage (from Taylor, 1989).

Left brain		*Right Brain*	
Female crying destructive lesion Male laughing irritative lesions		Hemispherectomy euphoria Male laughing destructive lesions	
Damage 'Dysphoria'	Despair Hopelessness Anger Self depreciation Fits of crying	*Damage* 'Indifference'	Minimization Placidity Jokes Elation Social disinhibition
Amytal	Dysphoria Tears	*Amytal*	Euphoria
ECT for depression	VIQ Loss	*ECT for depression*	PIQ Gain
Defective verbal mediation Faulty evaluation of nuances Bland Inappropriate symbolic process Reflective ruminative strategies Sombre Feeling coded in sterile intellectual terms Failure of matching to emotional scenes Neurolinguistic losses Catastrophic reaction		Reliance on emotional stimuli which are misperceived Disorders of affective speech and drive relevant cues from internal and external sources Affective tone Detection of horror expression Suppression of the unpleasant Inattention, denial, imperception, anosognosia, gesture, aprosodia	

were due to frequent limbic discharges without expression at the level of the scalp EEG and therefore in reality represent ictal events. These few patients showed complete normalization of their aberrant behaviour following resection of the epileptogenic area, whereas, in the large majority of operated TL epilepsy cases with concomittant TL personality and behavioural syndrome or paranoid psychosis, the psychopathology did not improve despite complete postoperative seizure control.

An even more puzzling phenomenon is the fortunately rare appearance of a so-called 'postoperative psychosis' following TL surgery. Personally I have seen such a postoperative psychosis only once (0.3%). This was a patient with a large resection involving not only the right TL, but also encroaching on the surrounding parieto-occipital area. Other authors, however, report a much higher incidence. Jensen and Larsen (1979a,b), for example, report that 9/94 cases (10%) experienced postoperative psychosis in TL epilepsy. Taylor (1975) in his study on the TL-ectomies of Falconer mentioned the following risk factors for postoperative psychosis: (i) the presence of small 'alien tissue' lesions; (ii) left hemisphere location; (iii) late onset of epilepsy; (iv) higher incidence in females than males; and (v) left handedness.

In a recent review, Taylor (1989) listed emotional and psychological effects of lateralized brain damage (Table 1), summarizing his and other authors' extensive experience.

PRE- AND POSTOPERATIVE 18F-FDG PET FINDINGS IN PATIENTS WITH AHE

We are presently conducting a comparison of pre- and postoperative 18F-FDG PET scans in patients who underwent selective AHE. Preoperatively all patients, except one, showed reduced CMRGlu in the operated TL. The interictal hypometabolic region usually comprized the entire TL. Following AHE, there was no normalization of energy metabolism in the lateral TL ipsilateral to the AHE in any of the hitherto pre- and postoperatively investigated patients (n=25). In fact, hypometabolism of 17±7% occurred in the lateral parts of TL, despite the fact that, on average, a total volume of only 7.2 ml was resected (consisting of removal of the amygdala, anterior hippocampus and parts of the parahippocampal gyrus) (Siegel *et al.*, 1990). The interictal hypometabolism in the affected TL persisted irrespective of the time since operation (postoperative PET scans were performed between 3 and 5 months following the operation, and the early 11 patients now having been studied for 12 months postoperatively) and irrespective of the patients' postoperative seizure outcome, i.e. irrespective of whether the operation led to complete seizure control or not (Leenders *et al.*, 1989; Hajek *et al.*, 1991). Whether the postoperative EEG activity correlates, at least to some degree, with the postoperative PET has to be studied more carefully by monitoring the EEG during PET scanning. However, EEG controls routinely performed 3 and 6 months postoperatively have shown that epileptiform activity had disappeared or is significantly decreased in most patients (Siegel and Wieser, 1989). It is therefore rather unlikely that epileptic activity in itself is responsible for the reduced brain tissue energy requirements in TLE with mesiobasal limbic seizure foci.

EPILEPTOLOGICAL OUTCOME OF AHE

Two hundred and ninety-three patients with medically refractory mesiobasal TL epilepsy have undergone selective TL surgery in the University Hospital of Zürich since 1975. Excluding patients who underwent selective TL resections outside the amygdala and hippocampus, 279 patients underwent selective AHE. Of these, 215 patients have been included in a follow-up study and classified according to the neuropathological findings of the resected specimen. A detailed list of histological findings is given elsewhere (Wieser, 1991). The male to female ratio was 120:95. In 114 patients the operation

Table 2. Most recent and year-by-year epileptological outcome of patients treated with selective amygdalohippocampectomy. The bottom part of the table shows the outcome of 58 non-lesional patients preoperatively classified into 'causal' and 'palliative' operations.

Follow-up groups	*Total*	*Outcome categories* *I*	*II*	*III* (%)	*IV*
Most recent follow-up ($\bar{x}$ 47; SD 30.8)	177	59	7	11	22
Year-by-year outcome					
1 year	177	65	5	11	19
2 years	138	59	7	12	22
3 years	106	59	4	12	25
4 years	91	63	4	13	20
5 years	73	59	7	12	22
6–8 years	34	59	3	12	26
9–13 years	10	70	10	10	10
Causal AHE ($\bar{x}$ 50.4; SD 35.3)	30	73	20	–	7
Palliative AHE ($\bar{x}$ 55.7; SD 31.0)	28	12	–	31	57

$\bar{x}$, mean in months; SD, standard deviation in months.

was on the right and in 101 patients on the left side. Mean age at the onset of the seizure disorder was 18.8 years (SD 15.3), and the mean age at operation was 29.7 years (SD 13.7). The calculated mean duration of the seizure disorder prior to operation was 11.0 years (SD 10.2). Patients with no microscopical pathology were operated earlier (mean 28.0 years; SD 8.8) than those with gliosis (slight gliosis: mean 30.1 years; SD 10.6; moderate gliosis: mean 32.2 years; SD 9.6; severe gliosis: mean 34.1 years; SD 7.3). Likewise the mean duration of epilepsy prior to surgery was 18.5 years (SD 8.1) in patients with slight gliosis, 21.9 years (SD 9.1) in cases with moderate gliosis, and 28.8 years (SD 4.5) in patients with severe gliosis.

The epileptological outcome was classified according to the recommendations of Engel (1987) into the following categories: I, seizure-free; II rare seizures (not more than 1–2 per year); III, worthwhile improvement (>90% reduction); and IV, no worthwhile improvement. A postoperative follow-up of at least 12 months was required prior to classification into one of the above categories.

The most recent epileptological outcome together with the follow-up period is reported in Table 2. The year-by-year outcome classification shows that the percentage of patients in each category remains fairly stable over time.

PRE-/POSTOPERATIVE MODIFICATIONS IN THE ANTIEPILEPTIC DRUG TREATMENT

It is well known that virtually all anticonvulsant medications can affect mental functions. Cognitive effects include deficits on neuropsychological tests, impaired short-term memory and memory concentration tasks, impaired attention, problem solving and visuomotor tasks. Behavioural effects include drowsiness, lethargy, disturbed sleep, irritability, aggressiveness, hyperactivity, disobedience, antisocial activities, alteration of emotional state and depressive symptoms. Drug reduction can result in a significant improvement of cognitive performance and behaviour (Durwen *et al.*, 1989).

In order to describe the neuropsychological and epileptological effects of the selective AHE it is therefore necessary to consider the pre-/postoperative modifications in the antiepileptic drug (AED) regimen. Whereas preoperatively all our patients had high doses of AEDs in polytherapy, postoperatively 49 out of 177 patients (28%) had a complete discontinuation of AEDs. AEDs are not required by 70% of the patients in the longest follow-up group (9–13 years, n=10), by 43% of the patients with a postoperative follow-up of 6–8 years (n=34), and by 42% of patients with a follow-up of 5 years (n=73). The mean postoperative period before discontinuation of the AEDs was 20.1 months (ranging from 6–60). Forty-six patients (94%)

remained seizure-free following AED discontinuation. Phenytoin was given in 56% of the 82 patients as monotherapy, phenobarbital or primidone in 22% and carbamazepine in 21%. When two AEDs were given (n=43) 79% of the patients received phenytoin, 44% phenobarbital or primidone, 37% carbamazepine, 26% valproate, and 14% diazepam or other AEDs.

PRE-/POSTOPERATIVE INTERICTAL SCALP EEG CHANGES FOLLOWING AHE

In a recently completed study we have examined the conventional interictal scalp EEGs (n=612) of 93 patients who underwent selective AHE over a period of 4 pre- and 4 postoperative years (Siegel and Wieser, 1989). In each EEG record the following parameters were visually assessed and quantitatively rated: background activity, ipsi- and contralateral focal slowing, ipsi- and contralateral epileptiform potentials, and generalized epileptiform abnormalities. There was a strong correlation between the amount of EEG improvement and the clinical seizure outcome. Patients with a good clinical outcome had, as a rule, an improved EEG by 3 months after the operation. Postoperatively, in the good outcome groups all parameters improved more, and most also earlier than in the bad outcome group. Most striking, however, was the difference between the outcome groups in the parameters contralateral and ipsilateral to the focal spiking (over TL region). Contralateral TL spiking ceased completely and ipsilateral TL spiking was much more reduced in the good outcome groups (I and II) than in the poorer outcome groups (III and IV).

DISCUSSION

Although it would be tempting to correlate directly pre- and postoperative performance changes with the site and extent of the therapeutic resection, this short review clearly shows that this is not advisable. The behavioural consequences of TL operations must be seen against the clinical background of our patients, who had suffered from years of severe drug-resistant TL epilepsy, the effects of treatment, and various psychosocial effects. Quite a large number of other factors must therefore be taken into account, e.g., outcome of seizures resulting from the operation, pre-/postoperative changes in AED treatment, pre-/postoperative EEG changes, pre-/postoperative vocational and social status, and, very importantly, family support. Several surgically active epilepsy centres have started to study their patients from these perspectives. Crandall *et al.* (1987), for example, listed the following characteristics of the best outcome group following TL surgery for epilepsy:

(i) younger than 30 years of age at surgery; (ii) strong family support; (iii) no or only mild psychopathology; and (iv) absence of an addictive personality. 'Good family support', of course, once again implies quite a large number of variables, including (a) early diagnosis, (b) early adequate AED treatment, and (c) early operation. This in turn implies (d) short seizure illness, (e) good post-surgical care, and (f) adequate rehabilitation, if necessary.

Since most of the above-mentioned factors depend on each other in one way or another, it is often difficult to decide what factors are more important in any given case. What counts clinically, however, is the final outcome, which has been satisfying in most of our patients. Nevertheless, from a scientific point of view it remains our hope that puzzling outstanding questions concerning the functions of the human hippocampus can be clarified by further studies. With regard to the notion that an impaired hippocampus means impaired memory and amnesia, three main mechanisms have been postulated and should be specifically addressed:

- *impaired consolidation* (short-term memory is intact, but long-term memory is impaired; Kornhuber (1973);
- *interference phenomena* (old memories interfere with consolidation of new ones; Warrington and Weiskrantz, 1970);
- *impaired retrieval* (new information can be acquired, but the retrieval of new information is impaired; Squire, 1982).

The existing bouquet of theories about the role and functions of the hippocampus clearly document that more human data must be collected before one or the other of these theories will become established. Without claiming completeness for the following list of hypotheses, the hippocampus has been viewed as:

- an *inhibitor* of diencephalic and midbrain systems (Kimble, 1968) and of the orienting response (Grastyan *et al.*, 1959);
- a *comparator* (Smythies, 1966; Gray's (1982) septo-hippocampal system): hippocampus filters and increases punishing, frustrating and new stimuli. The comparator is the subiculum; the entorhinal cortex projects the 'normal value' to the subiculum; and the 'effective value' is elaborated in the lamellar loop. A 'mismatch' in the subiculum activates inhibitory hippocampal forces;
- a *cognitive map* (O'Keefe and Nadal, 1978): 'egocentric', sensory and modality specific afferents reach the entorhinal cortex; from here topographically arranged projection to fascia dentata (synchronisator: 'time-locked-gate'); dependent on the theta-rhythm; via mossy fibres to CA3; activation of only those pyramidal cells which are on the peak of a theta-polarization wave; events and sensory stimuli are topographically stored; a similar stimulus-combination activates 'place neurons';

- a *RAM* (random access memory = machine memory for intermediate storage of results and data); hippocampal function required for nonspatial working memory (Olton and Feustle, 1981); hippocampus as a time and working memory (Rawlins and Tsaltas, 1983);
- a *register* of stacks or memory buffers (= 'sliding buffer' according to FILO (first in, last out) principle; Deadwyler *et al.*, 1988);
- a *planner for locomotion* (Vanderwolf and Robinson, 1981).

It is hoped that further work on patients with TLE, before and after surgery, especially selective lesions, will clarify some of these issues.

REFERENCES

Aeberli, R. (1990). *Emotionale entscheidungen bei hirnläsionen.* Thesis, University Zürich.

Aeberli, R., Regard, M., Landis, T. and Wieser, H.G. (1988). Emotional decisions before and after amygdalohippocampectomy (Abstr.). *J. Clin. Exp. Neuropsychol.*, **10**, 324.

Bear, D.M. (1979). Temporal lobe epilepsy. A syndrome of sensory-limbic hyperconnection. *Cortex*, **15**, 357–384.

Bear, D.M. and Fedio, P. (1977). Quantitative analysis of interictal behavior in temporal lobe epilepsy. *Arch. Neurol.*, **34**, 454–467.

Birri, R., Perret, E. and Wieser, H.G. (1982). Der Einfluss verschiedener Temporallappenoperationen auf das Gedächtnis bei epileptikern. *Nervenarzt*, **53**, 144–149.

Crandall, P.H., Rausch, R. and Engel Jr, J. (1987). Preoperative indicators for optimal surgical outcome for temporal lobe epilepsy. In: Wieser, H.G. and Elger, C.E. (Eds), *Presurgical Evaluation of Epileptics*, Springer-Verlag, Berlin, Heidelberg, New York, pp. 325–334.

Deadwyler, S.A., Hampson, R.E., Foster, T.C. and Marlow, G. (1988). The functional significance of long-term potentiation: relation to sensory processing by hippocampal circuits. In: Landfield, P.W. and Deadwyler, S.A. (Eds), *Long-term Potentiation: From Biophysics to Behavior*, Alan R Liss, New York, pp. 499–534.

Durwen, H.F., Elger, C.E., Helmstaedter, C. and Penin, H. (1989). Circumscribed improvement of cognitive performance in temporal lobe epilepsy patients with intractable seizures following reduction of anticonvulsant medication. *J. Epilepsy*, **2**, 147–153.

Engel Jr, J. (1987). Outcome with respect to epileptic seizures. In: Engel Jr, J. (Ed.), *Surgical Treatment of the Epilepsies*, Raven Press, New York, pp. 553–571.

Flor-Henry, P. (1972). Ictal and interictal psychiatric manifestations of epilepsy. Specific or non-specific? *Epilepsia*, **13**, 773–783.

Geschwind, N. (1979). Behavioral changes in temporal lobe epilepsy. *Psychol. Med.*, **9**, 217–219.

Girgis, M. and Kiloh, L.G. (Eds) (1980). *Limbic Epilepsy and the Dyscontrol Syndrome*, Elsevier/North-Holland Biomed Press, Amsterdam.

Gloor, P., Olivier, A., Quesney, L.F., Andermann, F. and Horowitz, S. (1982). The role of the limbic system in experiential phenomena of temporal lobe epilepsy. *Ann. Neurol.*, **12**, 129–144.

Gonser, A., Perret, E. and Wieser, H.G. (1986). Ist der Hippokampus für Lern- und Gedächtnisprozesse notwendig? *Nervenarzt*, **57**, 269–275.

Grastyan, E., Lissak, K., Madarasz, L. and Donhoffer, H. (1959). Hippocampal electric activity during the development of conditioned motor reflexes. *Electroencephalogr. Clin. Neurophysiol.*, **11**, 409–430.

Gray, J.A. (1982). *The Neuropsychology of Anxiety: an Enquiry into the Functions of the Septo-Hippocampal system*, Clarendon Press, Oxford.

Hajek, M., Wieser, H.G. and Leenders, K.L. (1991). PET Ergebnisse vor und nach selektiver Amygdala-Hippokampektomie. In: D. Scheffner (Ed.), *Epilepsie 90*, Einhorn Presse Verlag, D-Reinbek, Germany, pp. 309–312.

Jensen, I. and Larsen, J.K. (1979a). Mental aspects of temporal lobe epilepsy. *J. Neurol. Neurosurg. Psychiatry*, **42**, 256–265.

Jensen, I. and Larsen, J.K. (1979b). Psychoses in drug-resistant temporal lobe epilepsy. *J. Neurol. Neurosurg. Psychiatry*, **42**, 948–954.

Jones-Gotman, M. (1987). Comment: Psychological evaluation. In: Engel Jr, J. (Ed.), *Surgical Treatment of the Epilepsies*, Raven Press, New York, pp. 197–201.

Kimble, D.P. (1968). Hippocampus and internal inhibition. *Psychol. Bull.*, **70**, 285–295.

Kornhuber, H.H. (1973). Neural control of input into long term memory: limbic system and amnesic syndrome in man: In: Zippel, H.P. (Ed.), *Memory and Transfer of Information*, Plenum Press, New York.

Landolt, H. (1960). *Die Temporallappenepilepsie und ihre Psychopathologie*, Karger, Basel.

Leenders, K.L., Schmid, M., Antonini, A., Wyer, L., Fisch, R., Reist, H., Weinreich, R. and Wieser, H.G. (1989). Brain glucose utilisation in temporal lobe epilepsy before and after selective surgery. (Abstr.) *XIVth World Congress of Neurology*, New Delhi.

Milner, B. (1975). Psychological aspects of focal epilepsy and its neurosurgical management. In: Purpura, D.P., Penry, J.K. and Walter, R.D. (Eds), *Advances in Neurosurgery, Vol. 8: Neurosurgical Management of the Epilepsies*, Raven Press, New York, pp. 299–321.

Nadig, T., Wieser, H.G. and Perret, E. (1985). Learning and memory performance before and after unilateral selective amygdalohippocampectomy. In: Will, B.E., Schmitt, P. and Dalrymple-Alford, J.C. (Eds), *Brain Plasticity, Learning and Memory*, Plenum, New York, pp. 397–403.

O'Keefe, J. and Nadel, L. (1978). *The Hippocampus as a Cognitive Map*, Clarendon Press, Oxford.

Olton, D.S. and Feustle, W.A. (1981). Hippocampal function required for nonspatial working memory. *Exp. Brain Res.*, **41**, 380–389.

Penfield, W. and Jasper, H. (1954). *Epilepsy and the Functional Anatomy of the Human Brain*, Little, Brown, Boston.

Rawlins, N.J.P. and Tsaltas, E. (1983). The hippocampus time and working memory. *Behav. Brain Res.*, **28**, 335–344.

Schiess, R., Regard, M., Landis, T. and Wieser, H.G. (1990). Hemisphere dependent memory performance during selective amytal procedure and after amygdalohippocampectomy (Abstr.), *International Neuropsychology Society Symposium*, Innsbruck.

Siegel, A.M. and Wieser, H.G. (1989). Comparative pre- and postoperative interictal scalp electroencephalographic examinations in patients with selective amygdalohippocampectomy. *J. Epilepsy*, **2**, 65–72.

Siegel, A.M., Wieser, H.G., Wichmann, W. and Yasargil, M.G. (1990). Relationship between MR-imaged total amount of tissue removed, resection scores of specific mediobasal limbic subcompartments and clinical outcome following selective amygdalohippocampectomy. *Epilepsy Res.*, **6**, 56–65.

Slater, E., Beard, A.W. and Glithero, E. (1965). Schizophrenia-like psychosis of epilepsy. *Int. J. Psychiatry*, **1**, 6–8.
Smythies, J.R. (1966). *Brain Mechanisms and Behavior*, Academic Press, New York.
Squire, L.R. (1982). The neuropsychology of human memory. *Annu. Rev. Neurosci.*, **5**, 241–273.
Stevens, J. and Livermore, A. (1978). Kindling of the mesolimbic dopamine system: animal model of psychosis. *Neurology*, **28**, 36–46.
Stodieck, S.R.G., Regard, M., Landis, T. and Wieser, H.G. (1986). Seizure induced shift in hemispheric reading dominance (Abstr.), *International Conference on the Surgical Treatment of Epilepsy*, Palm Desert.
Taylor, D.C. (1975). Factors influencing the occurrence of schizophrenia-like psychoses in patients with temporal lobe epilepsy. *Psychol. Med.*, **5**, 249–254.
Taylor, D.C. (1989). Affective disorders in epilepsies: a neuropsychiatric review. *Behav. Neurol.*, **2**, 49–68.
Trimble, M.R. and Reynolds, E.H. (Eds) (1988). *Epilepsy, Behaviour and Cognitive Function*, Wiley, Chichester.
Vanderwolf, C.H. and Robinson, T.E. (1981). Reticulo-cortical activity and behavior: a critique of the arousal theory and a new synthesis. *Behav. Brain Sci.*, **4**, 459–514.
Wada, J. (1949). A new method for the determination of the side of cerebral speech dominance. A preliminary report on the intracarotid injection of Sodium Amytal in man. *Igaku to Seibutsugaku*, **14**, 221–222.
Warrington, E.K. and Weiskrantz, L. (1970). Amnesic syndrome: consolidation or retrieval? *Nature*, **228**, 628–630.
Waxman, S.G. and Geschwind, N. (1975). The interictal behavioral syndrome of temporal lobe epilepsy. *Ann. Gen. Psychiatry*, **32**, 1580–1586.
Wieser, H.G. (1979). Psychische Anfälle und deren stereo-elektroenzephalographisches Korrelat. *Z. EEG-EMG*, **10**, 197–206.
Wieser, H.G. (1980). Temporal lobe or psychomotor status epilepticus. *Electroencephalogr. Clin. Neurophysiol.*, **45**, 558–572.
Wieser, H.G. (1983a). *Electroclinical Features of the Psychomotor Seizure*, Gustav Fischer-Butterworths, Stuttgart, London.
Wieser, H.G. (1983b). Depth recorded limbic seizures and psychopathology. *Neurosci. Biobehav. Rev.*, **7**, 427–440.
Wieser, H.G. (1986). Selective amygdalohippocampectomy: indications, investigative technique and results. In: Symon, L. *et al.*. (Eds), *Advances and Technical Standards in Neurosurgery, Vol. 13*, Springer, Vienna, New York, pp. 39–113.
Wieser, H.G. (1991). Selective amygdalohippocampectomy: indications and follow-up. In: Quesney, L.F. *et al.* (Eds), Proceedings 50th Anniversary EEG Symposium, Montreal. *Can. J. Neurol. Sci.*, November.
Wieser, H.G. and Landis, T. (1983). Is the 'interictal behaviour syndrome of temporal lobe epilepsy' really an 'interictal' phenomenon? *Neurolog. Psychiatr.*, **6**, 70–78.
Wieser, H.G. and Yasargil, M.G. (1982). Selective amygdalohippocampectomy as a surgical treatment of mesiobasal limbic epilepsy. *Surg. Neurol.*, **17**, 445–457.
Wieser, H.G., Hailemariam, S., Regard, M. and Landis, T. (1985). Unilateral limbic epileptic status activity: stereo EEG, behavioral, and cognitive data. *Epilepsia*, **26**, 19–29.
Wieser, H.G., Valavanis, A., Roos, A., Isler, P. and Renella, R.R. (1989a). 'Selective' and 'superselective' temporal lobe Amytal tests: I. Neuroradiological, neuroanatomical, and electrical data. In: Manelis, J., Bental, E., Loeber, J.N. and Dreifuss, F. (Eds), *Advances in Epileptology, Vol. 17*, Raven Press, New York, pp. 20–27.

Wieser, H.G., Landis, T., Regard, M. and Schiess, R. (1989b). 'Selective' and 'super-selective' temporal lobe Amytal tests: II. Neuropsychological test procedure and results. In: Manelis, J., Bental, E., Loeber, J.N. and Dreifuss, F. (Eds), *Advances in Epileptology, Vol. 17*, Raven Press, New York, pp. 28–33.

Wieser, H.G., Landis, T. and Valavanis, A. (1989c). Selective Amytal memory tests: correlation with postoperative results (Abstr.), *Epilepsia*, **30**, 724.

Wittlieb-Verpoort, E. and Wieser, H.G. (1992). Tone discrimination in patients with temporal lobe lesions, in press.

Yasargil, M.G. and Wieser, H.G. (1987). Selective microsurgical resections. In: Wieser, H.G. and Elger, C.E. (Eds), *Presurgical Evaluation of Epileptics*, Springer, Berlin, Heidelberg, New York, pp. 352–360.

The Temporal Lobes and the Limbic System
Edited by M.R. Trimble and T.G. Bolwig

13

Cerebrovascular Diseases and Tumours in the Limbic System

OLAF B. PAULSON* and TOM G. BOLWIG**
*Departments of *Neurology and **Psychiatry, State University Hospital, Rigshospitalet, Copenhagen, Denmark*

INTRODUCTION

The limbic system consists of several structures which physiologically and anatomically are connected by pathways and synapses. They are located in quite different anatomical parts of the brain—frontal lobe, temporal lobe, hypothalamus, and diencephalon; however, all are near the base of the skull. Lesions in hippocampal area and amygdala in the temporal lobe are frequently encountered whereas other lesions in the limbic system are more rare. Neoplastic lesions appear with higher frequency than vascular lesions. Tumours may cause both focal symptoms due to the lesion itself and more diffuse (global) symptoms due to the mass effect of the space occupying lesion. With ischaemic vascular lesions the diffuse symptoms are of much less significance.

Lesions in the hippocampal area and amygdala frequently yield epileptic seizures of the partial complex type. With lesions in the olfactory bulb or tract, anosmia occurs. Otherwise lesions in the limbic system are characterized by a frequent occurrence of mental symptoms with memory disturbance, affective symptomatology, personality changes, in some cases psychosis and aphasia. A state of akinetic mutism may be seen in which the patient is apathetic, does not speak and is motionless, although not paretic. Thus, lesions in the limbic system often produce symptoms not only from limbic structures themselves but also from neighbouring brain tissue. These features of lesions in the limbic system due to tumours and cerebrovascular accidents are the topic of this chapter.

GENERAL ASPECTS OF SYMPTOMATOLOGY IN INTRACRANIAL TUMOURS AND CEREBROVASCULAR DISEASES

Intracranial tumours and intracranial haematomas are space occupying lesions. Accordingly, the symptoms arising from such lesions may have the nature of focal deficits due to damage of the tissue directly affected by the tumour or haematoma, or they may present as global, diffuse (or remote) symptoms due to tissue displacement by the space occupying lesion and due to increased intracranial pressure. Well known symptoms of the latter category are drowsiness and confusion, and in the extreme, symptoms of herniation. There is a tendency for slowly growing tumours to give more focal and fewer global symptoms compared with rapidly growing tumours. Also mental symptoms are more frequent with rapidly growing tumours than with slowly growing tumours (Keschner *et al.*, 1938; Busch, 1940), although slowly growing tumours may be more likely to present with mental symptoms alone.

Ischaemic lesions usually are of a more focal nature. In the acute phase a major ischaemic lesion can lead to the formation of brain oedema, which may spread to surrounding structures and act as a space occupying lesion. Otherwise the lesion ordinarily remains focal, corresponding to the area of complete or partial ischaemia. The focal nature of the lesion, however, does not exclude some remote effects in the central nervous system, but these are due to a mechanism other than that resulting from a space occupying lesion. It is thus well known that a major lesion in one cerebral hemisphere often results in a reduced neuronal output to the contralateral cerebellar hemisphere and hence to a demonstrably reduced blood flow and metabolism in this area, the so-called diaschisis (Meneghetti *et al.*, 1984). Diaschisis is most often asymptomatic, but it is of importance for the understanding and diagnosis of reduced function of structures not directly affected by the primary lesion.

GENERAL ASPECTS OF TUMOURS AND CEREBROVASCULAR DISEASES IN THE LIMBIC SYSTEM

Many tumours, e.g. metastatic brain tumours are distributed roughly in proportion to the weight of the different brain areas whereas others have a predilection for certain areas. With regard to the limbic system, extracerebral tumour tissue arising from the sphenoidal wing, the pituitary gland, the ethmoid sinus and the clivus of the base of the skull may compress and invade the neighbouring cerebral tissue and cause symptoms related to parts of the limbic system and from the visual pathways. Such tumours may be meningiomas, gliomas, pituitary adenomas, craniopharyngiomas, reticulomas as well as other types. Among the invading lesions are also the more uncommon such as sarcoidosis and Wegener's lymphogranulomatosis from the nasal cavity. Most tumours leading to symptoms predominantly from the limbic system are of the slowly growing type.

Cerebrovascular diseases affecting the limbic system appear to be more uncommon than tumours. Classical ischaemic strokes affecting the limbic system are quite rare or the stroke causes such extensive damage outside the limbic system that symptoms from these areas with, e.g. hemiplegia and aphasia completely dominate the clinical picture. However, ischaemic lesions in the mesial temporal regions may cause amnestic syndromes. Such lesions, unilateral, partial or transient probably represent one cause of the syndrome of transient global amnesia (TGA) in at least some of these patients.

Several patients with epilepsy arising from amygdala and the hippocampal region in the temporal lobe have no demonstrable structural lesion, and CT (X-ray computed tomography) and MRI (magnetic resonance imaging) are normal. However, the pathophysiological abnormality is often demonstrated with SPECT (single photon emission computed tomography) and PET (positron emission tomography) revealing reduced blood flow and metabolism in the involved area in the interictal state and increased flow and metabolism during the ictus with seizure activity (Andersen *et al.*, 1990). The cause of epilepsy in these patients is not well known, but it is generally recognized that the temporal–limbic system is composed of rather vulnerable structures which easily become affected in diseases involving the temporal lobes. In some patients with temporal lobe epilepsy without overt structural abnormalities the aetiology has been attributed to diffuse hippocampal 'gliosis' which might represent an extremely slow and diffusely growing 'tumour', or to post-ischaemic lesions during anoxic episodes, e.g. in connection with previous febrile convulsions in childhood. Ischaemic lesions as a result of arteriosclerotic vascular disease are not common, since the incidence of these, in contrast to stroke, does not increase with older age.

GENERAL SYMPTOMATOLOGY ACCOMPANYING LESIONS IN THE TEMPORAL LOBE LIMBIC SYSTEM

Cerebrovascular diseases

Specific implication of the temporal lobes in connection with haemorrhage or infarction from branches of the posterior cerebral artery, which together with the middle cerebral artery supply regions of the temporal lobe, has not been demonstrated. It is, however, noteworthy that occasionally psychosis with hallucinations and paranoid ideation may occur as a manifestation of cerebral vascular accidents involving the temporal lobe (Davison and Bagley, 1969), and amnesias are sometimes reported.

Neoplasms

Tumours located in the temporal lobes probably produce the highest incidence of mental disturbances when compared with tumours with other intracerebral localization. This may only in part be explained by the paroxysmal (epileptic) phenomena occasioned by temporal lobe epilepsy. Thus, in the careful study by Keschner *et al.* (1938), in which paroxysmal disturbances were excluded, temporal lobe tumours were associated with a higher percentage of mental symptoms than were tumours with other locations. It was also remarkable that a higher percentage of patients with early psychiatric symptomatology in the course of their illness was found in the temporal lobe tumour group. Similar observations were made by Hécaen and Ajuriaguerra (1956a,b), whose description of psychopathology in connection with tumours also included the occurrence of paroxysmal manifestations.

Dementia

Early onset and progression of dementia occurring in connection with temporal lobe tumours may be largely due to language disturbances accompanying tumours on the dominant side, while non-dominant temporal lobe tumours may remain clinically silent during their growth for a somewhat longer period of time (Lishman, 1987). One of the largest series of temporal lobe tumours described by Bingley (1958) pointed to a greater impairment of intellect with localization to the dominant side, both with regard to verbal and non-verbal functions. The liability of dominant lobe tumours to produce mental symptoms from that study seems further substantiated by the fact that psychopathology was even more pronounced during the course of illness, when no papillary oedema had developed and thus before obvious rise of the intracranial pressure.

Affective disturbance

Among the most common psychopathological features associated with temporal lobe tumours are affective symptomatology, with euphoria being as common with temporal as with frontal tumours (Keschner *et al.*, 1937; Schlesinger, 1950). This feature occurs mainly together with intellectual impairment. Depression, irritability and anxiety are found most commonly in cases of tumours on the dominant side and most often in association with language disturbances. In a later study by Bingley (1958), it was concluded that emotional changes were seen more frequently with dominant than with non-dominant tumours and often in association with a flattening of affect.

Personality disorder and psychosis

Changes of personality may be indistinguishable from those found with frontal lesions, and there do not appear to be any specific features described in association with temporal lobe tumours. Psychotic illness resembling schizophrenia has been described, and the psychosis may be the initial manifestation. Although such cases are rare, Davison and Bagley (1969) in their review of a number of reports came to the conclusion that the association of a diagnosis of schizophrenia and cerebral tumour exceeded chance. They found that, in 77 cases of 'schizophrenia' taken from 42 published reports compared with two large unselected series of tumours, a significantly higher proportion of temporal lobe localization and pituitary tumours was present in the 'schizophrenic' group. Of 245 cases of brain tumour, 11.5% were diagnosed as having functional disorder of which more than 60% were classified as having schizophrenia. All of these patients had involvement of the limbic system, especially the amygdaloid hippocampal region, the cingulate region, and the area of the third ventricle (Malamud, 1967).

Thus, a broad spectrum of psychiatric manifestations may result from lesions in the limbic system and generally they do not show a localization specificity. An exception are the features particular to temporal lobe epilepsy, the origin of which is most often unknown, but which may be paroxysmal manifestations of neoplasia including harmartomas, which are areas of abnormal tissue of developmental origin and include angiomas.

Taylor (1972), in a series of patients who had temporal lobectomy for temporal lobe epilepsy, looked at the pathology of the removed tissue. He noted a link between those with areas of focal 'alien tissue' including hamartomas and dysplasia, and the development of schizophrenia-like psychosis.

Strobos (1953) and Paillas and Tamalet (1950) found the occurrence of epilepsy in patients with temporal lobe tumours to be approximately 50%. The epileptic symptomatology most often presented in the form of seizures with complex partial symptomatology or with secondary generalization. The complex partial seizures may not only originate from the hippocampal area and amygdala, but also—although rather infrequently—from other parts of the grey matter of the limbic system. The term 'complex' is used because organized cerebral activity at a high level is affected. The manifestations of these seizures comprize a number of psychological phenomena such as changes in memory, ideation and affect, illusions and hallucinations and automatic behaviour (Gastaut and Broughton, 1972). These ictal disturbances have been described elsewhere in detail (see Trimble and Bolwig, 1986; Trimble, 1991). In cases of complex partial status (psychomotor status) the symptoms may be dominated by automatic behaviour and psychotic features, sometimes closely resembling schizophrenia with little obvious alteration of consciousness. Psychomotor and petit mal status may also lead to clouded states lasting hours and sometimes days. The former is surprisingly rare considering the frequency of complex partial seizures (Roger *et al.*, 1974), the latter is also infrequent although it is found especially in children and adolescents.

The phenomenology of interictal psychosis associated with temporal lobe epilepsy resembles that of the functional psychoses, and in contrast to an ictal psychosis arising from temporal lobe epilepsy with confusion, there is preserved clarity of consciousness. The interictal psychoses of epilepsy may be affective, paranoid or schizophrenia-like, the latter group best known from the description by Slater *et al.* (1963). These authors stressed that in patients who developed psychosis 12–20 years following their first seizure manifestation there was a preserved emotional response, and further they differed genetically from patients with schizophrenia. Among the patients with interictal psychosis, those with schizo-affective symptomatology, which seems to be the most commonly occurring form, show a trend to an intermittency in symptoms with a recurrent course (Perez *et al.*, 1985), while the schizophrenia-like or paranoid psychoses tend to have a more chronic course (for a review, see Trimble, 1991).

During recent years SPECT studies of regional cerebral blood flow in our institution have been applied in several psychiatric patients with somewhat unusual and uncharacteristic psychiatric symptoms raising suspicion of an organic background but with normal neurological examination and normal CT and MRI studies (personal unpublished observations) (Colour section, Plate 3). In some of these patients, unilateral flow abnormalities were revealed which could involve areas in the limbic system. These findings indicate that functional (metabolic) organic brain pathology may be an underlying association of psychopathology in at least some patients with psychiatric diseases in the absence of epilepsy. At present, the aetiology of these abnormalities remains unknown and it is also too early to speculate how frequently such abnormalities may be encountered.

SYMPTOMS ACCOMPANYING LESIONS IN SPECIFIC PARTS OF THE LIMBIC SYSTEM OUTSIDE THE TEMPORAL LOBE

Lesions in and symptoms from the limbic system are generally uncommon except for epilepsy arising from the limbic structures in the temporal lobe. Encephalitis has not been considered in this chapter, but it is well known that certain forms of encephalitis, for example that associated with herpes simplex, may localize to limbic structures and lead to psychopathology. In this section a brief description is given of symptoms and signs originating from the limbic system presented in a rostral-caudal direction, excluding the temporal lobe (see above).

Olfactory bulb and tract

This structure may be affected with basal frontal tumours especially seen with meningiomas of the sphenoidal wing. Lesions result in anosmia on the affected side. With advanced growth of the tumour the optic nerve may be compressed leading to optic atrophy on the side of the tumour, and simultaneous increase of the intracranial pressure may then result in papillary oedema on only the contralateral side.

Cingulate gyrus

Lesions are not frequent. They are accompanied by rather few symptoms but behavioural abnormalities with aggression, psychotic symptoms and bulimia have been encountered, especially with lesions in the anterior part of the cingulate gyrus. The same symptomatology as seen with lesions of the limbic system in the temporal lobe, i.e. acoustic, gustatory and visual hallucinations may be sometimes observed with frontal lobe tumours (Strauss and Keschener, 1935).

Diencephalon and mesencephalon

In contrast to tumours localized to the temporal lobe, neoplasms originating in the deep midline structures of the diencephalon (thalamus, hypothalamus and other structures located around the third ventricle) do not present with a great variety of psychopathological phenomena. Mental symptoms, however, are frequent especially the marked amnesic deficits typical of tumours in the region of the third ventricle (Delay *et al.*, 1964). The clinical picture is a pronounced inability to fixate current events, difficulty in learning new material and distortion of the recent past. Other cognitive functions including remote memory most often remain unaffected. Confabulation may be pronounced and, along with the amnesic features, the clinical picture may resemble a Korsakoff psychosis, in the absence of alcoholism (Williams and Pennybaker, 1954). Tumours of the diencephalon can lead to progressive dementia due to the chronic obstruction of the cerebral spinal fluid circulation.

Diencephalic tumours are associated with somnolence and hypersomnia, essentially an excess of normal sleep, from which the patient awakens normally in contrast to patients with torpor as a result of raised intracranial pressure. These disorders of sleep are due to lesions which afflict the hypothalamus especially the posterior part and adjacent regions of the upper mid-brain. Such tumours are often accompanied by other manifestations of hypothalamic disorder: amenorrhoea, impotence, diabetes insipidus and other endocrine problems or appetite disorder. A striking syndrome found with lesions in these regions is 'akinetic mutism', in which the patient without strict paresis, is apathetic, has no movements of voluntary character and does not speak, although alertness to a certain extent is preserved (Cairns, 1952). This condition must be distinguished from catatonic or depressive stupor.

Due to the close relationship to the optic chiasm, visual field defects may be seen with lesions in these regions, most often in the form of asymmetric bitemporal defects. With hypothalamic involvement slight pupillary abnormalities may rarely occur and disturbances of temperature regulation are seen.

Finally, anecdotal descriptions of affective disturbances with pronounced mood swings and lack of emotional control as a result of diencephalic tumours have been reported (Alpers, 1940; Reeves and Plum, 1969), as well as of personality changes resembling those found in patients with frontal lobe lesions: carelessness, flat euphoria and lack of concern for others (Lishman, 1987).

CONCLUSIONS

The limbic system consists of several connected structures spread from rostral to caudal parts of predominantly the basal supratentorial parts of the central nervous system. Vascular lesions and particularly neoplasms in the limbic system may cause a variety of neurological and psychiatric symptoms ranging from complex partial seizures, to psychosis, amnesia, disturbance of affect, personality disorders, disturbances of smell and vision, and alteration of consciousness.

REFERENCES

Alpers, B.J. (1940). Personality and emotional disorders associated with hypothalamic lesions. In: *The Hypothalamus and Central Levels of Autonomic Function. Research publication of the Association for Research in Nervous and Mental Disease, Vol. 20*, Williams and Wilkins, Baltimore.

Andersen, A.R., Waldemar, G., Dam, M., Fuglsang-Frederiksen, A., Herning, M., Kruse-Larsen, C. and Lassen, N.A. (1990). SPECT and EEG in focal epilepsy with and without normal CT and MRI scans. A preliminary study of 28 cases. In: Baldy-Moulinier, M., Askenazy, S., Lassen, N.A. and Engel, J. (Eds), *Focal Epilepsy, Clinical Use of Emission Tomography*, John Libbey, London, pp. 97–106.

Bingley, T. (1958). Mental symptoms in temporal lobe epilepsy and temporal lobe gliomas. *Acta Psychiatr. Neurol. Scand.*, **120** (Suppl.), 1–151.

Busch, E. (1940). Psychical symptoms in neurosurgical disease. *Acta Psychiatr. Neurol. Scand.*, **15**, 257–290.

Cairns, H. (1952). Disturbances of consciousness with lesion of the brainstem and diencephalon. *Brain*, **75**, 109–146.

Davison, K. and Bagley, C.R. (1969). Schizophrenia-like psychoses associated with organic disorders of the central nervous system: a review of the literature. In: Herrington, R.N. (Ed.), *Current Problems in Neuropsychiatry. Br. J. Psychiatry, Special Publication No. 4.*

Delay, J., Brion, S. and Derouesné, C. (1964). Syndrome de Korsakoff et étiologie tumorale. *Rev. Neurol.*, **111**, 97–133.

Gastaut, H. and Broughton, R. (1972). Epileptic seizures. Thomas, Springfield, IL.

Hécaen, H. and Ajuriaguerrra, J. de (1956a). *Troubles Mentaux au cours des Tumeurs Intracraniennes*, Masson, Paris.

Hécaen, H. and Ajuriaguerrra, J. de (1956b). Agnosie visuelle pour les objects inanimés par lésion unilatéral gauch. *Rev. Neurol.*, **94**, 222–233.

Keschner, M., Bender, M.B. and Strauss, I. (1937). Mental symptoms in cases of subtentorial tumour. *Arch. Neurol. Psychiatry*, **37**, 1–15.

Keschner, M., Bender, M.B. and Strauss, I. (1938). Mental symptoms associated with brain tumour: a study of 530 verified cases. *J. Am. Med. Assoc.*, **110**, 714–718.

Lishman, W.A. (1987). *Organic Psychiatry. The Psychological Consequences of Cerebral Disorder*, Blackwell Scientific Publications, Oxford.

Malamud, N. (1967). Psychiatric disorder with intracranial tumours of limbic system. *Arch. Neurol.*, **17**, 113–123.

Meneghetti, G., Vorstrup, S., Mickey, B., Lindewald, H. and Lassen, N.A. (1984). Crossed cerebellar diaschisis in ischemic stroke. A study of regional cerebral blood flow by ^{133}Xenon inhalation and single photon emission computer tomography. *J. Cereb. Blood Flow Metabol.*, **4**, 235–240.

Paillas, J.-E. and Tamalet, J. (1950). Les tumeurs temporales. *Presse Med.*, **58**, 550–554.

Perez, M.M., Trimble, M.R., Murray, N.N.F. and Reider, I. (1985). Epileptic psychosis: an evaluation of PSE profiles. *Br. J. Psychiatry*, **146**, 155–163.

Reeves, A.G. and Plum, F. (1969). Hyperphagia, rage and dementia accompanying a ventromedial hypothalamic neoplasm. *Arch. Neurol.*, **20**, 616–624.

Roger, J., Lob, H. and Tassarini, C.A. (1974). Status epilepsicus. In: Vinken, P.J. and Bruyn, G.W. (Eds), *Handbook of Clinical Neurology. Vol. 15*, Elsevier, Amsterdam.

Schlesinger, B. (1950). Mental changes in intracranial tumours, and related problems. *Confin. Neurol.*, **10**, 225–263; 322–355.

Slater, E., Beard, A.W. and Glithero, E. (1963). The schizophrenia-like psychoses of epilepsy. *Br. J. Psychiatry*, **109**, 95–150.

Strauss, I. and Keschener, M. (1935). Mental symptoms in cases of tumour of the frontal lobe. *Arch. Neurol. Psychiatry*, **33**, 986–1005.

Strobos, R.R.J. (1953). Tumours of temporal lobe. *Neurology*, **3**, 752–760.

Taylor, D.C. (1972). Mental state and temporal lobe epilepsy: a correlative account of 100 patients treated surgically. *Epilepsia*, **13**, 727–765.

Trimble, M.R. (1991). *The Psychoses of Epilepsy*, Raven Press, New York.

Trimble, M.R. and Bolwig, T.G. (1986). *Aspects of Epilepsy and Psychiatry*, Wiley, Chichester.

Williams, M. and Pennybacker, J. (1954). Memory disturbances in third ventricle tumours. *J. Neurol. Neurosurg. Psychiatry*, **17**, 115–123.

The Temporal Lobes and the Limbic System
Edited by M.R. Trimble and T.G. Bolwig

14

Memory and the Temporal Lobes

MICHAEL KOPELMAN
Division of Psychiatry, United Medical and Dental Schools of Guy's and St Thomas's Hospitals, St Thomas's Campus, London, UK

INTRODUCTION

The proper and peculiar place assigned and allotted for Memory is the Brayne, the mansion and dwelling house of Wit and all the Senses which being affected or . . . discrased, all the functions and offices of Nature are . . . passioned: insomuch that . . . there steppeth in place . . . forgetfulnes, amazedness, dotage, foolishness, lack of right wits, doltishnes, and idiocie.

Levinus Lemnius (1561)

The disorders and maladies of [memory], when classified and properly understood, are no longer to be regarded as a collection of . . . anecdotes of only passing interest. They will be found to be regulated by certain laws which constitute the very basis of memory, and from which its mechanism is easily laid bare.

T. Ribot (1882)

Levinus Lemnius attributed memory to the appropriate organ some 300 years before Alzheimer, and Ribot (1882) advocated the scientific approach to the study of memory at much the same time as Ebbinghaus (1885) and James (1890) were putting forward their strictly experimental and more theoretical ideas, respectively.

Despite these early forays, it is only in the last 25 years that a vast array of amnesia research has accumulated. Broadly speaking, a useful classification of the amnesic states seen in clinical practice consists of subdividing them into those which give rise to a discrete episode (or transient) amnesia and those which give rise to a more persistent memory impairment. These two main divisions can be further subdivided into those with a presumed organic basis and those in which an underlying psychological mechanism is postulated (Kopelman, 1987a). In this chapter, we shall only be considering the organic amnesias, which include transient global amnesia, on the one hand, and the so-called 'amnesic syndrome', on the other.

AETIOLOGY OF AMNESIAS

There are a variety of possible causes of the amnesic syndrome, including thiamine deficiency, resulting from alcohol abuse or severe malnutrition or malabsorption; head injury, which characteristically leads to damage in the anterior temporal lobes; post-herpes encephalitis, which can cause severe damage to the medial aspects of the temporal lobes as well as a lesser degree of frontal damage; severe hypoxia which, as we will see, can also affect the medial aspects of the temporal lobes; vascular lesions, which can also give rise to temporal lobe pathology; deep midline tumours; and the adverse consequences of temporal lobectomy. The fashionable way to classify these various amnesias is to subdivide them into diencephalic amnesia, temporal lobe amnesia, basal forebrain amnesia, and the frontal amnesias.

The classical example of a diencephalic amnesia is, of course, the alcoholic Korsakoff syndrome. However, vascular lesions affecting the anterior thalamus can also produce a severe amnesia (Winocur *et al.*, 1984; Von Cramon *et al.*, 1985). The critical lesions would appear to be in either the mamillary bodies, the mamillothalamic tract, the dorsomedial nucleus of the thalamus, the anterior thalamus, or some combination of these. Controversy still remains concerning which, if any, of these lesions is most critical (Victor *et al.*, 1971, 1989; Mair *et al.*, 1979; Mayes *et al.*, 1988).

Temporal lobe amnesia most typically occurs in herpes encephalitis, which can destroy much of the temporal lobes bilaterally but the hippocampus and amygdala are particularly implicated, both of which are components of Mishkin's limbic circuits (Mishkin, 1982). It can be postulated that Alzheimer's disease, in which there is considerable hippocampal damage (Tomlinson *et al.*, 1970) might also be considered a variety of temporal lobe amnesia.

Basal forebrain amnesia has been described more recently, and involves damage to cholinergic pathways projecting from the nucleus basalis to the neocortex and from the septal nucleus to the hippocampi, the latter pathology possibly being particularly critical in memory processes. Basal forebrain amnesia was first postulated in connection with Alzheimer's disease, but there have been a series of descriptions of patients with relatively 'pure' lesions of the basal forebrain who have suffered a moderately severe anterograde amnesia as a result (Damasio *et al.*, 1985a,b; Salazar *et al.*, 1986; Phillips *et al.*, 1987). There has also been a study involving lesions to the nucleus basalis in monkeys, which led to anterograde amnesia (Irle and Markowitsch, 1987), and another study showed that prolonged administration of alcohol to rats produced a reduced basal forebrain cell count associated with impaired learning (Arendt *et al.*, 1988). Furthermore, it can be shown that cholinergic blockade, administered to healthy subjects as a 'model' for cholinergic depletion within these pathways, mimics many aspects of anterograde amnesia in humans (Kopelman and Corn, 1988).

NEUROPSYCHOLOGICAL STUDIES OF MEMORY DEFICITS IN THE AMNESIC SYNDROME

Psychologists' models of memory processes used to be relatively simple. Twenty-five years ago, Waugh and Norman (1965) were proposing a model of memory, which was broadly consistent with that of James (1890). They postulated a 'short-term' or 'primary' memory store, which held information for a few seconds only, after which it was either held in primary memory by rehearsal or forgotten. An example is the way in which we may hold a telephone number until we have dialled it. After rehearsal has taken place on numerous occasions, the number will eventually be consolidated into a 'long-term' or 'secondary' memory store, from which the rate of forgetting is presumed to be much slower.

More recent models of memory are more complex, postulating a number of subdivisions in each of primary and secondary memory. Within secondary memory, so-called explicit memory involves the conscious recollection of events or incidents, semantic memory involves memory for facts or concepts, and implicit memory involves memory for skills or retained information for which we do not have conscious access or awareness (Fig. 1). Each of these subdivisions of memory can also be subdivided into a current or anterograde and a remote or retrograde component (Mayes, 1988; Baddeley, 1990). A particular area of recent research interest has been so-called implicit memory, which involves such procedures as classical conditioning and skill learning as well as the 'priming' of existing representations in semantic memory and of novel information or associations. Some of these aspects of memory are known to be preserved in organic amnesia, and others are currently under investigation (for a review, see Tulving and Schacter, 1990).

In many ways, the most intensively investigated form of amnesia is so-called diencephalic amnesia, such as occurs in the Korsakoff syndrome (for a review, see Butters and Cermak, 1980; Mayes, 1988; Butters and Stuss, 1989;

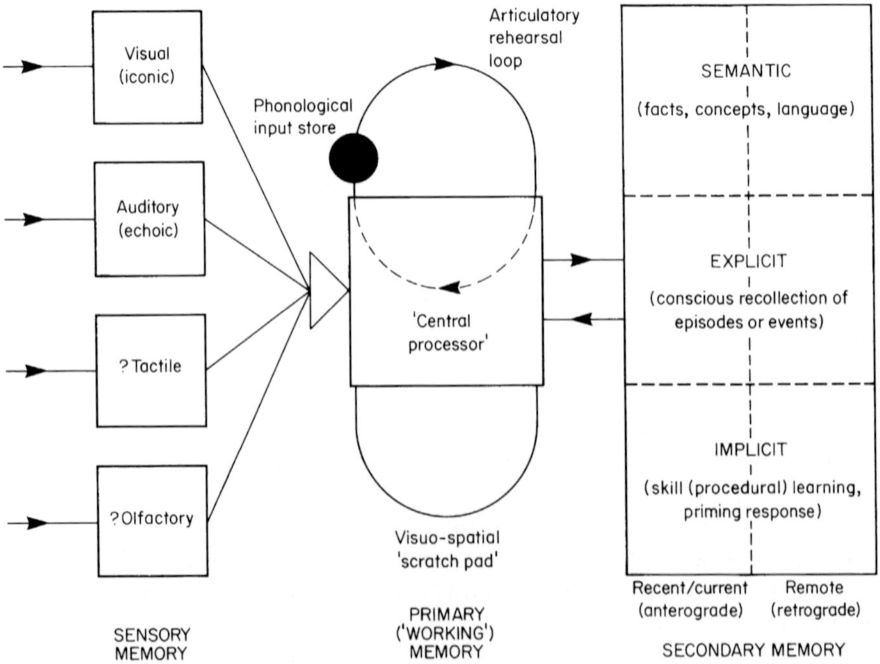

Figure 1. Current concepts of memory involve sensory registers in various modalities, primary or working memory which holds information for relatively brief periods of time, and secondary memory which can be subdivided into explicit, implicit and semantic subcomponents (see text).

Kopelman, 1991a,b). In this form of amnesia, primary memory is known to be relatively intact, as exemplified most typically on span tasks, e.g. digit span, block span. There are known to be deficits in the encoding of semantic or meaningful information (Butters and Cermak, 1980; Cutting, 1978) and also in the encoding of contextual information (Huppert and Piercy, 1976, 1978a; Mayes *et al.*, 1985; Meudell *et al.*, 1985), but it is controversial whether either of these impairments could account for the severity of the amnesia. More commonly, a deficit has been postulated in some process of 'physiological consolidation', and this is where depletions in neurotransmitters such as acetylcholine or abnormalities of the NMDA system may be important (Kopelman, 1987a; Kopelman and Corn, 1988). Various studies have suggested that the retention or storage of information is surprizingly normal if the information is learned adequately, which can be accomplished in experimental studies by a number of manipulations (Huppert and Piercy, 1978b; Squire, 1981; Kopelman, 1985; Martone *et al.*, 1986). Similarly, any deficits in retrieval processes are probably secondary to an underlying encoding or consolidation impairment (Meudell and Mayes, 1982). Various studies have shown that priming and the procedural learning of skills are surprizingly preserved in organic amnesia. For example, subjects may learn to play a new passage of music, without being aware that they have acquired this knowledge (Starr and Phillips, 1970). There is an extensive retrograde amnesia in the Korsakoff syndrome (Albert *et al.*, 1979; Kopelman, 1989), but this is not necessarily the case in amnesia resulting from thalamic infarction (Winocur *et al.*, 1984).

In temporal lobe amnesia, psychological research has found an essentially similar pattern of amnesia, with a severe learning deficit and relatively preserved immediate or primary memory, skill or procedural learning, and responses to priming. This pattern can also be produced by administering cholinergic blockade to healthy subjects as a 'model' of cholinergic depletion in the pathways passing from the septal nucleus to the hippocampus (Kopelman and Corn, 1988). Much of our knowledge of temporal lobe amnesia comes from the study of the patient HM, who was one of several patients who received bilateral temporal lobectomy in the 1950s, resulting in a profound global amnesia (Scoville and Milner, 1957; Milner, 1966). HM showed good immediate memory, and preserved intelligence, and was able to hold a sensible conversation. However, he would forget new information within a matter of a few seconds, unless he constantly rehearsed the information. In addition, he had a retrograde amnesia of approximately 3 years presurgery. He was able to show some skill learning, but he would cry afresh every time he was told that a particular uncle had died (Milner, 1966).

The principal way in which temporal lobe amnesia has been claimed to differ from diencephalic amnesia was that the rate of forgetting of new information may be accelerated. This hypothesis was first put forward by Huppert and Piercy (1978b, 1979) who showed pictures from magazines for prolonged intervals to Korsakoff patients, finding that, if they did this, the rate of forgetting was surprizingly normal. However, when they did this in HM, they found that his rate of forgetting appeared to be accelerated (Huppert and Piercy, 1979). However, this finding was not replicated in a more detailed study of HM conducted some years later (Freed *et al.*, 1987).

Nevertheless, the idea that 'temporal lobe' amnesics may forget faster than those with diencephalic amnesia is still fashionable. For example, Parkin and Leng (1988) compared the performance of a group of patients with temporal lobe lesions, resulting from either herpes encephalitis or vascular lesions, with the rate of forgetting of Korsakoff patients. On this task, there appeared to be accelerated forgetting of new information in the 'temporal lobe' group, relative to the Korsakoff group, between delays of 1–5 min. However, aside from the fact that they did not have any independent information on the sites of their patients' lesions apart from presumed aetiology, their result was confounded by a 'ceiling' effect at the first retention interval, which makes its interpretation very difficult. The forgetting curves at all subsequent intervals were in parallel. A similar claim was made by Levin *et al.* (1988), who used the Huppert–Piercy test to compare head injury patients who were within the period of post-traumatic amnesia (PTA) with those who had come out of PTA. These authors found that, after matching for initial recognition levels, the rate of forgetting was normal in those patients who were out of PTA, but was accelerated for those patients who were still within the period of PTA. The authors assumed that this result could be accounted for by a greater degree of temporal lobe damage in those patients who were still within PTA. However, in this case, they did publish CT scan evidence of the sites of their individual patients' lesions. Careful scrutiny of these data shows that it fails to support the authors' conclusion: some patients with temporal lobe pathology showed normal forgetting, whereas others who lacked temporal lobe pathology showed rapid forgetting. In short, there is not any good evidence that temporal lobe amnesics forget faster than diencephalic amnesic patients.

TRANSIENT GLOBAL AMNESIA

Transient global amnesia is a syndrome which has recently been attributed to possible hippocampal dysfunction (Hodges and Ward, 1989). These authors described transient global amnesia as a witnessed amnesia, occurring in clear consciousness without any focal signs or epilepsy and resolving clinically within 24 h. They obtained 114 cases (retrospective and prospective) in an Oxford survey, and estimated the annual incidence as 3.4 cases per 100 000 population. The mean age of their subjects was 62, and 61% of the subjects were male. The mean duration of the episode was 4.2 h, and it had been preceded by severe exercise in the previous 24 h in 18% of cases, a stressful life event in 14%, and medical and surgical procedures in 3%. An important finding was that there did not appear to be any association with transient ischaemic attacks or other evidence of vascular disease (Hodges and Warlow, 1990). The main association appeared to be with a past history of migraine, which was present in 25–30% of cases, and the attack itself was associated with headache in 10% of cases and with nausea in another 10%. In 7% of cases, the attack appeared to be the first manifestation of what subsequently proved to be complex partial seizures secondary to foci in the temporal lobes. In the remaining 60–70% of cases, no medical association was found.

Five of the cases were studied during and after the attack (Hodges and Ward, 1989). In these cases, the attack lasted 4–10 h, and clinically there appeared to be a permanent retrograde component to the amnesia of 0.5–2.0 h. During the attack, digit span was intact (as occurs in the amnesic syndrome discussed above), but there was severe impairment on such memory tasks as story recall, paired-associate learning, list learning, and the recall of a complex figure. On tests of retrograde memory, two out of five subjects were intact for the recall of famous faces from the past, whereas three out of five cases were impaired, showing a 'temporal gradient', i.e. relative sparing of earlier memories. On a further test, requiring subjects to produce so-called 'autobiographic memories' from their past to cue words, the subjects had to delve further into their past than did healthy control subjects, i.e. only 4% of memories in the TGA group came from the last five years against 25% in the control group. On follow-up of 41 cases at 6 months, Hodges and Oxbury (1990) found that there was no impairment of IQ or non-verbal memory, but there was still some evidence of impairment, relative to a comparison group, for story recall, famous faces, and the cued autobiographical memory test. This implied that recovery, although rapid and substantial, may not be complete.

RELATIONSHIP BETWEEN RETROGRADE AND ANTEROGRADE AMNESIA

The relationship between retrograde (R) memory loss and anterograde (A) amnesia has also been studied in patients with a 'persistent' organic amnesia. Shimamura and Squire (1986) found very low correlations between performance on anterograde and retrograde memory tests, although the correlation was significantly higher for anterograde tests and retrograde items from the most recent decade. Kopelman (1989) and Parkin *et al.* (1990) found somewhat higher correlations, but these still accounted for only a relatively small proportion of the total variance. For example, Kopelman (1989, 1991c) found that only 21% of the variance on retrograde tests could be predicted from anterograde test performance. In this study, an Autobiographical Memory Interview (Kopelman *et al.*, 1989, 1990) was employed, which required the recall of incidents or facts from the subject's own personal past; a Famous News Events Test assessing recall and recognition of pictures of past news events; and a Famous Personalities Test requiring subjects to identify the true names of famous people prominent at different time-periods in the past from fictitious names.

Kopelman (1991c) found that six out of eight 'frontal tests' correlated significantly with a retrograde memory quotient (RMQ), derived from overall performance on these five retrograde tests. Similarly, an R/A difference score, indicating relative sparing of retrograde memory, correlated significantly with five out of eight of the frontal tests. However, only one out of eight frontal tests correlated significantly with an anterograde memory quotient (AMQ), based on performance at four anterograde tests. This led Kopelman (1991c) to argue that, whereas limbic-diencephalic lesions give rise to an anterograde amnesia with a relatively brief and sometimes absent retrograde loss in mild or moderate head injury, localized thalamic infarction, and some cases of TGA, the combination of frontal dysfunction and limbic-diencephalic pathology (including the hippocampus) produces a disruption of the organization of retrieval processes, giving rise to an extensive retrograde loss.

In favour of the Kopelman (1991c) hypothesis, Della Sala *et al.* (1992) have recently described a sample of 16 patients with isolated frontal lesions, identified by CT scan. Six of these patients showed a striking impairment in the retrieval of autobiographical (retrograde) memories, which appeared to be particularly associated with a bilateral distribution of the frontal lesions. On the other hand, against this view, Kapur *et al.* (1992) have recently described a patient with a disproportionately severe loss of retrograde memories, in the presence of relatively mild anterograde impairment. Psychological test scores from a variety of retrograde tests, including the News Events Test, the Autobiographical Memory Interview, and Kapur's Dead-or-alive Test confirmed the severe retrograde loss. An MRI scan identified bilateral lesions in the anterior poles of the temporal lobes, and Kapur *et al.* (1992) argued that anterior temporal lesions must therefore be critical in producing an extensive retrograde loss.

Zola-Morgan *et al.* (1986) described a patient, RB, who exhibited a marked anterograde amnesia following repeated episodes of hypoxia with minimal retrograde loss. On this subject's death, a thorough pathological examination revealed bilateral, circumscribed lesions involving the entire CA1 fields of the hippocampi. It was argued that such lesions are critical for the anterograde impairment of memory. Squire *et al.* (1989) postulated that the CA1 and CA3 fields of the hippocampi are part of a circuit receiving multimodal and highly integrated information from the neocortex, registering relevant events and sending information back to the neocortex in a more diffuse manner. They argued that converging projections from cortical areas interact in the hippocampal formation to establish long-term potentiation in a particular subset of neurons. The potentiated subset of hippocampal neurons then generates a signal which emanates widely in the neocortex, reaching the neocortex through a series of stages involving the entorhinal cortex, parahippocampal gyrus and neocortical association areas. Synaptic change related to learning may occur at each of these stages between the hippocampus and neocortex, and these changes may also be facilitated by signals from the hippocampus. If the hippocampus is damaged before long-term potentiation has dissipated, memory for an event will to some degree to lost, i.e. a brief retrograde amnesia will occur. On the other hand, studies of retrograde amnesia show that remote memories are commonly preserved in patients with hippocampal damage, and consequently Squire *et al.* (1989) suggested that the sites of permanent representations must be elsewhere, probably in the neocortex. Such a view would be consistent with the notion that the frontal cortex is particularly critical for the retrieval of retrograde memories (Kopelman, 1991c) or that they are stored in the anterior temporal cortex (Kapur *et al.*, 1992)

CONFABULATION

It should also be mentioned that spontaneous or 'fantastic' confabulation probably results from coincidental frontal pathology rather than being a direct consequence of the temporal lobe pathology. Spontaneous confabulation refers to the fluent outpouring of erroneous, displaced memories and associations (Berlyne, 1972; Kopelman, 1987b) and a number of studies have found that it seems to be associated with clinical, psychometric, EEG or CT scan evidence of frontal pathology (Luria, 1976; Stuss *et al.*, 1978; Kapur and Coughlan, 1980; Baddeley and Wilson, 1986). By contrast, momentary or 'provoked' confabulation refers to fleeting distortions or intrusion errors, occurring in response to a challenge to the subject's memory, and there is evidence that this kind of confabulation may be a 'normal' response to a 'weak' or faulty memory (Kopelman, 1987b). As such, it can be seen in patients whose amnesia results from temporal lobe pathology. Kopelman (1987b) showed that, when tested at one week's delay, healthy subjects produced qualitatively similar distortions or intrusion errors in recalling a short paragraph to those produced by Korsakoff and Alzheimer patients at immediate recall.

SUMMARY

Summarizing what has been discussed so far, it appears that deficits of 'explicit' anterograde memory result from pathology within limbic-diencephalic circuits, which in turn are modulated by the basal forebrain, and that the hippocampal, particularly the CA1 and CA3 fields, are crucial for anterograde memory. There is evidence that retrograde memories require the mediation of other cortical regions, and these may include the frontal, cortex and/or the anterior or lateral regions of the temporal lobes. Skill learning may be dependent on subcortical processes, and other aspects of primary or 'implicit' memory may be particularly dependent upon other regions of the neocortex.

ASSESSMENT OF MEMORY

There are a variety of memory tests available to test anterograde memory performance. These include recall tasks, such as 'free' recall of a word list, story recall, paired-associate learning, and the recall of objects, pictures or designs. Such tests are included in a number of memory test batteries. Recognition tests are available for words, pictures, faces, and designs; and a commonly used test is the Warrington Recognition Memory Test (Warrington, 1984). Various 'special' tests are employed as research instruments by neuropsychologists—for example, in measuring rates of forgetting or memory for context. Commonly employed anterograde test batteries include the Wechsler Memory Scale—Revised (Butters *et al.*, 1988), the California Verbal Learning Test (Delis *et al.*, 1991), the Kendrick Object Learning Test (Kendrick, 1985), the Rivermead Behavioural Memory Test (Wilson, 1987), as well as the Warrington Recognition Memory Test.

All these tests have their advantages and disadvantages. For example, the Wechsler Memory Scale—Revised, although a considerable improvement on its predecessor, still lacks any recognition component. It is therefore sensible to combine it with the employment of the Warrington Recognition Memory Scale, although this makes a somewhat lengthy and unwieldy procedure.

As far as simple clinical testing is concerned, recall of a short paragraph, such as Logical Memory stories from the Wechsler Memory Test, can provide good discrimination between brain-damaged patients and healthy subjects or depressed patients (Kopelman, 1986). Adequate discrimination is also provided by a simple paired-associate learning test and by immediate and delayed recall of a name and address. On the other hand, supraspan tasks and the so-called Babcock Sentence provide poor discrimination, as elderly healthy subjects find these tasks stressful and commonly perform poorly (Kopelman, 1986).

There are also various research tests available to measure retrograde memory. These include tests about 'public information', such as Famous Faces, Famous Personalities, or the Famous News Events test. These tests are easy to score, but they need regular updating, and performance is related to IQ (Kopelman, 1989). An Autobiographical Memory Interview (Kopelman *et al.*, 1990) is now available which measures facts from the subject's own life as well as the recall of incidents or events from the subject's life.

MEMORY REMEDIATION

There are three possible components to memory remediation: (i) social and psychiatric needs, (ii) rehabilitation techniques, and (iii) pharmacological studies.

The social needs of the patient need assessment, and any preserved skills or abilities need to be noted. Other cognitive abilities should be addressed and obviously there may be a need for occupational placement and day care, accommodation, respite care for relatives, and advice and support for relatives.

The rehabilitation techniques (Wilson, 1987) generally employ the use of either external devices, such as prompts or cues, the use of diaries, or other memory aids or calculators. In addition, various 'internal' strategies can be used to improve memory encoding and retrieval. These include the use of visual imagery, the use of rhymes, using a story to retain components of memory, the use of preserved skills, etc. (Wilson, 1987).

As far as pharmacological strategies are concerned, there are various substances which have been used in dementing patients with very little success, such as hydergine, cyclandelate, and piracetam (Kopelman and Lishman, 1986). More specific treatments include the use of thiamine in Korsakoff patients, amantadine in Creutzfeldt–Jakob disease, and AZT in AIDS. The greatest degree of recent interest has been in neurotransmitter 'replacement' therapy and, although there is some evidence that THA (Tacrine) can be helpful, the degree of benefit is relatively small (Eagger *et al.*, 1991). Consequently, we remain only a little further on than was Levinus Lemnius, when he suggested in 1561:

> *When the weather is myelde and calme, and the Countrey temperate, I myslike not (as touchinge healthynesse of body) shavingeg of the crowne of the head. For thereby grosse vapours which hurt the Memory have more scope and liberty to evaporate and fume out.*
>
> Levinus Lemnius (1561)

REFERENCES

Albert, M.S., Butters, N., Levin, J. (1979). Temporal gradients in the retrograde amnesia of patients with alcoholic Korsakoff's disease. *Arch. Neurol. Chicago*, **36**, 211–216.

Arendt, T., Allen, Y., Sindon, J., Schugens, M.M., Marchbanks, R.M., Lantos, P.L. and Gray, J.A. (1988). Cholinergic-rich brain transplants reverse alcohol-induced memory deficits. *Nature*, **332**, 448–450.

Baddeley, A.D. (1990). *Human Memory: Theory and Practice*, Lawrence Erlbaum Associates, Hove and London.

Baddeley, A.D. and Wilson, B. (1986). Amnesia, autobiographical memory and confabulation. In: Rubin, D. (Ed.), *Autobiographical Memory*, Cambridge University Press, New York.

Berlyne, N. (1972). Confabulation. *Br. J. Psychiatry*, **120**, 31–39.

Butters, N. and Cermak, L.S. (1980). *Alcoholic Korsakoff's Syndrome: An Information-processing Approach to Amnesia*, Academic Press, New York and London.

Butters, N. and Stuss, D.T. (1989). Diencephalic amnesia. In: Boller, F. and Grafman, J. (Eds), *Handbook of Neuropsychology, Vol. 3*, Elsevier Science Publishers, Amsterdam.

Butters, N., Salmon, D.P., Munro Cullum, C., Cairns, P., Tröster, A.I. and Jacobs, D. (1988). Differentiation of amnesic and demented patients with the Wechsler Memory Scale–Revised. *Clin. Neurologist*, **2**, 133–148.

Cutting, J. (1978). A cognitive approach to Korsakoff's syndrome. *Cortex*, **14**, 485–495.

Damasio, A.R., Graff-Radford, N.R., Eslinger, P.J., Damasio, H. and Kassell, N. (1985a). Amnesia following forebrain lesions. *Arch. Neurol.*, **42**, 263–271.

Damasio, A.R., Eslinger, P.J., Damasio, H, van Hoesen, G.W. and Cornell, S. (1985b). Multimodal amnesic syndrome following bilateral temporal and basal forebrain damage. *Arch. Neurol.*, **42**, 252–259.

Delis, D.C., Massman, P.J., Butters, N., Salmon, D.P., Cermak, L.S. and Kramer, J.H. (1991). Profiles of demented and amnesic patients on the California Verbal Learning Test: implications for the assessment of memory disorders. *Psychol. Assess. J. Consult. Clin. Psychol.*, **3**, 19–26.

Della Sala, S., Laiacona, M., Spinnler, H. and Trivelli, C. (1992). Impaired autobiographical recollection in some frontal patients. Submitted for publication.

Eagger, S.A., Levy, R. and Sahakian, B.J. (1991). Tacrine in Alzheimer's disease. *Lancet*, **337**, 989–992.

Ebbinghaus, H. (1885). *Über das Gedächtnis*, Dunker, Leipsiz. (Translated by Ruyer, H. and Bussenius, C.E. (1913). *Memory*, Teachers College, Columbia University, New York.

Freed, D.M., Corkin, S. and Cohen, N.J. (1987). Forgetting in HM: a second look. *Neuropsychologia*, **25**, 461–472.

Hodges, J. and Oxbury, S.M. (1990). Persistent memory impairment following transient global amnesia. *J. Clin. Exp. Neurol.*, **12**, 904–920.

Hodges, J.R. and Ward, C.D. (1989). Observations during transient global amnesia: a behavioural and neuropsychological study of five cases. *Brain*, **112**, 595–620.

Hodges, J. and Warlow, C.P. (1990). The aetiology of transient global amnesia. *Brain*, **113**, 639–657.

Huppert, F.A. and Piercy, M. (1976). Recognition memory in amnesic patients: effect of temporal context and familiarity of material. *Cortex*, **12**, 3–20.

Huppert, F.A. and Piercy, M. (1978a). The role of trace strength in recency and frequency judgements by amnesic and control subjects. *Q. J. Exp. Psychol.*, **30**, 347–354.

Huppert, F.A. and Piercy, M. (1978b). Dissociation between learning and remembering in organic amnesia. *Nature*, **275**, 317–318.

Huppert, F.A. and Piercy, M. (1979). Normal and abnormal forgetting in organic amnesia: effect of locus of lesion. *Cortex*, **15**, 385–390.

Irle, E. and Markowitsch, H.J. (1987). Basal forebrain-lesioned monkeys are severely impaired in tasks of association and recognition memory. *Ann. Neurol.*, **22**, 735–743.

James, W. (1890). *Principles of Psychology, Vol. 1*, Holt, New York.

Kapur, N. and Coughlan, A.K. (1980). Confabulation and frontal lobe dysfunction. *J. Neurol. Neurosurg. Psychiatry*, **43**, 461–463.

Kapur, N., Ellison, D., Smith, M., McLellan, L. and Burrows, E.H. (1992). Focal retrograde amnesia following bilateral temporal lobe pathology: a neuropsychological and magnetic resonance study. *Brain*, in press.

Kendrick, D. (1985). *Cognitive Tests for the Elderly*, NFER-Nelson, Windsor.

Kopelman, M.D. (1985). Rates of forgetting in Alzheimer-type dementia and Korsakoff's syndrome. *Neuropsychologia*, **23**, 623–638.

Kopelman, M.D. (1986). Clinical tests of memory. *Br. J. Psychiatry*, **148**, 517–525.

Kopelman, M.D. (1987a). Amnesia: organic and psychogenic. *Br. J. Psychiatry*, **150**, 428–442.

Kopelman, M.D. (1987b). Two types of confabulation. *J. Neurol. Neurosurg. Psychiatry*, **50**, 1482–1487.

Kopelman, M.D. (1989). Remote and autobiographical memory, temporal context memory, and frontal atrophy in Korsakoff and Alzheimer patients. *Neuropsychologia*, **27**, 437–460.

Kopelman, M.D. (1991a). Alcoholic brain damage. In: Glass, I.B. (Ed.), *The International Handbook of Addiction Behaviour*, Tavistock/Routledge, London.

Kopelman, M.D. (1991b). The 'new' and the 'old': components of the anterograde and retrograde memory loss in Korsakoff and Alzheimer patients. In: Squire, L.R. and Butters, N. (Eds), *The Neuropsychology of Memory; 2nd edn.*, Guildford, New York.

Kopelman, M.D. (1991c). Frontal dysfunction and memory deficits in the alcoholic Korsakoff syndrome and Alzheimer-type dementia. *Brain*, **114**, 117–137.

Kopelman, M.D. and Corn, T.H. (1988). Cholinergic 'blockade' as a model for cholinergic depletion: a comparison of the memory deficits with those of Alzheimer-type dementia and the alcoholic Korsakoff syndrome. *Brain*, **111**, 1079–1110.

Kopelman, M.D. and Lishman, W.A. (1986). Pharmacological treatments of dementia (non-cholinergic). *Br. Med. Bull.*, **42**, 101–105.

Kopelman, M.D., Wilson, B.A. and Baddeley, A.D. (1989). The Autobiographical Memory Interview: a new assessment of autobiographical and personal semantic memory in amnesic patients. *J. Clin. Exp. Neuropsychol.*, **11**, 724–744.

Kopelman, M.D., Wilson, B.A. and Baddeley, A.D. (1990). *The Autobiographical Memory Interview*, Thames Valley Test Company, Bury St Edmunds.

Lemnius, L. (1561). The touchstone of complexions. Translated Hunter, R. and Macalpine, I. (Eds), (1963) *Three Hundred Years of Psychiatry: 1535–1860*, Oxford University Press, Oxford.

Levin, H., High, W.M. and Eisenberg, H.M. (1988). Learning and forgetting during post-traumatic amnesia in head-injured patients. *J. Neurol. Neurosurg. Psychiatry*, **51**, 14–20.

Luria, A.R. (1976). *The Neuropsychology of Memory*, Wiley, New York.

Mair, W.G.P., Warrington, E.K. and Weiskrantz, L. (1979). Memory disorder in Korsakoff's psychosis; a neuropathological and neuropsychological investigation of two cases. *Brain*, **102**, 149–183.

Martone, E., Butters, N. and Trauner, D. (1986). Some analyses of forgetting of pictorial material in amnesic and demented patients. *J. Clin. Exp. Neuropsychol.*, **8**, 161–178.

Mayes, A.R. (1988). *Human Organic Memory Disorders*, Cambridge University Press, Cambridge.

Mayes, A.R., Meudell, P.R. and Pickering, A. (1985). Is organic amnesia caused by a selective deficit in remembering contextual information? *Cortex*, **21**, 167–202.

Mayes, A.R., Meudell, P.R., Mann, D. and Pickering, A. (1988). Location of lesions in Korsakoff's syndrome: neuropsychological and neuropathological data on two patients. *Cortex*, **24**, 36.

Meudell, P. and Mayes, A. (1982). Normal and abnormal forgetting: some comments on the human amnesic syndrome. In: Ellis, A.W. (Ed.), *Normality and Pathology in Cognitive Functions*, Academic Press, London.

Meudell, P.R., Mayes, A.R., Ostergaard, A. and Pickering, A. (1985). Recency and frequency judgements in alcoholic amnesics and normal people with poor memory. *Cortex*, **21**, 487–511.

Milner, B. (1966). Amnesia following operation on the temporal lobes. In: Whitty, C.W.M. and Zangwill, O. (Eds), *Amnesia, 1st edn*, Butterworths, London.
Mishkin, M. (1982). A memory system in the monkey. *Phil. Trans. R. Soc. London B*, **298**, 85–95.
Parkin, A.J. and Leng, N.R.C. (1988). Comparative studies of human amnesia: syndrome or syndromes? In: Markokwitsch, H. (Ed.), *Information Processing by the Brain*, Hans Huber, Toronto.
Parkin, A.J., Montaldi, D., Leng, N.R.C. and Hunkin, N.M. (1990). Contextual cueing effects in the remote memory of alcoholic Korsakoff patients and normal subjects. *Q. J. Exp. Psychol.*, **42A**, 585–596.
Phillips, S., Sangalang, V. and Sterns, G. (1987). Basal forebrain infarction—a clinicopathological correlation. *Arch. Neurol.*, **44**, 1134–1138.
Ribot, T. (1882). *Diseases of Memory*, Appleton, New York.
Salazar, A.M., Grafman, J., Schlesselman, S., Vance, S..C., Mohr, J.P., Carpenter, M., Pevsner, P., Ludlow, C. and Weingartner, H. (1986). Penetrating war injuries of the basal forebrain: neurology and cognition. *Neurology*, **36**, 459–465.
Scoville, W.B. and Milner, B. (1957). Loss of recent memory after bilateral hippocampal lesions. *J. Neurol. Neurosurg. Psychiatry*, **20**, 11–21.
Shimamura, A.P. and Squire, L.R. (1986). Korsakoff's syndrome: a study of the relation between anterograde amnesia and remote memory impairment. *Behav. Neurosci.*, **100**, 165–170.
Squire, L.R. (1981). Two forms of human amnesia: an analysis of forgetting. *J. Neurosci.*, **1**, 635–640.
Squire, L.R., Shimamura, A.P. and Amaral, D.G. (1989). Memory and the hippocampus. In: Byrne, J. and Berry, W. (Eds), *Neural Models of Plasticity*, Academic Press, New York.
Starr, A. and Phillips, L. (1970). Verbal and motor memory in the amnesic syndrome. *Neuropsychologia*, **8**, 75–88.
Stuss, D.T., Alexander, M.P., Liberman, A. and Levine, H. (1978). An extraordinary form of confabulation. *Neurology*, **28**, 1166–1172.
Tomlinson, B.E., Blessed, G. and Roth, M. (1970). Observations on the brains of demented old people. *J. Neurol. Sci.*, **11**, 205–242.
Tulving, E. and Schacter, D.L. (1990). Priming and human memory systems. *Science*, **247**, 301–306.
Victor, M., Adams, R.D. and Collins, G.H. (1971). *The Wernicke-Korsakoff Syndrome, 1st edn*, F.A. Davis Co., Philadelphia.
Victor, M., Adams, R.D. and Collins, G.H. (1989). *The Wernicke-Korsakoff Syndrome, 2nd edn*, F.A. Davis Co., Philadelphia.
Von Cramon, D.Y., Hebel, N. and Schuri, U. (1985). A contribution to the anatomical basis of thalamic amnesia. *Brain*, **108**, 997–1008.
Warrington, E.K. (1984). *The Recognition Memory Test*, NFER-Nelson, Windsor.
Waugh, N.C. and Norman, D.A. (1965). Primary memory. *Psychol. Rev.*, **72**, 89–104.
Wilson, B.A. (1987). *Rehabilitation of Memory*, Guildford Press, New York.
Winocur, G., Oxbury, S., Roberts, R., Agnetti, V. and Davis, C. (1984). Amnesia in a patient with bilateral lesions to the thalamus. *Neuropsychologia*, **22**, 123–143.
Zola-Morgan, S., Squire, L.R. and Amaral, D.G. (1986). Human amnesia and the medial temporal region: enduring memory impairment following a bilateral lesion limited to field CA1 of the hippocampus. *J. Neurosci.*, **6**, 2950–2967.

The Temporal Lobes and the Limbic System
Edited by M.R. Trimble and T.G. Bolwig

15

Neuropathology of Psychoses: Towards a Common Biology

GARETH WYN ROBERTS and KATHERINE HORTON
Serious Mental Afflictions Research Team, St Mary's Medical School, Imperial College of Science, Technology and Medicine, London, UK

INTRODUCTION

The pathology of psychosis, in particular of the schizophrenias and the schizophrenia-like psychosis of temporal lobe epilepsy, has been the subject of considerable investigation and debate. After decades of controversy the data from disparate lines of enquiry are beginning to fuse into an emerging consensus on the basic principles and parameters of the alterations to brain structure which generate psychosis.

In this chapter we will review the data on the neuropathology of schizophrenia and the schizophrenia-like psychoses (SLP) of temporal lobe epilepsy, examine the similarities and discuss the basic mechanisms and principles involved.

NEUROPATHOLOGY OF SCHIZOPHRENIA

Schizophrenia is enormously costly, both in human and financial terms. The lifetime risk for the population is about 1% and it is a lifelong debilitating condition for 40% of those given the diagnosis.

At any one time there are approximately 250 000 sufferers in the UK, occupying 20% of psychiatric beds at an annual cost of £2–3 billion (authors' estimate). Despite the presence of delusions, hallucinations and cognitive impairment, the diagnostic hallmarks of schizophrenia, life expectancy is not altered (except for the significantly increased risk of suicide), and case histories spanning five or six decades are not uncommon.

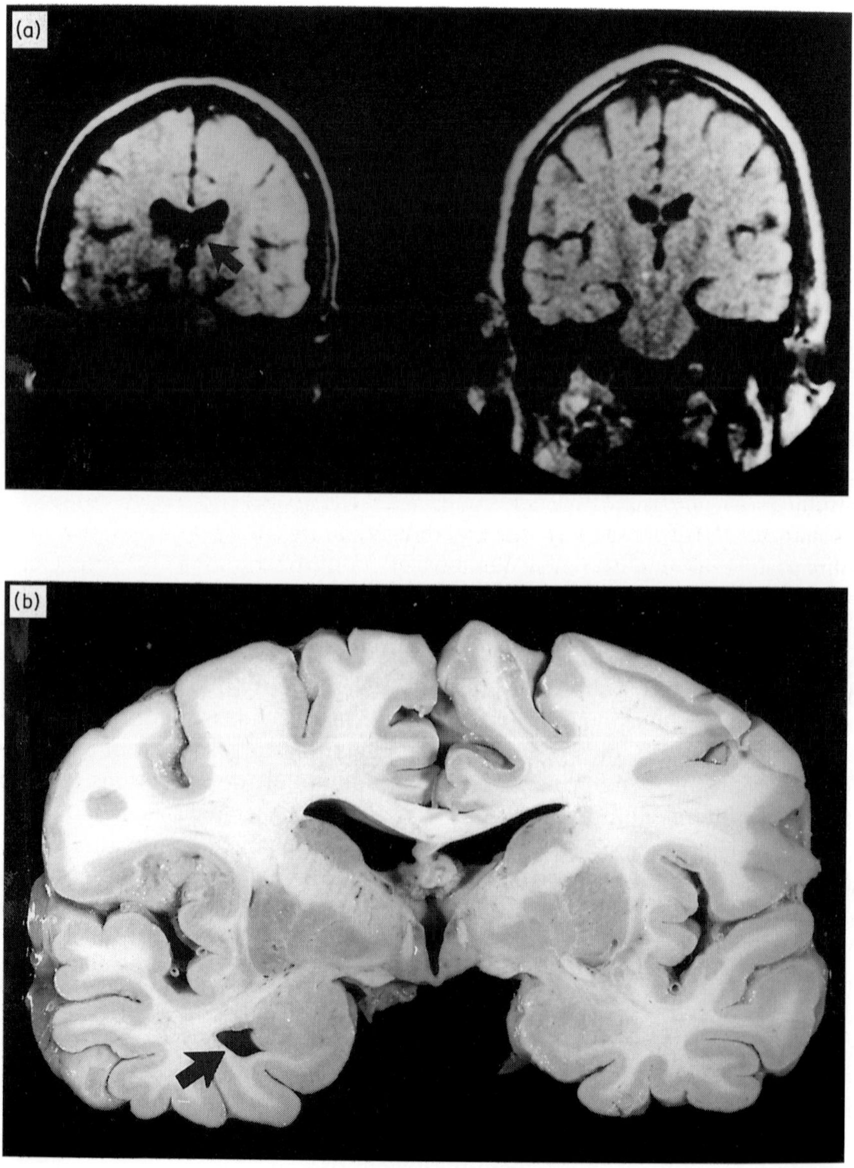

Figure 1. (a) CT scan of a patient with schizophrenia compared with an age and sex matched control. Note enlargement of lateral ventricle. (b) Coronal slice through brain of a patient with chronic schizophrenia. Note enlargement of temporal horn on left side (arrow).

Schizophrenia is generally viewed as a 'functional' psychosis, a label implying a condition arising from the activity of neurons with no basis of structural or pathological alteration of brain substance. Clinicians place considerable emphasis on the differential diagnosis of functional psychoses from the dementias (chronic organic psychoses) in which structural changes in the brain are known to relate to cognitive and intellectual impairment. Despite the clinical evidence of brain dysfunction in schizophrenia, little progress was made in determining its organic parameters for most of this century and early neuropathological studies were conflicting and controversial.

The renaissance of neuropathological investigations into schizophrenia dates from a 1976 study which used the emerging technology of computed tomography (CT) (Johnstone *et al.*, 1976) to re-examine the issue of ventricular enlargement (Fig. 1). It demonstrated ventricular enlargement in schizophrenics which was correlated with cognitive impairment but was unrelated to physical treatment (e.g. electroconvulsive therapy). Magnetic resonance (NMR) studies have confirmed these findings (Crow and Johnstone, 1987; Shelton and Weinberger, 1986; Bachneff, 1991) thus firmly establishing the presence of an underlying structural abnormality in the brains of many schizophrenic subjects. However, the degree of ventricular enlargement is variable and is not diagnostic (e.g. ventricular enlargement is also seen in Huntington's chorea and Creutzfeldt–Jakob disease).

Brain structure in schizophrenia

Recent studies on brain weight in schizophrenic patients have produced consistent results. Each has found a significant decrease of approximately 6% in brain weight in schizophrenic patients compared with controls, accounting for such factors as height, weight, sex and year of birth (Brown *et al.*, 1986; Pakkenberg, 1987; Bruton *et al.*, 1990). In the study of Bruton *et al.* (1990) further analysis revealed that both male and female schizophrenics had reductions of a similar magnitude and losses in brain weight were found in both left and right cerebral hemispheres. Other parameters of gross brain structure are also altered. Significant (4%) reductions in brain length (maximum antero-posterior length of formalin fixed cerebral hemispheres) in both male and female schizophrenics (approx. 7 mm) have been shown (Bruton *et al.*, 1990). Again separate analysis indicated that both left and right hemispheres were shorter (cf. brain weight, above). Studies on the volume of brain structures also show significant reductions in the volume of the cerebral hemispheres (8% loss), cerebral cortex (12% loss), and central grey matter (6% loss) (Pakkenberg, 1987).

White matter volumes are generally not changed. Morphometric and MRI studies indicate loss of cortical grey matter which is most pronounced in the temporal lobe (Suddath *et al.*, 1990). Post-mortem studies have also replicated the finding of ventricular enlargement with an increase of 33% (10 ml) in the total volume of the ventricular system (Pakkenberg, 1987) and significant increases in the cross-sectional area of the anterior horn (+19%) and temporal horn (+97%) of the lateral ventricles (Brown *et al.*, 1986, Fig. 1).

These data confirm the presence of structural abnormalities in the brains of schizophrenics and provide some indication as to which brain regions are particularly affected. Cortical regions are preferentially affected and the data on ventricle size and cortical morphometry suggest that the ventricular enlargement may be regional in that the temporal lobes are the most affected area.

Which brain areas are affected?

Planimetric studies of archival material revealed considerable volume reductions of temporal lobe structures (hippocampal formation, amygdala, parahippocampal gyrus) and a moderate reduction of the inner pallidal segment (–20%) in schizophrenic subjects (Bogerts *et al.*, 1985). The parahippocampal cortex was also significantly thinner (11% reduction) (Brown *et al.*, 1986; cf. MRI study of Suddath *et al.*, 1990).

These changes were of a lesser degree than those found in other brain diseases such as Alzheimer's disease or Huntington's chorea. None of the studies provides much support for the notion of homogeneous cortical atrophy or that the basal ganglia are particularly affected. The temporal lobe, specifically the medial temporal lobe structures (hippocampus and parahippocampal gyrus), are preferentially involved (Fig. 2). These post-mortem studies are supported by several MRI studies (Suddath *et al.*, 1989) which used image analysis to quantify temporal lobe size and the amounts of grey and white matter in the brains of schizophrenics. In the last study, significant reductions were seen in the amount of temporal lobe grey matter (reduced by 18% right hemisphere, 21% left hemisphere) in schizophrenics. These reductions correlated inversely with ventricular enlargement in the same sample. No differences were seen in the amount of temporal lobe white matter. The reductions in temporal lobe grey matter were most pronounced at the level of the amygdala and anterior hippocampus.

Cell counts have been made in the hippocampal formation, pyramidal cell bands, hippocampal segments and entorhinal cortex in the brains of schizophrenics (Falkai and Bogerts, 1986; Falkai *et al.*, 1988a; Jeste and Lohr, 1989). Each study showed reduced numbers of neuronal cells but there was no evidence of gliosis (as would be indicated by increased glial cell numbers).

A qualitative description of gross and microscopic morphological changes in the temporal lobe of schizophrenics has been presented by Jakob and Beckman (1986). The changes included cell loss from cortical lamina of the ventral insula (claustrocortex) and parahippocampal gyrus. These changes

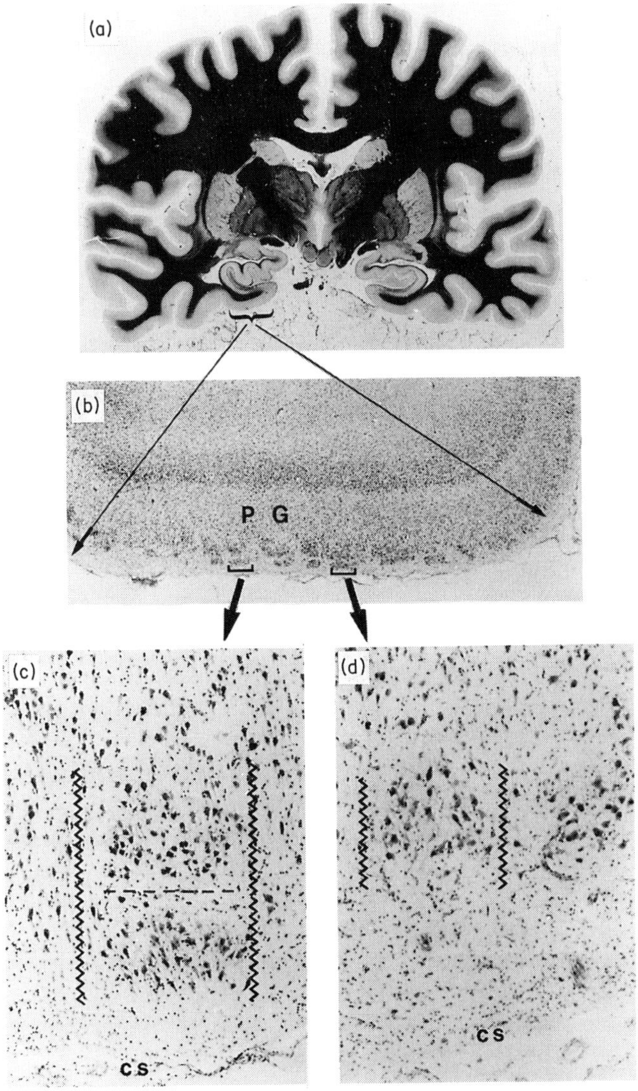

Figure 2. Aberrant development in the parahippocampal gyrus in schizophrenia. The parahippocampal gyrus (PG) located close to the hippocampus (a) has a characteristic pattern of cell formations (b). In this region of cortex 'pre-α-clouds' of neurons (cortical layer II, bracketed) lie close to the cortical surface. A high-power view (c) of one of the 'clouds' in a control (zig-zag lines) shows it to be formed of two cell clusters separated by a cellular gap (dashed line). In schizophrenics (d) the 'pre-clouds' are poorly developed, separate cell clusters not being discernable, and the whole formation lies deeper from the cortical surface (CS). (Reproduced with permission, from Roberts, 1991.)

did not extend anterior to the prepiriform cortex nor posterior to occipital level of the temporal cortex (cf. Kovelman and Scheibel, 1984; Suddath *et al.*, 1989). The presence of these cytoarchitectonic disturbances has been confirmed by other workers (Conrad *et al.*, 1991; Arnold *et al.*, 1991). The cytoarchitecture of the remaining temporal neocortex was normal. The abnormalities were present in both hemispheres but were more conspicuous in the left hemisphere. Of interest was the tendency for patients with marked pathological abnormalities to have an earlier age of onset of psychotic symptoms. These findings were considered to indicate abnormal ontogenetic development of a small part of the entorhinal cortex. A preliminary semi-quantitative study of the cytoarchitectonics of the pre-alpha cells of the parahippocampal gyrus has confirmed the report of cytoarchitectural abnormalities (Falkai *et al.*, 1988a) (Fig. 2).

In conclusion, the medial temporal lobe in patients suffering from chronic schizophrenia appears to have a different organization of architecture to that seen in the brains of people not suffering from a psychotic illness.

What causes the architectural folly?

The early CT findings were regarded as evidence for an underlying degenerative process in schizophrenia and led to a reappraisal of Kraepelin's (1919) earlier concept of schizophrenia as an organic dementia (dementia praecox). This view fitted with the correlation between ventricular enlargement and cognitive impairment, a finding to be expected in a neurodegenerative condition. However, the correlation between length of illness and increasing ventricular size seen in other neurodegenerative diseases failed to emerge (Weinberger, 1984, 1987; Crow and Johnstone, 1987). Further, changes of a similar degree were found in patients only weeks or months after the onset of their first psychotic episode and subsequent proposals hypothesized that changes in brain structure in schizophrenia were caused by a variety of factors. Subgroups of schizophrenics were associated with various aetiological factors, of which family history (genetic) and obstetric or perinatal complications (environmental) emerged as the most important (Murray *et al.*, 1985, 1988; Roberts, 1991; Jones and Murray, 1991).

In an effort to disentangle the relevance or otherwise of these factors, the types of process which could underlie the structural changes in schizophrenia have been examined in recent neuropathological studies. Attention has focused on gathering evidence on the nature of the pathological changes and ascertaining when these changes could have occurred.

Disturbed brain development—neuropathological evidence

All types of disease process which cause neuronal damage result in glial reaction marked by proliferation of glial cells and rises in associated glial protein (such as glial fibrillary acidic protein GFAP) and enzymes (e.g. monoamine oxidase-B) (Roberts *et al.*, 1987). Finding a constant pattern of such reactivity in brains of schizophrenics would signal a neurodegenerative process and indicate the location of the damage.

Recent quantitative studies using a variety of methods have failed to demonstrate the presence of gliosis or evidence of systematic neurodegenerative changes in the brain of schizophrenics (for reviews, see Roberts and Bruton, 1990; Roberts, 1991). Foetal brain tissue does not show an adult glial response until after 6 months (Larroche, 1984) and an early destructive lesion might not have a gliotic trace. However, the type of cytoarchitectonic changes reported in the schizophrenic brain (Jacob and Beckman, 1986) indicates that they originate in the last trimester before birth, a period when an adult-like glial response to injury does occur (Larroche, 1984; Volpe, 1989).

Are the neuropathological data compatible with the intrusion of external environmental events, such as those caused by obstetric or birth complications or infection on the development of the brain around the time of birth? Birth difficulties can give rise to intraventricular haemorrhages and infarcts which lead to enlarged ventricles and small brains (Gilles and Green, 1985; Volpe, 1989). Such pathologies are accompanied by gliosis, cyst formation and periventricular leukomalacia. These birth related and perinatal lesions can be detected years after the event by neuropathological investigation (Kuchna and Kozlowski, 1991). However, although the brains of schizophrenics have structural changes, the white matter volume is not reduced, gliosis and inflammatory responses are absent (for reviews, see Roberts and Bruton, 1990; Roberts, 1991) and there is little evidence for traumatic injury (Bruton *et al.*, 1990). On the whole, neuropathological studies do not suggest that brain damage due to birth injury or perinatal infection is a major factor in the genesis of the structural abnormalities in schizophrenia.

Thus, the available pathological evidence indicates that the structural changes in such brains are not the result of a neurodegenerative process or a destructive lesion. Rather the data fit the profile of a disturbance in brain development (Roberts *et al.*, 1987). Although ideas of abnormal development in schizophrenia have a long history (see Lewis, 1989a,b) it is only recently that this idea has been substantiated by data obtained from direct observation of the neuropathology of the condition.

Schizophrenia—a developmental disorder

If schizophrenia is a neurodevelopmental anomaly of the medial temporal lobes then it follows that several other predictions might be made about the disease (Roberts *et al.*, 1987). The lesion should be present from birth. It should precede the onset of clinical symptoms and should probably be constant and not progressive. Only a few studies have addressed these questions. Ventricular enlargement has been reported in a 10 year-old diagnosed as schizophrenic (Woody *et al.*, 1987) and in two teenagers scanned before the onset of their schizophrenic symptoms (O'Callaghan *et al.*, 1988; Weinberger, 1988). There is little or no evidence of progressive structural changes. In the first such study to examine the problem in the 1930s, only 20% of patients were reported as showing progressive ventricular enlargement over a 4 year period (Lemke, 1935) and three recent studies show no evidence of progression in groups of patients scanned over 5–8 years (Illowsky *et al.*, 1988; Reverly *et al.*, 1988; Vita *et al.*, 1988). Why a developmental lesion present from birth gives rise to a clinical syndrome 20 years later is an unexplained mystery at the present time.

Conclusions

Neuropathological studies indicate that the brains of schizophrenics suffer from a developmental abnormality which preferentially, but not exclusively, affects the medial temporal lobe (parahippocampal gyrus, hippocampus and amygdala). Medial temporal lobe structures are believed to have a crucial role in the integration and processing of the input from association cortex (Fig. 3). Dysfunction of this system could result in the clinical symptoms which form the core of the schizophrenia syndrome. The cause of the anomaly is probably genetic in the vast majority of cases and affects brain development during the third trimester.

The asymmetrical pattern of development in the normal human brain can explain why such a defect affecting both hemispheres simultaneously will disproportionately affect the left (dominant) hemisphere (Roberts, 1991).

The span of a decade has seen a spectacular paradigm shift from believing that schizophrenia had no organic basis to localizing the brain regions primarily involved (medial temporal lobe) and uncovering the main aetiological factor responsible for the structural changes (aberrant brain development). The 1990s should see the final unveiling of the precise disorder in the mechanisms regulating brain development which result in schizophrenia. This knowledge will give us the identity of the gene(s) responsible and thus pave the way for genetic screening, more effective therapy and, ultimately, a cure.

TEMPORAL LOBE EPILEPSY AND SCHIZOPHRENIA-LIKE PSYCHOSIS

Since the early report of Falret (1854) there has been interest in the association between psychosis and epilepsy (see Chapter 11). Temporal lobe

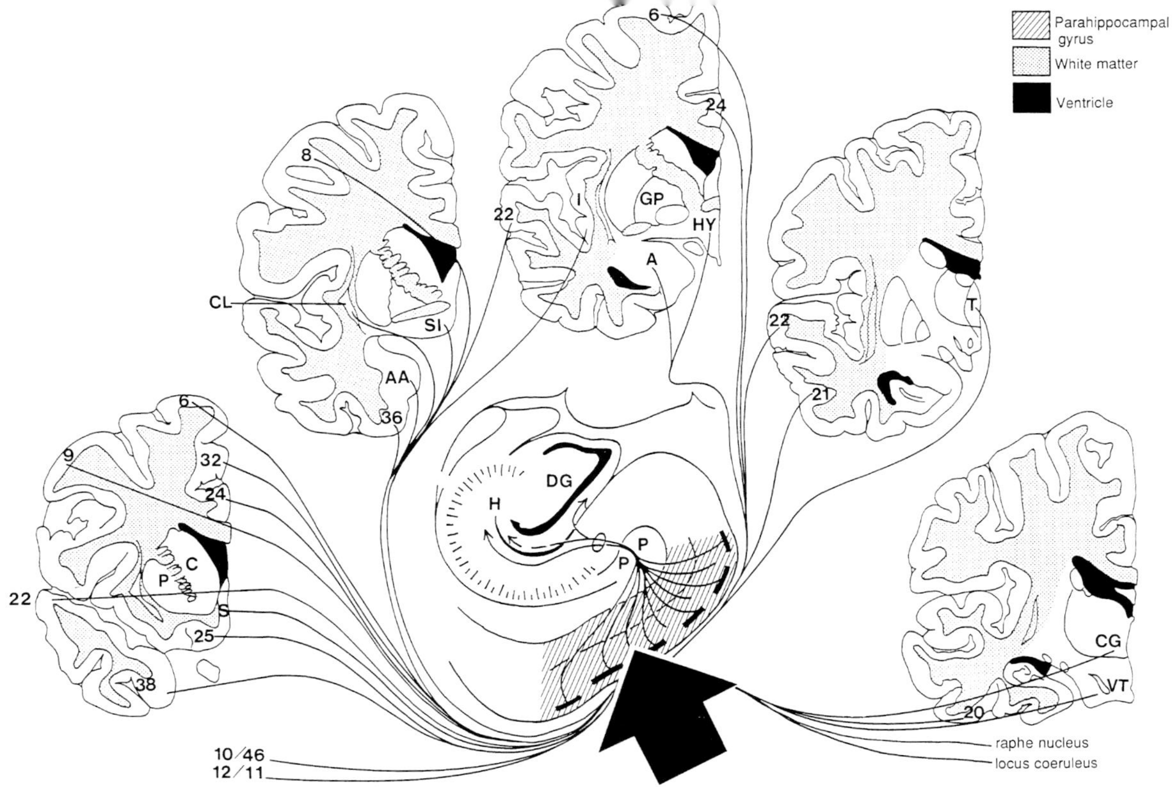

Figure 3. Projections to the parahippocampal gyrus. The links between various cortical and subcortical areas and the parahippocampal gyrus are shown diagrammatically. The projections shown are those from the same hemisphere but it should be noted that similar (but smaller) projections from the opposite hemisphere are also present. The terminal regions of the projections are topographically organized and often separate projections arise from subdivisions of one area (e.g. amygdala). (A, amygdala; AA, anterior amygdala; C, caudate; CG, central grey; CL, claustrum; DG, dentate gyrus; GP, globus pallidus; H, hippocampus; HY, hypothalamus; I, insula; P, putamen; PP, perforant path; S, septum; SI, substantia inominata; T, thalamus; VT, ventral tegmentum; 6–46, Brodman areas.) (Reproduced with permission, from Roberts, 1991.)

epilepsy (TLE) is particularly associated with the schizophrenia-like psychoses of epilepsy (SLP) (Slater and Beard, 1963). Patients with TLE have higher rates of psychosis than the general population (Trimble, 1981). The psychosis develops in the course of the epilepsy rather than the reverse with a time lag of some 10–15 years observed between the onset of TLE and the development of psychotic symptoms (Slater and Beard, 1963). This observation is not explained by the relative ages of onset of the two conditions when occurring independently of each other. TLE has a wide range of onset but only a quarter of cases develop recurrent seizures before age 15 (Currie *et al.*, 1971). For schizophrenia 60–75% of cases have their first admission between 20 and 40 years of age (Bleuler, 1978). A series of studies (Hill, 1953; Pond, 1957; Slater and Beard, 1963) examined the clinical phenomenology of epileptic psychotics and outlined a schizophrenia-like syndrome with delusions, hallucinations and thought disorder. This syndrome was considered to differ from 'true' schizophrenia in several ways. Cases showed a relative lack of schizoid premorbid personality, preservation of affect and little evidence of a genetic predisposition to psychiatric illness. However, individual cases were often phenomenologically indistinguishable from 'true' schizophrenia (Toone *et al.*, 1982; Stoudemire *et al.*, 1983).

Flor-Henry observed no excess of abnormal childhood experience in his psychotic group, Bruens also reported a normal premorbid personality in 16 of 19 cases and Jensen and Larsen's psychotic epileptics (combining affective and schizoaffective psychoses) had higher levels of intelligence and better academic attainment compared with non-psychotic controls.

This is not to say that premorbid personalities in patients with epilepsy are normal. It is clear that in many cases (where it could be assessed) patients suffered considerably from presumed epilepsy-related personality change (aggression, paranoia, obsessions). No excess of major psychiatric illness in the families of psychotic epileptics was reported by Slater and Beard (1963) or by Flor-Henry (1969). Jensen and Larsen (1979) did report such an excess amongst the families of their cases of patients with temporal lobe epilepsy undergoing lobectomy but no information was given regarding the diagnosis of these relatives.

Pathology of SLP in temporal lobe epilepsy

Only a limited number of studies have attempted to correlate the schizophrenia-like psychoses of TLE with anatomical, pathological or physiological parameters. Flor-Henry (1969) reported that schizophrenia-like states predominate in epileptics with left or bilateral temporal foci, a finding subsequently replicated (Sherwin, 1981; Sherwin *et al.*, 1982; Trimble, 1986).

Attempts at correlating seizure activity or seizure type with psychopathology have proven inconclusive (Toone, 1981). There is some evidence of a negative correlation between medial temporal sclerosis and psychosis and a positive correlation between alien tissue lesions and psychosis (Taylor, 1975). Jensen and Klinken (1976) reported an association between focal lesions and psychosis. Whether one or more of the structural, physiological or biochemical bases of TLE will relate to the underlying defect in schizophrenia is uncertain.

In view of progress made in uncovering the biological basis of schizophrenia, the underlying biology of SLP in temporal lobe epilepsy needs investigation. The putative relationship is worth pursuing on the assumption that 'like effects commonly have similar causes' and 'it is as a mock-up of genuine schizophrenia that the schizophrenic-like epileptic is worth special study' (Slater and Beard, 1963).

The pathological parameters of material from patients who underwent temporal lobectomy and who had or subsequently developed schizophrenia-like psychoses have been investigated in a large study (for details, see Bruton, 1988; Roberts *et al.*, 1990). The data from this study have been assessed in relation to our previous studies on the pathology of schizophrenia. By comparing the two phenomenologically related syndromes we have identified common pathological factors present which might help us begin to define the neuropathology of psychosis.

For each case the medical notes were obtained and examined for evidence of pre-operative or post-operative psychiatric symptoms. Patients were seen and assessed by different clinicians over several decades (1950–1975) and, as a result, some inconsistencies are inevitable. The presence of schizophrenia-like psychoses was only accepted on the basis of a firm casenote diagnosis and followed criteria previously used in similar studies. Briefly—patients were examined by an experienced psychiatrist and schizophrenia would have been the diagnosis of choice in the absence of epilepsy. Diagnosis was based on the presence of hallucinations, delusions, thought disorder and affective disturbance in a setting of clear consciousness. In addition the schizophrenia-like state existed for a considerable time (months). Patients with transient psychotic states or psychotic states which were accompanied by alterations in consciousness or confusion were excluded.

Basic parameters of TLE

Laterality and sex

TLE shows an even division between left and right sided foci and a preponderance of males to females in all categories of pathology (see Bruton, 1988 for further discussion). The male to female ratio of the entire series was 1.68:1 ($p < 0.0001$) and similar sex ratios were found for right or left foci. This increased ratio, has been reported in other studies (Jensen, 1976).

Table 1. Pathology and age at first seizure.

Pathological group	*Age of first seizure, (years) SD (range)*	*Age at operation (years)*
1. Developmental	22.8 ± 16.4 (4–47)	38.2 ± 7.8 (30–48)
2. Trauma	17.3 ± 13.1 (0–39)	33.1 ± 13.1 (17–48)
3. AT astrocytic	27.3 ± 19.0 (2–54)	34.6 ± 17.1 (15–54)
4. AT ganglioglial	6.4 ± 5.3 (0–12)	17.6 ± 9.2 (7–30)
5. AT cortical dysplasia	14.7 ± 13.2 (3–39)	26.9 ± 13.2 (17–49)
6. AT oligodendrocytic	26.0 ± 18.4 (6–49)	38.2 ± 15.1 (19–56)
7. AT mixed glial	11.1 ± 10.1 (1–23)	19.7 ± 11.8 (2–38)
8. AT vascular	16.0 ± 10.8 (7–28)	23.7 ± 12.7 (14–38)
9. AHS	5.2 ± 7.9 (0–30)	22.6 ± 9.3 (5–54)
10. Inflammatory	8.6 ± 6.3 (0–19)	24.8 ± 10.2 (9–46)
11. Indefinite	14.7 ± 10.7 (1–35)	31.2 ± 9.5 (14–50)
12. No lesion	15.4 ± 11.7 (0–47)	28.6 ± 11.7 (9–54)

AT, alien tissue; AHS, Ammon's horn sclerosis.

Onset of first seizure

The mean age of first seizure was closely associated with type of pathology, (Table 1) with Ammon's horn sclerosis (AHS) and gangliogliomas having significantly earlier mean age of first seizure (5.2 and 6.4 years, respectively) than other pathologies (p <0.05). Age of first seizure for most other types of pathology was in middle to late teens. Surprisingly the 'developmental' group had an older mean age of onset (22.8 years).

Basic parameters of SLP

Sex

Of the series of 249 referred for lobectomy, 16 had a pre-operative diagnosis of TLE and SLP (6.4% of sample, 10 male, six female).

SLP and laterality

Approximately 10% of the cases with TLE developed SLP pre- or post-operatively (Lindsay *et al.*, 1979; Roberts *et al.*, 1990). In the total series of SLP cases there were 15 left and 10 right sided foci. Although the bias towards left sidedness is maintained, this difference is not significant (p = 0.1 one tailed sign test).

Pre-operatively 16 of the TLE series had a diagnosis of SLP (these were cases operated on early in the series, in the latter period selection procedures were altered to exclude TLE cases with psychoses). The majority of these cases (11 of 16) had a left sided focus (p=0.1 one tailed sign test), this trend has been found in other studies and has been discussed (Sherwin *et al.*, 1982; Flor-Henry, 1983).

There was no discernable bias in the laterality of the focus of those with TLE developing SLP *post-operatively* (five right and four left lobectomies developed SLP).

Interest in the side of the focus and the nature of the psychopathology seen in association with temporal lobe epilepsy dates from Flor-Henry's (1969) report of a highly significant association between a lesion on the left side and a schizophrenia-like rather than affective disturbance. Subsequent work (e.g. Taylor, 1975; Sherwin *et al.*, 1982; Perez *et al.*, 1985) has further documented this association. Most impressive in this respect is the prospective follow-up by Lindsay *et al.* (1979) of 87 children with temporal lobe seizures: of nine patients who developed psychoses, seven had a left side focus and two had bilateral foci. The effect of side of lesion is of interest since studies of the brain in schizophrenia have reported reduced width of the left hemisphere in early onset, by comparison with later onset patients with schizophrenia, and controls (Crow *et al.*, 1989) and a relative reduction in temporal lobe area and volumes on the left side. Most strikingly in a post-mortem study (Crow *et al.*, 1989) temporal horn enlargement in schizophrenia but not in Alzheimer-type dementia was found to be selective to the left side of the brain (Fig. 1). These findings reinforce the case that the disease process in schizophrenia is associated with a defect of development of the left temporal lobe. It has been suggested that the mechanisms of brain development which are disturbed in schizophrenia give rise to a more pronounced disturbance of the left temporal lobe (Roberts, 1991).

Trimble (1986) suggests that the first rank symptoms of Schneider signify dysfunction in dominant temporo-limbic areas. Perhaps such dysfunction arises in the psychoses associated with temporal lobe epilepsy because a lesion which happens to be on the left side of the brain interferes with function at a critical stage of development. Such asymmetries and their developmental timing may be critical for the differentiated functions of the human brain.

Taylor (1975) and Orsini and Satz (1986) have pointed out that biases in left handedness or laterality could be viewed as an index of unusual cerebral organization and that an early seizure onset could bias towards left handedness. Our data on early age of first fit in the SLP group could explain the marked prevalence of left handedness seen in other studies (Taylor, 1975). Of interest is the fact that all four of the cases which 'lost' their schizophrenic symptoms after lobectomy had left sided foci and left lobectomy, three cases had an AHS lesion and one an alien tissue astrocytic lesion and two of these cases had a record of birth injury.

Environmental factors

Of the cases with SLP, some had recorded incidents of birth injury (three cases, 12%), head injury (two cases, 8%) and or febrile convulsions (six cases, 24%). No fewer than eight of these cases had AHS. Of the two remaining cases, one had a ganglioglioma and AHS (birth injury). These factors were not significantly over represented compared with the total sample where birth injuries were found in 13%, head injuries in 15% and febrile convulsions in 22%. In the total sample, 80% of cases with AHS lesions had a history of birth injury, head injury or febrile convulsions. From our data, birth injury, head injury and febrile convulsions are present in the cases with SLP to the same degree as in the total sample, these factors are also associated with the same type of pathology as in the total sample (i.e. AHS). Thus the environmental factors, birth injury, febrile convulsions and head injury do not appear to be associated with SLP.

Pathology associated with SLP

The two types of pathology most often seen in SLP in our study were Ammon's horn sclerosis and gangliogliomas (Table 2). In the total series of over 250 cases there were approximately equal numbers of left and right AHS cases (54 to 53), SLP was found more often in the cases with left sided foci (eight left, two right in total series, $p = 0.05$, Fisher exact one tailed test). Patients with alien tissue gangliogliomas and no lesion each accounted for about 20% of the SLP cases. No lesion was found in 15% of the total series. It is worth noting that gangliogliomas were relatively rare (found in 3.3% of the total sample). The latter is a surprizingly low figure considering the percentage of cases with gangliogliomas who developed SLP (80% of patients with gangliogliomas).

The association of AHS and SLP is at odds with the negative correlation previously reported. The marked association of gangliogliomas and SLP whilst supporting the positive correlation reported by Taylor (1975) in relation to alien tissue lesions was not seen in any of the other alien tissue pathologies, and runs counter to his suggestion that 'intrinsic' properties of the lesion do not influence the risk of psychosis.

On the basis of our study there is a strong association between two types of pathology (AHS and gangliogliomas) and SLP.

AHS and gangliogliomas

There are similarities between AHS and gangliogliomas in the anatomical location of the lesion and in the age of first seizure. The youngest mean age of first attack is found in the AHS group (5.2 years). Surprizingly a similar

Table 2. Incidence of schizophrenia according to neuropathological group.

Pathological group	*Side of focus*	*No.*	*Pre-operative schizophrenic*	*Post-operative schizophrenic*
1. Developmental	L	4	1	–
	R	2	–	–
2. Trauma	L	4	–	–
	R	6	–	–
3. AT astrocytic	L	6	1	–
	R	3	–	–
4. AT ganglioglial	L	3	–	1
	R	6	–	3
5. AT cortical dysplasia	L	5	–	–
	R	3	–	–
6. AT oligodendrocytic	L	4	–	–
	R	2	–	–
7. AT mixed glial	L	5	–	1
	R	8	1	–
8. AT vascular	L	2	–	–
	R	2	–	–
9. AHS	L	54	6	2
	R	53	2	–
10. Inflammatory	L	5	–	–
	R	6	–	–
11. Indefinite	L	11	–	–
	R	14	1	1
12. No lesion	L	25	3	–
	R	16	1	1

mean age of first seizure was found in the ganglioglioma group (6.4 years). This was in marked contrast to the mean age of first seizure of most of the other pathology groups which come under the common rubric of alien tissue lesions (see Table 1). Other alien tissue lesions had much later onsets of first seizure (27.3 years for glial lesions and 14.7 years for neuronoglial lesions).

Location of lesion

The anatomical location of lesions also differed within the alien tissue groups (Fig. 4). Ganglioglial lesions preferentially affected medial temporal lobe (hippocampus, amygdala, uncus and hippocampal gyrus) and rarely affected lateral temporal lobe structures (cf. AHS), whereas neuronoglial lesions primarily affected the lateral temporal cortex (Fig. 4). A similar preference of gangliogliomas for medial temporal lobe structures has recently been reported by others (Armstrong *et al.*, 1988). The ganglioglioma group showed a marked tendency to develop SLP post-operatively. This effect may well be the result of bias due to the early age of onset of seizures and consequent operation (mean age at operation 17.6 years) in this group, given that the peak incidence of schizophrenia lies between 20 and 40 years of age.

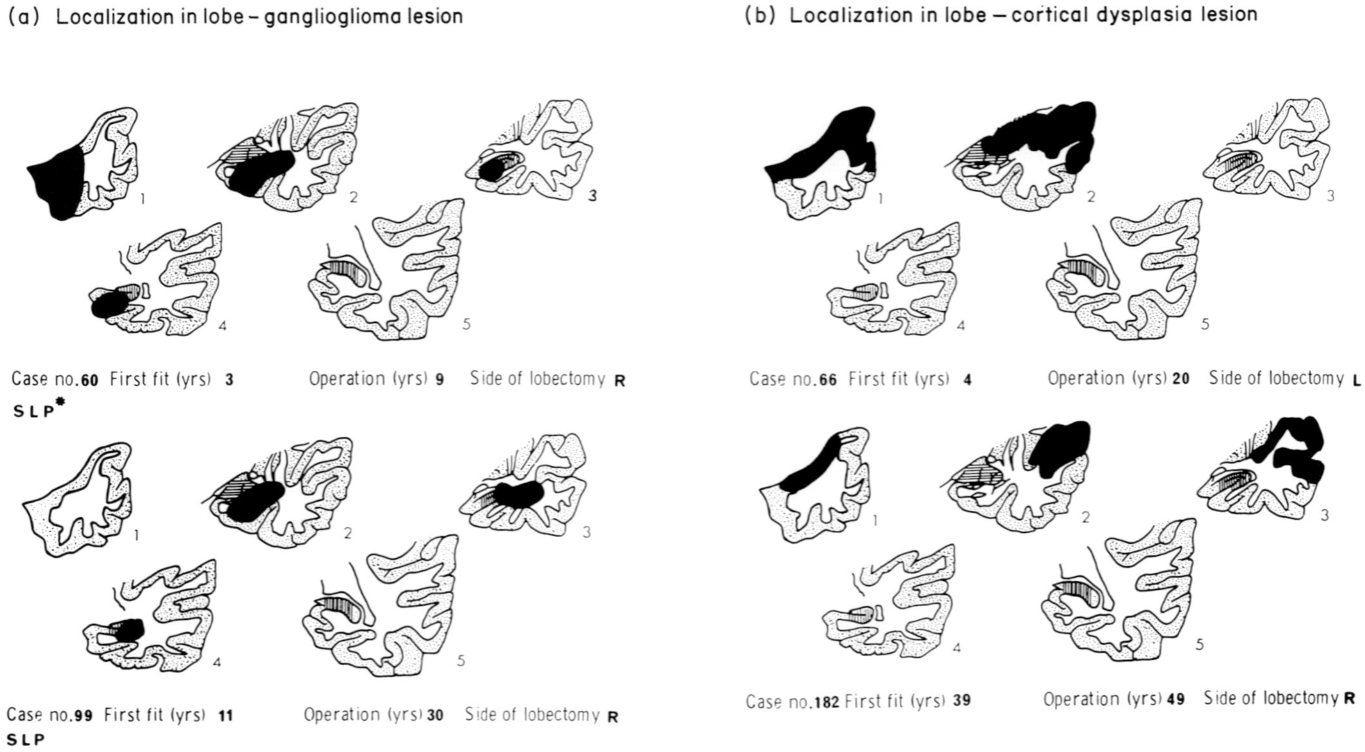

Figure 4. Location of alien tissue lesions in the temporal lobe. Representation of localizations of the different types of neuroglial and glial lesions. Ganglioglial lesions (a) are found in the medial temporal lobe and are associated with SLP. Cortical dysplasia lesions (b) are generally found in the lateral temporal cortex and are not associated with SLP. Astrocytic (c) and oligodendrocytic (d) lesions do not contain aberrant neurons, are randomly located in the temporal lobe and are not associated with SLP.

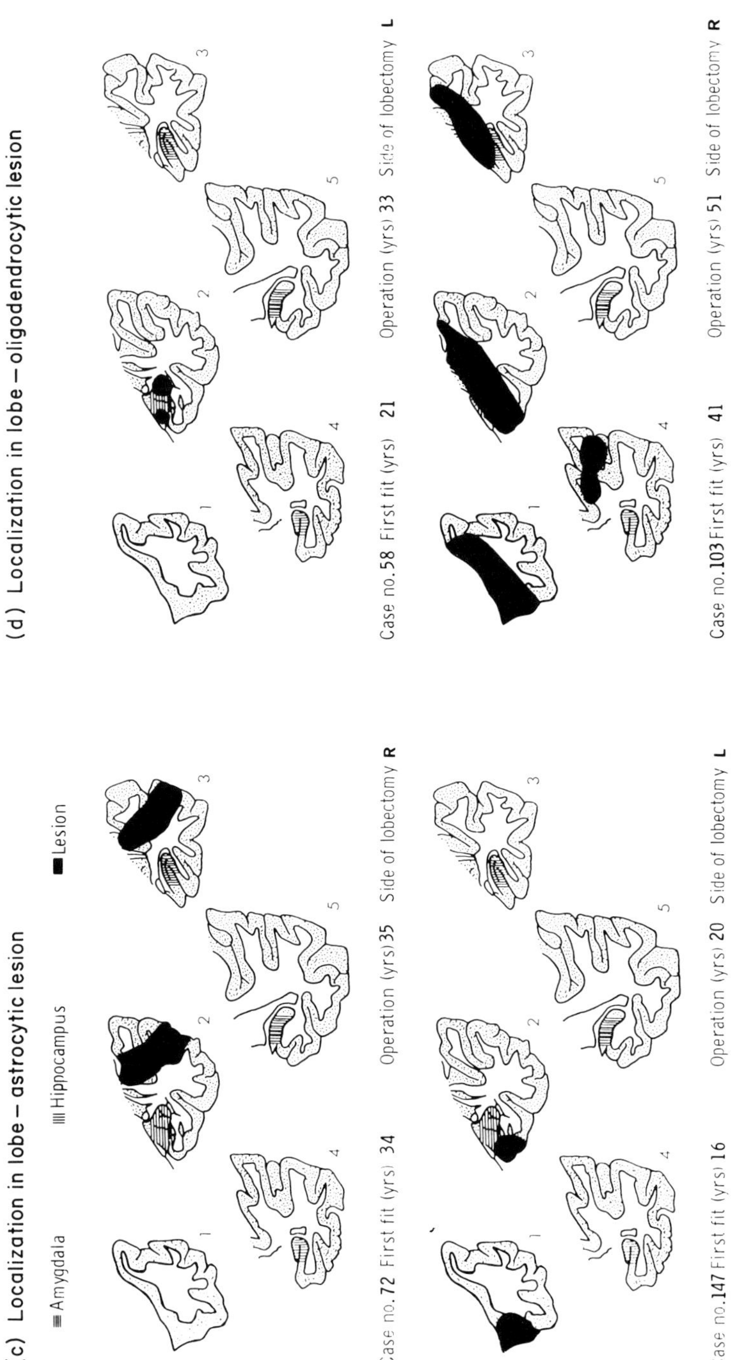

Figure 4. *Continued.*

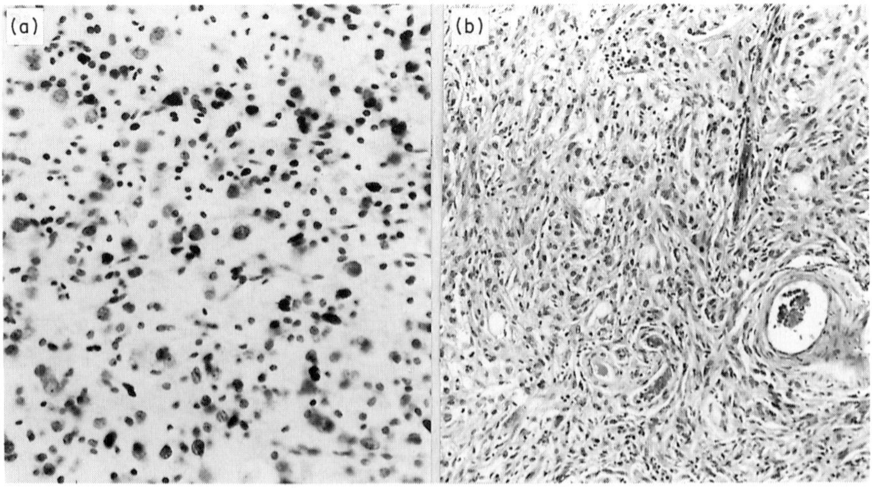

Figure 5. Morphology of alien tissue lesions in temporal lobe epilepsy. (a) Ganglioglioma—aberrant ganglion cells are scattered throughout the lesion. Abnormal astrocytes and oligodendrocytes are also present (×160, van Gieson). (b) Astrocytic glial—the lesion is composed primarily of spindle shaped fibrillary astrocytes (×10, H and E). (Reproduced by courtesy of Dr C.J. Bruton.)

However, this bias does not change the observation that proportionately a larger percentage of patients with ganglioglial lesions develop SLP than any other pathological group.

Morphology of SLP lesions

Several useful comments can be made concerning the morphology of lesions associated with SLP. Alien tissue astrocytic and oligodendrocytic lesions occurred in the medial temporal lobe (Fig. 5) but neither of these was associated with SLP. Gangliogliomas also contained astrocytes and oligodendrocytes but have, in addition, numerous ganglion cells (neurons, Fig. 5). It is probable that this neuronal component of gangliogliomas is responsible for the association with SLP since astrocytes and oligodendrocytes did not show such an association either separately or together.

Gangliogliomas, AHS and SLP—functional considerations

Gangliogliomas are small well circumscribed lesions classified as neoplasias (Russell and Rubenstein, 1989). They occur most frequently in children and young adults and are often thought to have been present from birth—even in adult cases there is usually a characteristic history of longstanding seizures suggesting that the lesion had its onset in early life. The most frequently affected site in the brain is the temporal lobe and the lesions are common in males (male to female ratio, 3:2).

The lesions are composed of neuronal and glial cells (Fig. 5). The neuronal cells resemble aberrant ganglion cells which may show abnormal shape, orientation or processes. Although classified as neoplasia the growth and development of gangliogliomas suggests a hamartomatous origin (Armstrong and Bruton, 1987; Bruton, 1988; Cavanagh, 1958; Russell and Rubenstein, 1989). Hamartomas are considered to be tumour-like but primarily non-neoplasic malformations or errors ('architectural follies'—Taylor *et al.*, 1971) in tissue development. Support for such a view is found in studies in which gangliogliomas are found in conjunction with microscopic lesions some of which were maldevelopmental in nature (Cavanagh, 1958; Armstrong *et al.*, 1988). Other reports have also noted the association of gangliogliomas with ectopic lesions or developmental anomalies (partial agenesis of the corpus callosum, micropolygyria, etc.; see Russell and Rubenstein, 1989).

Gangliogliomas are rarely malignant and their association with congenital structural abnormalities underlines the relationship between gangliogliomas and malformation. The clinical and biological evolution of gangliogliomas suggests a neoplasm in which the fraction of tumour cells actively growing is very low and natural history is one of progressive maturation not invasive growth (Russell and Rubenstein, 1989). The glial element is an occasional exception to this, they can undergo anaplastic change and subsequent malignant progression.

The origin and predilection for the temporal lobe of gangliogliomas could be related to the fact that in the subgranular zone of the dentate gyrus, neurogenesis of granule cells continues after birth (Rakic, 1985). The gangliogliomas cause localized disruption of the normal cortical layers disrupting cortical cytoarchitecture. It would be reasonable to suppose that such physical disruption early in life would also give rise to physiological abnormalities resulting in disruption of *function*; a prospect made more probable by electron microscopic studies (Rubenstein and Herman, 1972) which demonstrate that synaptic contact between ganglioglioma cells and adjacent (normal?) cells exists and that dense core vesicles are present in the cytoplasm and processes of the ganglion cells. Such vesicles are similar to those found in peptide and catecholamine containing neurons. It may be that gangliogliomas are capable of neuronal-type functions and signal transduction and do not merely act as space-occupying lesions. The potential effect of such functions (or dysfunctions) could be far reaching particularly during development.

Such a marked association between pathology and SLP effect was not seen in the AHS group (where only 10% of the cases with AHS lesions developed SLP), which had similar parameters of early onset of seizures and early operations. In the AHS group of the total sample, 80% had recorded birth injuries and/or febrile convulsions ($p < 0.02$ and 0.0001, respectively).

In respect of temporal lobe epilepsy it may be expected that the area of maximum abnormality (as located by EEG) is excised. Although the most abnormal regions of cortex may have been removed it is possible that other electrically 'less ostentatious' areas of cortical abnormality may be left behind. This possibility is strongly supported by the fact that even within the limits of the resected lobes abnormality is disseminated rather than confined to a single patch. The degree to which other areas or the other hemisphere of the brain may have been affected either structurally or functionally is uncertain.

Early abnormality and early onset of seizures is likely to disturb normal function in other brain areas and the opposite hemisphere (Margerison and Corsellis, 1986; Engel *et al.*, 1982; Babb *et al.*, 1984). Damage to both hemispheres would explain why lobectomy and removal of the seizure focus whilst reducing seizure frequency does not in itself generally alter the clinical manifestations of SLP in temporal lobe epilepsy (cf. Jensen and Larsen, 1979; Pakalnis *et al.*, 1987).

RELEVANCE OF SCHIZOPHRENIA-LIKE PSYCHOSIS TO 'REAL' SCHIZOPHRENIA

The studies on the pathology of schizophrenia and SLP suggest that a series of factors are common to the neuropathology of these conditions.

The work on the neuropathology of SLP suggests that certain types of lesions of the medial temporal cortex, which arise during critical phases of brain development and cause early disruption of neuronal function (early age of first seizure) are associated with the development of SLP. Such developmental anomalies may be more common than previously realized since the presence of subtle disturbances in the cortical cytoarchitecture of many epileptic brains has been reported (Meencke and Janz, 1984; Hardiman *et al.*, 1988; Kaufman and Galaburda, 1989) although the extent and significance of this phenomenon is uncertain (Lyon and Gastaut, 1985; Meencke and Janz, 1984). Neuropathological studies of schizophrenia support the view that the pathological basis for the structural changes found in the brains of schizophrenics is a developmental anomaly arising early in life, disrupting neuronal architecture and affecting both left and right medial temporal lobe (Roberts *et al.*, 1987; Weinberger, 1987; Roberts, 1988).

Thus neuropathological studies on the brains of schizophrenics and analysis of the pathology associated with SLP point to common crucial factors—the age and site at which disruption of the neuronal architecture takes place and the type of lesion causing the disruption. Developmental anomalies or (to a lesser extent) early onset of seizures in TLE can cause the same kind of neuronal disruption or 'architectural folly' (Taylor *et al.*, 1971) in the neuronal organization of the medial temporal lobe that is believed to occur in schizophrenia (Jacob and Beckman, 1986; Falkai *et al.*, 1988b). If this was the case then SLP may be a phenocopy of the genetically inspired architectural folly in schizophrenia (as proposed by Davison, 1983).

Explaining how an early fixed lesion can give rise to a psychosis with a fluctuating course 20 years later has been the subject of considerable discussion (Weinberger, 1987; Roberts, 1991). Feinberg (1983) has argued that vulnerability to schizophrenia may be an emergent phenomenon. Huttenlocher (1979) has shown that cortical synaptic density rises to a maximum at ages 2–3 (150% of adult levels) and then declines steeply in late childhood and adolescence to levels that persist throughout adulthood into old age. Such changes in synaptic density could be the anatomical substrate for changes in electrical properties of the cerebral cortex that occur in late childhood and which include maturation of EEG patterns and an increase in seizure threshold (Thatcher *et al.*, 1987). The extensive rationalization of brain function that takes place during adolescence could uncover a developmental anomaly in brain structure previously compensated for (Taylor, 1975) and explain the emerging potential to developing schizophrenic symptoms. It is obvious that in TLE the extent of disruption in brain structures is much more severe than that seen in schizophrenia. So how are psychosis and epilepsy related aetiologically? Medial temporal lobe structures are amongst the most epileptogenic in the brain and it is likely that disorderly neuronal activity which may give rise to schizophrenia-like symptoms is of a kind which if above a certain threshold is likely to cause seizures (Slater and Beard, 1963).

SLP cases may well be a good 'mock-up' of schizophrenia (Roberts *et al.*, 1990) as many of the factors thought to be important in schizophrenia are present in SLP cases. In some respects the study of SLP cases may give additional advantages.

Within the cases described above some pathologies are seen not to be associated with schizophrenia despite being developmental in origin (e.g. alien tissue cortical dysplasia lesions) and careful comparison of these cases with 'schizophrenogenic' ganglioglial lesions may lead to a more careful definition of the parameters associated with increased risk of schizophrenia-like psychoses.

Integrating the results of studies on the pathology of schizophrenia and the pathology of SLP seen in temporal lobe epilepsy has already given us several insights into the parameters delineating the biology of psychosis. Additional work in this field will undoubtedly uncover the irreducible minimum of altered brain structure which forms the substrate of psychosis.

ACKNOWLEDGEMENTS

This work was supported by The Wellcome Trust and by The Stanley Foundation.

REFERENCES

Armstrong, D.D. and Bruton, C.J. (1987). Postscript: what terminology is appropriate for tissue pathology? In: Engle, J. (Ed.), *Surgical Treatment of the Epilepsies*, Raven Press, New York, pp. 541–551.

Armstrong, D.D., Rouah, E., Zhu, Z., Rutecki, P., Mizrahi, E. and Grassman, R. (1988). The spectrum of histopathology of gangliogliomas in patients with complex partial epilepsy. *J. Neuropathol. Exp. Neurol.*, **47**, 373.

Arnold, S.E., Hyman, B.T., Van Hoesen, G.W. and Damasio, A.R. (1991). Some cytoarchitectural abnormalities of the entorhinal cortex in schizophrenia. *Arch. Gen. Psychiatry*, **48**, 625–632.

Babb, T.L., Brown, W.J., Pretorius, J., Davenport, C., Leib, J.P. and Crandall, P.H. (1984). Temporal lobe volumetric cell densities in temporal lobe epilepsy. *Epilepsia*, **25**, 729–740.

Bachneff, S.A. (1991). Positron emission tomography and magnetic resonance imaging: a review and a local circuit neurons hypo(dys)function hypothesis of schizophrenia. *Biol. Psychiatry*, **30**, 857–886.

Bleuler, M. (1978). *The Schizophrenic Disorders*, Yale University Press, New Haven and London.

Bogerts, B., Meertz, E. and Schonfeldt-Bausch, R. (1985). Basal ganglia and limbic system pathology in schizophrenia: a morphometric study of brain volume and shrinkage. *Arch. Gen. Psychiatry*, **42**, 784–791.

Brown, R., Colter, N., Corsellis, J.A.N., Crow, T.J., Frith, C.D., Jagoe, R., Johnstone, E.C. and Marsh, L. (1986). Post-mortem evidence of structural brain changes in schizophrenia: differences in brain weight, temporal horn area and parahippocampal gyrus compared with affective disorder. *Arch. Gen. Psychiatry*, **43**, 36–42.

Bruton, C.J. (1988). *The Neuropathology of Temporal Lobe Epilepsy*, Maudsley Monograph 31, Oxford University Press, Oxford.

Bruton, C.J., Crow, T.J., Frith, C.D., Johnstone, E.C., Owens, D.G.C. and Roberts, G.W. (1990). Schizophrenia and the brain: a prospective clinico-neuropathology study. *Psychol. Med.*, **20**, 285–304.

Cavanagh, J.B. (1958). On certain small tumours encountered in the temporal lobe. *Brain*, **81**, 389–405.

Conrad, A.J., Abebe, T., Austin, R., Forsythe, S., Scheibel, A.B. (1991). Hippocampal pyramidal cell disarray in schizophrenia as a bilateral phenomenon. *Arch. Gen. Psychiatry*, **48**, 413–417.

Crow, T.J. and Johnstone, E.C. (1987). Schizophrenia: nature of the disease process and its biological correlates. In: Plum, F. (Ed.), *Handbook of Physiology—The Nervous System V*, American Physiological Society, Baltimore, pp. 843–869.

Crow, T.J., Ball, J., Bloom, S.R., Brown, R., Bruton, C.D., Colter, N., Frith, C.D., Johnstone, E.C., Owens, D.G.C. and Roberts, G.W. (1989). Schizophrenia as an anomaly of development of cerebral asymmetry: a post-mortem study and proposal concerning the genetic basis of the disease. *Arch. Gen. Psychiatry*, **46**, 1145–1150.

Currie, S., Heathfield, K.W.G., Henson, R.A. and Scott, D.F. (1971). Clinical course and prognosis of temporal lobe epilepsy. *Brain*, **94**, 173–190.

Davison, K. (1983). Schizophrenia-like psychoses associated with organic cerebral disorders: a review. *Psychiatr. Dev.*, **1**, 1–34.

Engel Jr, J., Brown, W.J., Kuhl, D.E., Phelps, M.E., Mazziotta, J.C. and Crandall, P.H. (1982). Pathological findings underlying focal temporal lobe hypometabolism in partial epilepsy. *Ann. Neurol.*, **12**, 518–528.

Falkai, P. and Bogerts, B. (1986). Cell loss in the hippocampus of schizophrenics. *Eur. Arch. Psychiatr. Neurol. Sci.*, **236**, 154–161.

Falkai, P., Bogerts, B. and Rozumek, M. (1988a). Limbic pathology in schizophrenia: the entorhinal region—a morphometric study. *Biol. Psychiatry*, **24**, 515–521.

Falkai, P., Bogerts, B., Roberts, G.W. and Crow, T.J. (1988b). Measurement of the alpha-cell-migration in the entorhinal region: a marker for the developmental disturbances in schizophrenia? *Schizophrenia Res.*, **1**, 157–158.

Feinberg, I. (1983). Schizophrenia: caused by a fault in programmed synaptic elimination during adolescence? *J. Psychiatr. Res.*, **17**, 319–334.

Flor-Henry, P. (1969). Psychosis and temporal lobe epilepsy. *Epilepsia*, **10**, 363–395.

Flor-Henry, P. (1983). Determinants of psychosis in epilepsy; laterality and forced normalization. *Biol. Psychiatry*, **18**, 1045–1057.

Gilles, F.H. and Green, B.E. (1985). Neuropathologic indicators of abnormal development. In: Freeman, J.M. (Ed.), *Prenatal and Perinatal Factors Associated with Brain Disorders*, NIH, Bethesda.

Hardiman, O., Burke, T., Philips, J., Murphy, S., O'Moore, B., Staunton, H. and Farrell, M.A. (1988). Microdysgenesis in resected temporal neocortex; incidence and clinical significance in focal epilepsy. *Neurology*, **38**, 1041–1047.

Hill, D. (1953). Discussion of surgery in temporal lobe epilepsy. *Proc. R. Soc. Med.*, **46**, 965–976.

Huttenlocher, P.R. (1979). Synaptic density in human frontal cortex—developmental changes and effects of aging. *Brain Res.*, **163**, 195–205.

Illowsky, B.N., Juliano, D.M., Bigleow, L.B. and Weinberger, D.R. (1988). Stability of CT scan findings in schizophrenia: results of an 8 year follow-up study. *J. Neurol. Neurosurg. Psychiatry*, **51**, 209–213.

Jakob, H. and Beckman, H. (1986). Prenatal developmental disturbances in the limbic allocortex in schizophrenics. *J. Neural. Transm.*, **65**, 303–326.

Jensen, I. (1976). Temporal lobe epilepsy. Etiological factors and surgical results. *Acta. Neurol. Scand.*, **53**, 103–118.

Jensen, I. and Klinken, L. (1976). Temporal lobe epilepsy and neuropathology. *Acta. Neurol. Scand.*, **54**, 391–414.

Jensen, I. and Larson, J.K. (1979). Mental aspects of temporal lobe epilepsy. Follow-up of 74 patients after resection of a temporal lobe. *J. Neurol. Neurosurg. Psychiatry*, **42**, 256–265.

Jeste, D. and Lohr, J.B. (1989). Hippocampal pathologic findings in schizophrenia. A morphometric study. *Arch. Gen. Psychiatry*, **46**, 1019–1024.

Johnstone, E.C., Crow, T.J., Frith, C.D., Husband, J. and Kreel, L. (1976). Cerebral ventricular size and cognitive impairment in chronic schizophrenia. *Lancet*, **ii**, 924–926.

Jones, P. and Murray, R.M. (1991). The genetics of schizophrenia is the genetics of neurodevelopment. *Br. J. Psychiatry*, **158**, 615–623.

Kaufman, W.E. and Galaburda, A.M. (1989). Cerebrocortical microdysgenesis in neurologically normal subjects: a histopathologic study. *Neurology*, **39**, 238–244.

Kovelman, J.A. and Scheibel, A.B. (1984). A neurohistological correlate of schizophrenia. *Biol. Psychiatry*, **191**, 1601–1621.

Kraepelin, E. (1919). *Dementia Praecox and Paraphrenia*, Churchill Livingstone, Edinburgh. Translated: Barclay, R.M. and Robertson, G.M. (1971), R.E. Krieger, New York.

Kuchna, I. and Kozlowski, P.B. (1991). The sequels of perinatal central nervous system damage after long-term survival. *Clin. Neuropathol.*, **10**, 203.

Larroche, J.C. (1984). Malformations of the nervous system. In: Adams, J.M., Corsellis, J.A.N. and Duchen, L.W. (Eds), *Greenfields Neuropathology, 4th edn*, Edward Arnold, London, p. 385.

Lemke, R. (1935). Untersuchungen uber die soziale Prognose der Schizophrenia unter besonderer Beruckichtigung des encephalographischen Befundes. *Arch. Psychiatr. Nervenk.*, **104**, 89–135.

Lewis, M.S. (1989a). Age incidence and schizophrenia: Part I. The season of birth controversy. *Schizophrenia Bull.*, **15**, 59–73.

Lewis, M.S. (1989b), Age incidence and schizophrenia: Part II. Beyond age incidence. *Schizophrenia Bull.*, **15**, 75–80.

Lindsay, J., Ounstead, C. and Richards, P. (1979). Long-term outcome in children with temporal lobe seizures. III. Psychiatric aspects in childhood and adult life. *Dev. Med. Child Neurol.*, **21**, 630–636.

Lyon, G. and Gastaut, H. (1985). Considerations on the significance attributed to unusual cerebral histological findings recently described in eight patients with primary generalised epilepsy. *Epilepsia*, **26**, 365–367.

Margerison, J.H. and Corsellis, J.A.N. (1966). Epilepsy and the temporal lobes: a clinical and electroencephalographic and neuropathological study of the brain in epilepsy with particular reference to the temporal lobes. *Brain*, **89**, 499–530.

Meencke, H.J. and Janz, D. (1984). Neuropathological findings in primary generalised epilepsy: a study of eight cases. *Epilepsia*, **25**, 8–21.

Murray, R.M., Lewis, S.W. and Revely, A.M. (1985). Towards an aetiological classification of schizophrenia. *Lancet*, **ii**, 1023–1026.

O'Callaghan, E., Larkin, C., Remond, O., Stack, J., Ennis, J.T. and Waddington, J.L. (1988). 'Early onset schizophrenia' after teenage head injury. A case report with magnetic resonance imaging. *Br. J. Psychiatry*, **153**, 394–396.

Orsini, D.L. and Satz, P. (1986). A syndrome of pathological left-handedness: correlates of early left hemisphere injury. *Arch. Neurol.*, **43**, 333–337.

Pakalnis, A., Drake Jr, M.E., Kuruvilla, J. and Kellum, J.B. (1987). Forced normalisation. Acute psychosis after seizure control in seven patients. *Arch. Neurol.*, **44**, 289.

Pakkenberg, B. (1987). Post-mortem study of chronic schizophrenic brains. *Br. J. Psychiatry*, **151**, 744–752.

Perez, M.M., Trimble, M.R., Murray, N.M.K. and Reider, I. (1985). Epileptic psychoses: an evaluation of P.S.E. profiles. *Br. J. Psychiatry*, **146**, 155–163.

Pond, D.A. (1957). Psychiatric aspects of epilepsy. *J. Indian Med. Prof.*, **3**, 1441–1451.

Rakic, P. (1985). Limits of neurogenesis in primates. *Science*, **227**, 227–1054.

Reveley, M.A., Chitkara, B. and Lewis, S.W. (1988). Ventricular and cranial size in schizophrenia: a 4–7 year follow-up. *Proceedings of IVth Winter Workshop on Schizophrenia, Badgastein, Austria.*

Roberts, G.W. (1988). Abnormalities in brain structure in schizophrenia. *Curr. Opinion Psychiatry*, **1**, 83–89.

Roberts, G.W. (1991). Schizophrenia: a neuropathological perspective. *Br. J. Psychiatry*, **158**, 8–17.

Roberts, G.W. and Bruton, C.J. (1990). Notes from the graveyard: schizophrenia and neuropathology. *Neuropath. Appl. Neurobiol.*, **16**, 3–16.

Roberts, G.W., Colter, N., Lofthouse, R.M., Johnstone, E.C. and Crow, T.J. (1987). Is there gliosis in schizophrenia? Investigation of the temporal lobe. *Biol. Psychiatry*, **22**, 1459–1468.

Roberts, G.W., Done, D.J., Bruton, C.J. and Crow, T.J. (1990). A 'mock-up of schizophrenia'. Schizophrenia-like psychoses and temporal lobe epilepsy. *Biol. Psychiatry*, **28**, 127–143.

Rubenstein, L.J. and Herman, M.M. (1972). A light- and electron-microscopic study of a temporal lobe ganglioglioma. *J. Neurol. Sci.*, **16**, 27–48.

Russell, D.S. and Rubenstein, L.J. (1989). *Pathology of Tumours of the Nervous System*, Edward Arnold, London.

Shelton, R. C. and Weinberger, D.R. (1986). X-ray computerised tomography studies of schizophrenia; a review and synthesis. In: Nasrallah, H.A. and Weinberger, D.R. (Eds), *The Neurology of Schizophrenia*, Elsevier, Amsterdam.

Sherwin, I. (1981). Psychosis associated with epilepsy: significance of the laterality of the epileptogenic lesion. *J. Neurol. Neurosurg. Psychiatry*, **44**, 83–85.

Sherwin, I., Person-Magnon, P., Bancaud, J., Bonis, A. and Talairach, J. (1982). Prevalence of psychosis in epilepsy as a function of the laterality of the epileptogenic lesion. *Arch. Neurol.*, **39**, 621–625.

Slater, E. and Beard, A.W. (1963). The schizophrenia-like psychoses of epilepsy. *Br. J. Psychiatry*, **109**, 95–150.

Stoudemire, A., Nelson, A., Houpt, J.L. (1983). Interictal schizophrenia-like psychoses in temporal lobe epilepsy. *Psychosomatics*, **24**, 331–339.

Suddath, R.L., Casanova, M.F., Goldberg, T.E., Daniel, D.G., Kelsoe, J.R. and Weinberger, D.R. (1989). Temporal lobe pathology in schizophrenia: a quantitative magnetic resonance imaging study. *Am. J. Psychiatry*, **146**, 464–472.

Suddath, R.L., Christison, G.W., Torrey, E.F., Casanova, M.F. and Weinberger, D.R. (1990). Anatomical abnormalities in the brains of monozygotic twins discordant for schizophrenia. *N. Engl. J. Med.*, **322**, 789–794.

Taylor, D.C. (1975). Factors influencing the occurrence of schizophrenia-like psychosis in patients with temporal lobe epilepsy. *Psychol. Med.*, **5**, 249–254.

Taylor, D.C., Falconer, M.A., Bruton, C.J. and Corsellis, J.A.N. (1971). Focal dysplasia of cerebral cortex in epilepsy. *J. Neurol. Neurosurg. Psychiatry*, **34**, 369–387.

Thatcher, R.W., Walker, R.A. and Guidice, S. (1987). Human cerebral hemispheres develop at different rates and ages. *Science*, **236**, 1110–1113.

Toone, B.K. (1981). Psychoses of epilepsy. In: Reynolds, E.H. and Trimble, M.R. (Eds), *Epilepsy and Psychiatry*, Churchill Livingstone, London, pp. 113–137.

Toone, B.K., Garralda, M.E. and Ron, M.A. (1982). The psychoses of epilepsy and the functional psychoses: a clinical and phenomenological comparison. *Br. J. Psychiatry*, **141**, 256–261.

Trimble, M.R. (1981). *The Psychopathology of Epilepsy*, Geigy Pharmaceuticals, UK, pp. 218–278.

Trimble, M.R. (1986). Positive and negative symptoms in psychiatry. *Br. J. Psychiatry*, **148**, 587–589.

Vita, A., Sacchetti, E., Valvassori, G. and Cazzullo, C.L. (1988). Brain morphology in schizophrenia: a 2-5 year CT scan follow-up study. *Acta Psychiatr. Scand.*, **78**, 618–621.

Volpe, J.J. (1989). Intraventricular haemorrhage in the premature infant—current concepts. Part 1. *Ann. Neurol.*, **25**, 3–11.

Weinberger, D.R. (1984). Computed tomography (CT) findings in schizophrenia: speculations on the meaning of it all. *J. Psychiatr. Res.*, **18**, 477–490.

Weinberger, D.R. (1987). Implications of normal brain development for the pathogenesis of schizophrenia. *Arch. Gen. Psychiatry*, **44**, 660–669.
Weinberger, D.R. (1988). Premorbid neuropathology in schizophrenia. *Lancet*, **ii**, 959–960.
Woody, R.C., Bolyard, K., Eisenhauer, G. and Altshuler, L. (1987). CT scan and MRI findings in a child with schizophrenia. *J. Child Neurol.*, **2**, 105–110.

The Temporal Lobes and the Limbic System
Edited by M.R. Trimble and T.G. Bolwig

16

Quantification of Human Brains from Schizophrenics

BENTE PAKKENBERG
Neurological Research Laboratory, Bartholin Institute, Copenhagen, Denmark

INTRODUCTION

Stereological techniques have been introduced in which micro- and macroscopic brain volumes may be estimated in an unbiased way by the use of the Cavalieri principle of volume measurement (Gundersen and Jensen, 1987; Regeur and Pakkenberg, 1989). The use of a recent stereological method, the dissector, as applied to human brain tissue to give an estimate of numerical density combined with the Cavalieri principle, has made it possible to use unbiased principles to estimate the total number of neurons in any brain area that can be defined. These methods have been applied to post-mortem brains from schizophrenics and controls.

MACROSCOPIC BRAIN VOLUMES IN POST-MORTEM SCHIZOPHRENIC BRAINS

Johnstone and coworkers (1976) were the first to show enlarged ventricles in schizophrenia using computerized axial tomography (CT). A great number of CT-scan investigations have emerged since then (for reviews, see Weinberger *et al.*, 1983; Seidman, 1983) in which the size of the ventricular system has been compared with a number of parameters such as intellectual and neuropsychological impairment (Johnstone *et al.*, 1976; Rieder *et al.*, 1979; Donnelly *et al.*, 1980; Pearlson *et al.*, 1984; Owens *et al.*, 1985; Obiols *et al.*, 1987), negative schizophrenic features (Andreasen *et al.*, 1982; Takahashi *et al.*, 1981), difference in response to medication (Luchins *et al.*,

1984; Nasrallah *et al.*, 1983; Weinberger *et al.*, 1980), the possible role of biological treatments (Johnstone *et al.*, 1976; Weinberger *et al.*, 1979; Owens *et al.*, 1985), age of onset, duration of illness and severity of illness (Nasrallah *et al.*, 1983; Andreasen *et al.*, 1982; Woods and Wolf, 1983). No consistent correlations between ventricular size and any of the above factors have been clearly identified in schizophrenics.

Several investigators studied whether ventricular enlargement predates the onset of disease or changes in size during the course of the disease. In 1982, Weinberger *et al.* reported a CT scan study of 35 patients with first-episode schizophreniform disorder, 17 with chronic schizophrenia, 23 with affective disorders, together with 27 with other psychiatric disorders and 26 controls. Both the schizophreniform patients and chronic schizophrenics had significantly larger cerebral ventricles compared with other psychiatric patients or control subjects. Seven of the 35 patients with first-episode schizophreniform disorders had cerebral ventricle areas larger than expected for the second and third decades of life according to ventricle/brain ratio (VBR), taken from the CT slice with the largest ventricular profile.

Schulz *et al.* (1983) studied the VBRs of 15 teenage schizophrenic/schizophreniform patients and eight borderline patients compared with age-matched controls (n=18) and reported the schizophrenic group to have significantly larger ventricles. This finding was subsequently confirmed by Turner *et al.* (1986) who studied the VBRs of 30 patients fulfilling DSM-III criteria for schizophrenia and were within 2 years of presentation. This group was compared with 26 age-matched normal volunteers and it was found that VBR was significantly greater in the schizophrenic group.

Contrasting their results with the pneumoencephalographic (PEG) findings of Huber (1964) and Haug (1963), Illowsky *et al.* (1988) found no progression of VBR in 15 schizophrenic patients (age 32 to 40 years) over an interval of 7–9 years. This finding is in agreement with other reports of unchanged ventricular enlargement over 2–5 years, after the onset of disease (Nasrallah *et al.*, 1986; Vita *et al.*, 1988).

THE DANISH STUDIES

The macroscopic structures of the brain were studied by division into the cortex, white matter, central grey matter and ventricles. Using the previously described stereological methods, volume estimations were done on a collection of brains from 29 chronic schizophrenic patients (14 males and 15 females), mean age 73.8 years (range 41 to 91 years) and compared with 30 controls in the same age range (Pakkenberg, 1987). Differences between groups were tested by comparing two regression lines, schizophrenic versus control, taking into account the fact that brain volumes in humans are correlated to body height.

The volumes of the hemispheres, the cortex and the central grey matter were found to be significantly reduced while the volume of the ventricles (the only variable not related to body height) was significantly enlarged in the schizophrenics compared with the control group. There was no statistically significant difference between the volume of the white matter in the two groups. The average ventricular volume in the control group was 26.3 ml, and in the schizophrenics 35.1 ml. In the older age group (65 to 91 years), no statistically significant difference was found in the volumes of the ventricles.

Using the same principle, a post-mortem study was carried out on 19 brains from leucotomized schizophrenic patients and 20 age-matched controls (Pakkenberg, 1989). Brains from patients with leucotomy represent a special problem in the evaluation of the volume of the ventricles, since the defect left by leucotomy often connects the ventricles to the cerebral surface through the frontal lobe. Since this lesion allows CSF to escape through the frontal lobe, it is either difficult or impossible to measure the ventricular system by volume displacement. With the Cavalieri method this is no longer a problem and furthermore it is also possible to estimate the volume of the defect left by the leucotomy. Compared with controls, the volumes of the hemispheres, the cortex, the white matter and the central grey structures were all significantly reduced in brains from schizophrenic patients. No statistically significant difference was found between the volumes of the ventricles in the leucotomized schizophrenics and the control group, which may be due to the rather high age of the individuals (72.4 years). The white matter and the central grey structures were significantly reduced compared with a group of non-leucotomized schizophrenic brains. No difference was found in the size of the lesions in patients who improved compared with the patients who remained unchanged, and the outcome was unrelated to lesional asymmetry.

A major limitation is the problem of interpreting results obtained from fixed brain tissue. Volume changes induced by post-mortem events, time from death to fixation, the fixatives used etc., all are potential confounding variables which may influence brain volumes. A second major problem in the interpretation of these data is that the sample consists of brains from elderly, institutionalized, chronic patients heavily treated with neuroleptics, ECT and/or insulin. The reduced volumes found for almost every parameter of the macroscopic data may therefore not be a result of the disease itself but at least partly a combination of disease and the life conditions of this schizophrenic population.

TOTAL NEURON NUMBER IN SCHIZOPHRENIC BRAINS COMPARED WITH A CONTROL GROUP

The major problems in estimating the total neuronal number in any defined brain region include the following: (i) how to estimate, in an unbiased way,

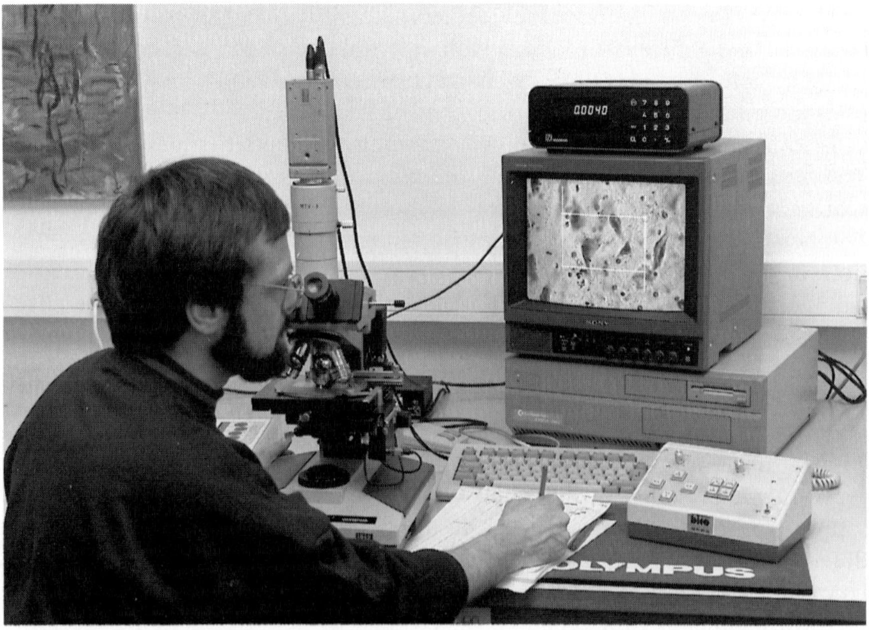

Figure 1. The basic equipment consists of a BH-2 Olympus microscope equipped with motorized stage movement, an electronic microcater with digital readout for measuring movements in the Z-axis, an AMIGA 2000 computer, and a colour video camera/monitor. On the screen is seen an unbiased counting frame superimposed on neocortical neurons.

the volume of the organ; (ii) how to sample uniformly in the complex and very irregularly shaped cortex; (iii) how to estimate numerical density of neurons.

The Cavalieri theorem together with systematic sampling and point-counting can be applied to any organ that can be cut into slices and it is independent of the size or shape of the organ. The second and third problems listed above have recently been overcome with the advent of unbiased stereology and the principles have been applied to human brains (for practical details and analyses of sampling designs, see Gundersen and Jensen, 1987; Gundersen *et al.*, 1988a,b; Pakkenberg and Gundersen, 1988; Pakkenberg *et al.*, 1989; West and Gundersen, 1990). Recently Williams and Rakic (1988, 1989) have applied the same technique but used the three-dimensional counting frame (Gundersen, 1981; Howard *et al.*, 1985) in order to get unbiased neuronal numerical densities. A method for uniform sampling in human neocortex combined with a modification of the dissector principle, the optical dissector, has recently been introduced (Gundersen, 1986; Brændgaard *et al.*, 1990) (Fig. 1).

The remarkable efficiency of systematic sampling combined with unbiased counting methods is the most recent breakthrough in the quantification of the central nervous system. The dissector principle of particle counting to estimate total cell numbers was first applied to estimate total cell numbers in human brain tissue in 1988 (Pakkenberg and Gundersen, 1988).

A number of qualitative and semi-quantitative changes in central brain regions in schizophrenia have been described. The supranucleus medialis-dorsalis thalami were studied by Hempel (1958) who reported a 44% reduction in nerve cell density in schizophrenics. A qualitative estimate by Bäumer (1954) reported reduced density in nucleus medialis thalami in 17 brains of schizophrenic patients compared with a control group. Dom *et al.* (1981) compared five brains from catatonic schizophrenic cases with five controls and found no difference in numerical nerve cell density in thalamus medialis and nucleus accumbens. In 1986, Falkai and Bogerts, using cell density estimates corrected with a conventional correction formula, reported a significant loss of neurons in the hippocampus of 13 schizophrenics compared with 11 controls. No nerve cell loss was found in the granular cells of the dentate fascia or any region of the subiculum. Heckers *et al.* (1991) using an in principle unbiased counting method, found no difference in the estimates of the total number of neurons in hippocampal subdivisions in 13 brains of schizophrenics and 13 control brains closely matched for sex and age.

The dissector method was applied to 12 brains from chronic schizophrenic patients, eight males and four females (average age 62 years), in order to obtain an unbiased estimate of the total neuronal number in the mediodorsal thalamic nucleus (MD), ventral pallidum (VP), nucleus accumbens (NA) and the basolateral nucleus of amygdala (BLA). The results revealed a 40% decrease in nerve cell number from 1.81×10^6 to 1.08×10^6 in the MD in the schizophrenics compared with controls. In the nucleus accumbens a 50% reduction in the total number of nerve cells was found in the eight brains from schizophrenics which were studied. In the same brains no significant difference was observed in total neuron number in the ventral pallidum. In five brains no significant difference was found in the total neuronal number in the basolateral nucleus of amygdala compared with an equal number of controls (Pakkenberg, 1990).

SUMMARY

Within recent years, the quantification of the central nervous system has shown great progress. Meaningful biological interpretations of volumetric measurements have the limitation that they may not always reflect pathological processes affecting neurons in various brain diseases, for example, the caudate nucleus is severely affected in patients with Huntington's chorea but shows no signs of atrophy at early stages of disease. Accordingly, diagnostic insight in this and other disorders is often limited to patients in whom the disease is already obvious.

The major advance in stereology during recent years is the ability to obtain unbiased estimates of total neuron number in any part of the central nervous system that can be defined. The remarkable objectivity of these methods will enable neuroscientists to use these new tools to efficiently quantify brains obtained from both normal and diseased individuals. In our studies we have shown changes in certain nuclei in schizophrenia, especially in the thalamus and nucleus accumbens, which may have a bearing on the pathogenesis of the disease.

REFERENCES

Andreasen, N.C., Smith, M.R. Jacoby, C.G., Dennert, J.W. and Olsen, S.A. (1982). Ventricular enlargement in schizophrenia: definition and prevalence. *Am. J. Psychiatry*, **139**, 292–296.

Bäumer, H. (1954). Veränderungen des thalamus bei schizophrenie. *J. Hirnforsch.*, **1**, 156–169.

Brændgaard, H., Evans, S.M., Howard, C.V. and Gundersen, H.J.G. (1990). The total number of neurons in the human neocortex unbiasedly estimated using optical dissectors. *J. Microsc.*, **157**, 285–304.

Dom, R., De Saedeleer, J., Bogerts, J. and Hopf, A. (1981). Quantitative cytometric analysis of basal ganglia in catatonic schizophrenics. *Biol. Psychiatry*, 723–726.

Donnelly, E.F., Weinberger, D.R., Waldman, I.N. and Wyatt, R.J. (1980). Neuropsychological prediction of structural brain abnormalities on computed tomography in a group of chronic schizophrenic patients. *J. Nerv. Ment. Dis.*, **168**, 305–308.

Falkai, P. and Bogerts, B. (1986) Cell loss in the hippocampus of schizophrenics. *Eur. Arch. Psychiatr. Neurol. Sci.*, **236**, 154–161.

Gundersen, H.J.G. (1981). Stereologi—Eller hvordan tal for rumlig form og indhold opnås ved iagttagelse af strukturer på snitplaner. *Lægeforeningens forlag, Copenhagen*, pp. 1–25 (Thesis in Danish).

Gundersen, H.J.G. (1986). Stereology of arbitrary particles. *J. Microsc.*, **143**, 3–45.

Gundersen, H.J.G. and Jensen, E.B. (1987). The efficiency of systematic sampling in stereology and its prediction. *J. Microsc.*, **147**, 229–263.

Gundersen, H.J.G., Bendtsen, T.F., Korbo, L., Marcussen, N., Møller, A., Nielsen, K., Nyengaard, J.R., Pakkenberg, B., Vesterby, A. and West, M.J. (1988a). Some new, simple and efficient stereological methods and their use in pathological research and diagnosis. *Acta Pathol. Microbiol. Scand.*, **96**, 379–394.

Gundersen, H.J.G., Bagger, P., Bendtsen, T.F., Evans, S.M., Korbo, L., Marcussen, N., Møller, A., Nielsen, K., Nyengaard, J.R., Pakkenberg, B., Sørensen, F.B., Vesterby, A. and West, M.J. (1988b). The new stereological tools: dissector, fractionator, nucleator, and point sampled intercepts and their use in pathological research and diagnosis. *Acta Pathol. Microbiol. Scand.*, **96**, 857–881.

Haug, J.O. (1963). Pneumoencephalographic studies in mental disease. *Norwegian Monographs on Medical Science*, Universitetsforlaget, pp. 1–104.

Heckers, S., Heinsen, H., Geiger, B. and Beckmann, H. (1991). Hippocampal neuron number in schizophrenia. A stereological study. *Arch. Gen. Psychiatry*, **48**, 1002–1008.

Hempel, K.-J. (1958). Histopathologische untersuchungen am supranucleus mediodorsalis thalami bei schizophrenie. *J. Hirnforsch*, **4**, 205–253.

Howard, V., Reid, S., Baddeley, A. and Boyde, A. (1985). Unbiased estimation of particle density in the tandem scanning reflected light microscope. *J. Microsc.*, **138**, 203–212.

Huber, G. (1964). Neuroradiologie und Psychiatrie. *Psychiatrie der Gegenwart, Forschung und Praxis, Vol. 1/lB*, Grundlagenforschung zur Psychiatrie, Part B, Springer-Verlag, Berlin.

Illowsky, B.P., Juliano, D.M., Bigelow, L.B. and Weinberger, D.R. (1988). Stability of CT scan findings in schizophrenia: results of an 8 year follow-up study. *J. Neurol. Neurosurg. Psychiatry*, **51**, 209–213.

Johnstone, E.C., Crow, T.J., Frith, C.D., Husband, J. and Kreel, L. (1976). Cerebral ventricular size and cognitive impairment in chronic schizophrenia. *Lancet*, **ii**, 924–926.

Luchins, D.J., Lewine, R.R.J. and Meltzer, H.Y. (1984). Lateral ventricular size, psychopathology, and medication response in the psychoses. *Biol. Psychiatry*, **19**, 29–44.

Nasrallah, H.A., Kuperman, S., Hamra, B.J. and McCalley-Whitters, M. (1983). Clinical differences between schizophrenic patients with and without large cerebral ventricles. *J. Clin. Psychiatry*, **44**, 407–409.

Nasrallah, H.A., Olson, S.C., McCalley-Whitters, M., Chapman, S. and Jacoby, C.G. (1986). Cerebral ventricular enlargement in schizophrenia: a preliminary follow-up study. *Arch. Gen. Psychiatry*, **43**, 157–159.

Obiols, J.E., Marcos, T. and Salamero, M. (1987). Ventricular enlargement and neuropsychological testing in schizophrenia. *Acta Psychiatr. Scand.*, **76**, 199–202.

Owens, D.G.C., Johnstone, E.C., Crow, T.J., Frith, C.D., Jagoe, J.R. and Kreel, L. (1985). Lateral ventricular size in schizophrenia: relationship to the disease process and its clinical manifestations. *Psychol. Med.*, **15**, 27–41.

Pakkenberg, B. (1987). Post-mortem study of chronic schizophrenic brains. *Br. J. Psychiatry*, **151**, 744–752.

Pakkenberg, B. (1989). What happens in the leucotomised brain? A postmortem morphological study of brains from schizophrenic patients. *J. Neurol. Neurosurg. Psychiatry*, **52**, 156–161.

Pakkenberg, B. (1990). Pronounced reduction of nerve cell number in mediodorsal thalamic nucleus and nucleus accumbens in schizophrenics. *Arch. Gen. Psychiatry*, **47**, 1023–1028.

Pakkenberg, B. and Gundersen, H.J.G. (1988). Total number of neurons and glial cells in human brain nuclei estimated by the dissector and the fractionator. *J. Microsc.*, **150**, 1–20.

Pakkenberg, B., Evans, S.M., Møller, A., Brændgaard, H. and Gundersen, H.J.G. (1989). Total number of neurons in human neocortex related to age and sex estimated by way of optical dissectors. *Acta Stereologica*, **8**, 251–256.

Pearlson, G.D., Garbacz, D.J., Breakey, W.R., Ahn, H.S. and DePaulo, J.R. (1984). Lateral ventricular enlargement associated with persistent unemployment and negative symptoms in both schizophrenia and bipolar disorder. *Psychiatry Res.*, **12**, 1–9.

Regeur, L. and Pakkenberg, B. (1989). Optimizing sampling designs for volume measurements of components of human brain using a stereological method. *J. Microsc.*, **155**, 113–121.

Rieder, R.O., Donnelly, E.F., Herdt, J.R. and Waldman, I.N. (1979). Sulcal prominence in young chronic schizophrenic patients: CT scan findings associated with impairment on neuropsychological tests. *Psychiatry Res.*, **1**, 1–8.

Schulz, S.C., Koller, M.M., Kishore, P.R., Hamer, R.M., Gehl, J.J. and Friedel, R.O. (1983). Ventricular enlargement in teenage patients with schizophrenia spectrum disorder. *Am. J. Psychiatry*, **140**, 1592–1595.

Seidman, I.J. (1983). Schizophrenia and brain dysfunction: an integration of recent neurodiagnostic findings. *Psychol. Bull.*, **94**, 195–238.

Takahashi, R., Inanaga, V., Kato, N. *et al.* (1981). CT scanning and the investigation of schizophrenia. In: Perris, C., Struwe, G. and Jansson, B. (Eds), *Biological Psychiatry*, Elsevier, Amsterdam, pp. 259–268.

Turner, S.W., Toone, B.K. and Brett-Jones, J.R. (1986). Computerized tomographic scan changes in early schizophrenia—preliminary findings. *Psychol. Med.*, **16**, 219–225.

Vita, A., Sacchetti, E., Valvassori, G. and Cazzullo, C.L. (1988). Brain morphology in schizophrenia: a 2- to 5-year follow-up study. *Acta Psychiatr. Scand.*, **78**, 618–621.

Weinberger, D.R., Torrey, E.F., Neophytides, A.N. and Wyatt, R.J. (1979). Structural abnormalities in the cerebral cortex of chronic schizophrenic patients. *Arch. Gen. Psychiatr*, **36**, 935–939.

Weinberger, D.R., Bigelow, L.B., Kleinman, J.E., Klein, S.T., Rosenblatt, J.E. and Wyatt, R.J. (1980). Cerebral ventricular enlargement in chronic schizophrenia. *Arch. Gen. Psychiatry*, **37**, 11–13.

Weinberger, D.R., DeLisi, L.E., Perman, G.P., Targum, S. and Wyatt, R.J. (1982). Computed tomography in schizophreniform disorder and other acute psychiatric disorders. *Arch. Gen. Psychiatry*, **39**, 778–783.

Weinberger, D.R., Wagner, R.L. and Wyatt, R.J. (1983). Neuropathological studies of schizophrenia: a selective review. *Schizophrenia Bull.*, **9**, 193–212.

West, M.J. and Gundersen, H.J.G. (1990). Unbiased stereological estimation of the number of neurons in the human hippocampus. *J. Comp. Neurol.*, **296**, 1–22.

Williams, R.W. and Rakic, P. (1988). Three-dimensional counting: an accurate and direct method to estimate numbers of cells in sectioned material. *J. Comp. Neurol.*, **278**, 344–352.

Williams, R.W. and Rakic, P. (1989). Erratum and Addendum. Three-dimensional counting: an accurate and direct method to estimate numbers of cells in sectioned material. *J. Comp. Neurol.*, **281**, 335.

Woods, B.T. and Wolf, J. (1983). A reconsideration of the relation of ventricular enlargement to duration of illness in schizophrenia. *Am. J. Psychiatry*, **140**, 1564–1570.

The Temporal Lobes and the Limbic System
Edited by M.R. Trimble and T.G. Bolwig
1992 Wrightson Biomedical Publishing Ltd

17

The Temporal Lobes and Affective Disorders

ROBERT M. POST, SUSAN R.B. WEISS, TERENCE A. KETTER, MARK S. GEORGE, MIKE CLARK and JEFFREY ROSEN
Biological Psychiatry Branch, National Institute of Mental Health, Bethesda, Maryland, USA

INTRODUCTION

A variety of methodological approaches have linked temporal lobe function and dysfunction to affective symptomatology. Stimulation and ablation studies in animals provide important evidence for the role of the temporal lobe in affective behaviour (Post, 1986). At the same time, these studies in animals raise a number of methodological concerns about the nature of the relationship of the temporal lobe to affective behaviour.

For example, a variety of seizure inductions which generate similar types of motor convulsions may evoke very different kinds of behaviour. While it was initially reported that amygdala-kindled seizures would enhance aggression in the studies of Pinel and associates (1977), this was subsequently not confirmed by Bawden and Racine (1979) and Weiss *et al.* (1986 and unpublished observations) following amygdala kindling in rats. Pharmacologically kindled seizures with lidocaine are highly similar in appearance to those achieved by electrical stimulation of the amygdala and yet are associated with marked instances of interictal aggression (Post *et al.*, 1984a). However, lidocaine-injected animals that did not develop seizures did not show this aggression. In contrast, intracerebroventricular (i.c.v.) administration of corticotropin releasing hormone (CRH) can produce limbic-type seizures virtually identical to those seen with amygdala- and lidocaine-kindling, yet aggression can be evoked independently of the experience of a seizure (Ehlers *et al.*, 1983; Weiss *et al.*, 1986). The mild irritability following amygdala-kindled seizures lasts for only several minutes, while the interictal behavioural disturbance following lidocaine can be profound and long-lasting, with aggression directed towards laboratory personnel and noted in a 'resistance to capture' measure. In contrast, aggression associated with CRF administration occurs reciprocally between bouts of seizures (or in the absence of seizures as noted above) and tends to be directed towards conspecifics with vicious defensive biting and attack behaviour (Weiss *et al.*, 1986). (We have also noted that animals housed alone have appeared to be more aggressive following lidocaine-kindled seizures than those that are housed in groups.)

The studies of Kopa *et al.* (1968) and Belenkov and Shalkovskaya (1980) further highlight the role of environmental contingencies in the behavioural response to electrical stimulation of the brain. Animals receiving the same brain stimulation current through the same electrode show very different behavioural effects depending on both environmental contingencies, as illustrated in the Valenstein effect (Valenstein *et al.*, 1970), and on learned associations to these environments. That is, cats that receive brain stimulation while they are in an environment associated with presentation of food may show positive response such as purring, but when stimulated on a shelf that has been previously associated with mild foot shock, demonstrate hissing and other negative affective responses.

These data are also convergent with the seminal studies of Porrino and colleagues (1984) who demonstrated that self-stimulation of a variety of brain sites could be rewarding and increase glucose utilization in temporal lobe, ventral-striatal, and cortical areas of brain, but that the same stimulation parameters recorded on tape and re-administered to the same animals (i.e. induced now by the experimenter) evoked different patterns of brain-glucose utilization. Thus, the contingencies, 'meaning', and degree of control over the brain stimulation may produce vastly different effects on the animals' behavioural and affective repertoire.

In addition to these methodological considerations, we would also emphasize two other levels of concern for this analysis. To the extent that critical functional behaviours in brain are represented and rerepresented at many hierarchical levels in the central nervous system, the question might be reformulated from 'whether the temporal lobes play a role in the modulation of affective behaviour' to 'at what level of control do they play the key role in modulating affective behaviour'. That is, the control of temperature regulation may be modulated in a progressively more complex and refined fashion at successively higher levels of the CNS from brain stem to hypothalamus to forebrain and limbic structures and, finally, at the cortex (Satinoff, 1978). A similar hierarchical control of affect may exist in the CNS, and the level of impact of temporal lobe dysfunction on affective behaviour then becomes the critical question. For an excellent review of this hierarchical conception of brain function in relationship to affect, see MacLean (1990).

Dysfunction in temporal lobe structures may also interact importantly with other areas of the brain involved in the modulation of affective behaviour. In particular, we would focus on the role of the temporal lobe in modulating ventral striatal structures most closely associated with psychomotor activation, reward, and hedonic processes crucial to the affective disorders, as well as interactions with frontal lobe structures which may be critically involved in the affective disorders.

As a final caveat, we would re-emphasize the point made by others of the heterogeneity of structures within the limbic system and even within specific nuclei such as the amygdala. That is, a variety of evidence exists to support opposing functions of amygdala and hippocampus on affective behaviour, aggression, autonomic behaviour, and neuroendocrine output (see Table 6 in Post, 1986). In addition, Flynn and associates (1970) among others have emphasized the opposing functions of the cortico-medial versus baso-lateral amygdala, and Adamec and Stark-Adamec (1983) have found very different impacts on behaviour by stimulating the dorsal versus ventral hippocampus.

Thus, any general notion of the impact of limbic system function and dysfunction on affective behaviour certainly must be viewed in the context of the complexity and diversity of the systems involved, their interconnectedness, and their critical interactions with the contingencies of the ongoing behaviour of the organism. With this series of caveats in mind, we will focus our exploration on two general types of methodological strategies aimed at elucidating the role of temporal lobe structures in the affective disorders. The first set of studies will deal with the effects of stimulation of limbic structures in animals and man on affective behaviour. This will also include information derived from endogenous stimulation of limbic structures which occurs in complex partial seizures. These data will then be reflected back on the preliminary but rapidly growing database on alterations in temporal lobe and associated brain structures as assessed with glucose utilization and cerebral blood flow by positron emission tomography (PET) and related brain imaging studies.

COMPLEX PARTIAL SEIZURES OF THE TEMPORAL LOBE AND LIMBIC STRUCTURES: RELATIONSHIP WITH AFFECTIVE SYMPTOMATOLOGY

While the specificity of the relationship of complex partial seizures (CPS) of the temporal lobe (TL) with affective symptomatology may be argued, it is nonetheless clear that a large proportion of patients presenting with CPS experience affective symptoms some time during their lives (for reviews, see Robertson and Trimble, 1983; Altshuler, 1991). (CPS will be assumed to refer to a TL substrate throughout.) While it has not been precisely delineated for the affective psychoses, there appears to be a lag in onset of psychotic disturbances following the onset of the seizure disorder. In many studies this duration averages about 11 years (Slater *et al.*, 1963; see review in Post *et al.*, 1986b). Many of the psychoses of epilepsy have prominent affective features (Slater *et al.*, 1963; Edeh and Toone, 1987). What might be the critical pathophysiological links and reasons for this long lag from the onset of the seizure disorder to the emergence of affective psychoses? Is it related to the biological and psychosocial impact of a progressively developing epileptogenic process that eventually becomes partially refractory to treatment with affective symptomatology as a consequence? Clearly, longitudinal prospective studies of the relationship of affective disorder to CPS, its course, and drug responsivity would be most helpful in sorting out the various options.

The complexity of the potential relationships is also highlighted by the observations that marked affective disturbances can occur either simultaneously with the occurrence of major runs of CPS (either associated with drug refractoriness or drug withdrawal) or inversely with the expression of seizures (Flor-Henry, 1969; Dongier, 1960; Kristensen and Sindrup, 1978). That is, in some patients an inverse relationship between seizures and affective dysfunction may exist, either as a general phenomenon or occurring more specifically in the context of forced normalization (von Meduna, 1935; Landolt, 1958; Pakalnis *et al.*, 1987; Wolf, 1991). In this light, it is useful to recall that the major motor seizures of electroconvulsive therapy are the most effective treatment for the primary affective psychoses of the depressive type (Fink, 1984) and are highly effective in treating manic episodes as well (Milstein *et al.*, 1987; Mukherjee *et al.*, 1988). These data reaffirm the potential inverse relationship between seizures and affective symptomatology. Moreover, the conundrum is further illustrated by the recent observations of Engel (personal communication, 1988) and others (Mizrahi *et al.*, 1990) that temporal lobe surgery (even associated with complete remission of the CPS) may be followed by the occurrence of major affective disorders some months after the successful surgery. Adding further complexity to the problem of associative patterns between seizures and affective and psychotic disturbances is that anticonvulsants may either alleviate (carbamazepine, valproate) (Post, 1990a) or exacerbate (primidone, ethosuximide, phenobarbital) (Robertson and Trimble, 1983; Brent *et al.*, 1990) affective emotions.

How could we begin to place these complex relationships into a series of comprehensible and perhaps testable frameworks? We suggest that lessons learned from a model of complex partial seizures in animals may help structure several conceptual approaches that might elucidate the subtleties of these interrelationships. Lessons from amygdala and hippocampal kindling may thus be enlightening.

AMYGDALA KINDLING: IMPLICATIONS FOR THE PROGRESSIVE INVOLVEMENT OF NEURAL STRUCTURES IN BRAIN AND INTERRELATIONSHIP WITH NEUROPEPTIDES

While the details of amygdala kindling development and evolution have been described elsewhere (Goddard *et al.*, 1969; Racine, 1978; Adamec, 1990; Pinel and Rovner, 1978; Pinel, 1981; Sato *et al.*, 1990; Wada and Sato, 1974; Wada *et al.*, 1976), as well as in Chapter 5 of this volume, a refocusing on several elements of this paradigm pertinent to the discussion of affective disorders may nonetheless be useful in the context of this chapter. Specifically, we wish to highlight the issue of progressive treatment of structures both within and outside of the limbic system that occur over the course of amygdala kindling, and to emphasize the potential impact of such a seizure evolution on alterations in gene expression. Such effects may also alter a variety of classical neurotransmitter and neuropeptide substrates which may play a role in modulating affective function.

Early investigators using electrical recording techniques and regional glucose utilization suggested that there was a progressive evolution in structures sequentially incorporated into the kindled process as a function of amygdala kindling development (Pinel and Rovner, 1978; Wada and Sato, 1974; Racine, 1978; Engel *et al.*, 1982; Ackermann *et al.*, 1986). Recently, Clark and associates (1991a) in our laboratory have reinvestigated this phenomenon using the proto-oncogene *c-fos* as a marker of neuronal cell bodies activated in the process of electrical stimulation of the brain (Sagar *et al.*, 1988; Douglas *et al.*, 1988; Dragunow *et al.*, 1989; Shin *et al.*, 1990; Dragunow and Robertson, 1987). Using *in situ* hybridization, one labels complementary strands of mRNA for the proto-oncogene *c-fos* and ascertains what areas of brain undergo transient induction of this proto-oncogene.

c-fos may be induced by a variety of receptor and second messenger-activated processes occurring through both cyclic AMP and calcium-dependent mechanisms associated with neurotransmission. Once the mRNA for *c-fos* is so induced in the nucleus, it is transported to the ribosomes where the Fos protein is synthesized. Other Fos-related antigens (Fras) and protein products of different proto-oncogenes, such as *c-jun*, *jun-B*, *jun-D*, etc., are also synthesized in a similar manner. These proteins are then transported to the nucleus where they form homo- and hetero-dimers with various binding strengths for regulatory domains in initiating further DNA transcription. For example, the Fos-Jun heterodimer is more potent than the Fos homodimer in binding at the AP1 binding site of target genes and increases the synthesis of new proteins, peptides, and receptors. The 'mix' of oncogenes binding at the AP1 site is thought to differ over time, providing the fine tuning of transcriptional regulation by both activation and repression (Morgan and Curran, 1988).

In this fashion, it is thought that the transient inductions of *c-fos* and related oncogenes may be one of the first steps in a process of altering gene expression in a long-lasting fashion, which could result in alteration in the pattern of proteins and neuropeptides affected as a consequence of prior electrical stimulation of the brain (Morgan and Curran, 1989; Dragunow *et al.*, 1989). Thus, one can conceptualize the *in situ* mapping of *c-fos*, both as a tool for elucidating anatomical pathways activated by stimulation of the amygdala-kindled focus, and as a potentially important biological substrate in a cascade of effects critical to creating the 'memory trace' for the kindled process.

During amygdala kindling, Clark and associates (1991a) have observed that two different pathways may be affected in the early stages of the process. They have found that either the pyriform cortex or the dentate gyrus may be activated unilaterally, but with successive numbers of stimulations or longer afterdischarges (ADs) these structures may then be bilaterally activated, as revealed by the pattern of *c-fos* induction. It appears that the duration of the AD in part determines which pathway is initially utilized, with shorter ADs being associated with the pyriform cortex pattern and longer ADs generating marked unilateral and then bilateral inductions of the dentate gyrus of the hippocampus. At this point one could only surmise the potential differential impacts for cognition, affect, and behaviour that might be associated with the different pathways to the onset of amygdala kindling. As kindling progresses, not only does the process become bilateral, but many other areas of brain are incorporated into the kindled seizure, as revealed by *c-fos* induction in pyriform, frontal, parietal, insular, temporal, perirhinal, occipital, and entorhinal cortices, as well as the amygdala. Regardless of the initial pattern of *c-fos* expression (pyriform or dentate gyrus) in the early stages of amygdala kindling, the pattern in the latter stages was a combination of the two initial patterns (pyriform and dentate gyrus) extending to include the cortical regions listed above and the amygdala.

These data clearly illustrate that a process that is initially confined to the amygdala and its overlying cortices rapidly expands unilaterally and then bilaterally to incorporate not only other limbic areas such as dentate gyrus, but many areas of brain outside of the 'temporal lobe' and limbic system. Thus, we are now in a position to ask whether this process of expansion of the kindled focus (if it is paralleled by similar evolution in the course of CPS), is critically associated with the emergence of affective symptomatology and dysfunction.

When temporal lobes and their underlying amygdala and hippocampal structures are directly stimulated in man, a variety of affective and experiential phenomena are elicited (Penfield and Perot, 1963; Halgren *et al.*, 1978; Halgren, 1981; Gloor *et al.*, 1982; Stevens *et al.*, 1969; Ervin *et al.*, 1969). Are sufficient numbers of stimulations of these structures induced endogenously in the course of CPS to elicit longer term affective symptomatology? Or does the process require a spread to other areas of brain before the symptoms reach a threshold for major affective dysfunction?

The clinical studies using deoxyglucose and related PET methodology in patients with CPS reveal evidence of widespread interictal hypometabolism in many instances in areas far beyond the temporal lobe structures originally involved in the seizure focus (Engel *et al.*, 1982; Theodore *et al.*, 1987; Engel *et al.*, Chapter 7 this volume; Post *et al.*, 1987a). Bromfield *et al.* (1992) have attempted to utilize this methodology to assess areas of the brain showing altered glucose utilization in patients with CPS, with and without prominent affective symptomatology. Trimble and associates used this methodology to elucidate prominent differences in temporal lobe metabolism in those with and without psychotic symptomatology (Ring and Trimble, 1992). Bromfield and associates (1992) found, in a small series of patients with left temporal lobe seizure foci, that those with depressive symptoms (as assessed by the Beck Depression Inventory) had greater degrees of frontal lobe hypometabolism than patients without such affective symptomatology. These data are of considerable interest from the perspective that frontal lobe hypometabolism not only appears to be a consistent correlate of schizophrenic psychosis, but also commonly occurs in patients with affective disturbances of various aetiologies, including primary affective disorder (Buchsbaum *et al.*, 1984, 1986; Baxter *et al.*, 1985, 1989; O'Connell *et al.*, 1989), and affective disorders secondary to parkinsonism (Mayberg *et al.*, 1990a) and Huntington's disease (Mayberg *et al.*, 1990b). The studies of Schwartz and associates (1987, 1990) are particularly interesting, as they found that the severity of depression as measured by the Hamilton Depression Inventory was significantly correlated with the degree of frontal hypometabolism. Post *et al.* (1987a) found decreases in maximal glucose utilization in the temporal lobes (R > L) of depressed patients compared with normal volunteers. Thus, these studies raise the perspective that temporal lobe dysfunction itself, associated with either the ictal process or its local compensatory mechanisms, or processes extending beyond the temporal lobe into synaptically-related areas of brain such as the frontal lobe, may be critical to the emergence of affective symptomatology. How might these local and distant reactions be evoked?

PEPTIDE CHANGES IN AMYGDALA KINDLING: IMPLICATIONS FOR AFFECTIVE SYNDROMES

As noted above, pathways elucidated by *c-fos* induction may develop long-term alterations in biochemical or even structural adaptations following the repeated induction of kindled seizures. For example, Smith and associates (1991) have found that amygdala-kindled seizures lead to the transient induction of mRNA for corticotropin releasing hormone (CRH) in the dentate hilus. Both amygdala-kindled ADs alone, and full-blown seizures appear capable of inducing this CRH mRNA in neurons previously expressing low levels of the mRNA, and in new neurons where the substance had not previously been expressed. mRNA for CRH is increased at 24 h after the last amygdala-kindled seizure, but returns to normal levels by 3 weeks. Kubek and associates (1984, 1990) and Meyerhoff *et al.* (1990) have observed increases in TRH mRNA and TRH levels following the induction of electroconvulsive seizures or amygdala-kindled seizures. Rosen *et al.* (1992) in our laboratory have mapped the induction of TRH mRNA in detail following amygdala-kindled seizure evolution using *in situ* hybridization. They have observed (as in the case of *c-fos*) that in brain areas with negligible baseline levels of TRH mRNA, substantial inductions can occur first unilaterally in either dentate gyrus or pyriform cortex, and then bilaterally, with either repetition of amygdala-kindled stimulations or increasing length of afterdischarge. With full-blown stage 4 or 5 seizures, TRH mRNA induction appears more widespread with dentate gyrus, pyriform and entorhinal cortices all becoming activated bilaterally. TRH and its analogues have anticonvulsant properties against feline amygdala-kindled seizures (Sato *et al.*, 1984). Shinoda *et al.* (1989) have described increases in mRNA for somatostatin, and Higuchi *et al.* (1985) and Kato *et al.* (1983) have reported sustained increases in somatostatin immunoreactivity in brain following a series of amygdala-kindled or lidocaine-kindled seizures. Rosen and associates (1992) have observed increases in enkephalin mRNA in the entorhinal and pyriform cortices following stage 1 and 5 seizures, as well as decreases in mRNA for dynorphin in the dentate gyrus following stage 5 amygdala-kindled seizures. Much work remains to be conducted in order to clarify the spatio-temporal evolution of changes in the mRNA, and peptides themselves in brain, following amygdala kindling. Nonetheless, these preliminary data raise a number of intriguing perspectives of possible relevance to the affective disorders. In particular, could acute seizures induce longer-lasting changes in neurotransmitters and peptides that are critically dysregulated in affective illness?

A highly consistent body of literature has now documented activation of the hypothalamic-pituitary-adrenal axis in approximately 40% of patients with severe endogenous depression (Carroll *et al.*, 1980; Rubinow *et al.*, 1984b). This is typically manifested by increases in cortisol secretion measured either directly in blood or urine, or indirectly through the escape from dexamethasone suppression, or as revealed by a blunted ACTH response to CRF (Gold *et al.*, 1984; Holsboer, 1989). These data are convergent with a growing body of data indicating that the abnormality may be at the level of increased secretion of CRH itself since several studies (Nemeroff *et al.*, 1984; Risch *et al.*, 1990) have reported increased levels of CRH in the spinal fluid of endogenously depressed patients. Moreover, intrathecal administration of CRH in the rhesus monkey appears to yield a pattern of behaviour that is highly similar to that observed during the despair phase of the separation reaction in this primate species (Kalin, 1986), and i.c.v. CRH elicits *c-fos* induction in the same areas of brain as observed with amygdala kindling (Clark *et al.*, 1991b).

There is also evidence from Nemeroff and associates that TRH may be hypersecreted in depression, with elevated levels in CSF being reported (Banki *et al.*, 1988). Rubinow and associates (1984a) reported decreased levels of somatostatin in the cerebrospinal fluid of depressed patients, a finding that has been widely replicated by more than six investigative groups (for reviews, see Rubinow *et al.*, 1991; Post *et al.*, 1986a).

Thus, one is now in a position to question whether complex partial seizures of the temporal lobe and limbic system, as in the kindling model described above, are associated with the induction of neuropeptides in critical limbic and hypothalamic areas, as well as in related cortical structures that might then be associated with the emergence of affective symptomatology. If a similar spatio-temporal evolution of biological changes associated with kindled seizures and their excitatory and compensatory–inhibitory neuropeptide concomitants could be outlined in CPS then potential mechanisms relating to the complexities of the interrelationships between CPS and affective disorders noted above could be clarified.

One could propose a highly preliminary schema that could be directly tested. For example, transient inductions of CRH following a series of seizures could help 'explain' the appearance of depression, irritability, and other affective dysregulation immediately following a series of seizures. At the same time, either focal seizures or generalized seizures of electroconvulsive therapy can increase TRH secretion, perhaps as a compensatory anticonvulsant mechanism (Sato *et al.*, 1990; Kubek *et al.*, 1990). Depending upon whether the TRH hypersecretion of depression is of primary pathophysiological significance, or reflects a compensatory opposing mechanism (associated with anticonvulsant effects), one could conceptualize long-term neuropeptide alterations following seizures that could play either a facilitating or inhibitory role in the generation of affective symptomatology. Additionally, as the increases in somatostatin (SRIF) following a series of seizures dissipate, this could provide a biochemical substrate for the late-developing depression in some patients with CPS or those with an inverse relationship between seizures and affective experiences. These late changes in somatostatin or other peptides could even be a factor in the late onset of affective disorders following a temporal lobectomy and successful treatment of CPS.

While all of these propositions remain to be directly explored in subsequent clinical and basic laboratory studies, the conceptual paradigm offered here may provide a substrate for considering how acute convulsive events may lead to longer-lasting changes in the biochemical systems known to be linked to affective disturbances; i.e. increases in CRH, TRH and decreases in SRIF. Since these alterations occur both as a function of space and time and may be related to numbers, severity, and intervals between seizures, they provide a potential substrate for considering how the complexities of the relationships between seizures and affective disorders could be integrated into a single comprehensive framework. As more becomes known as to which neural substrates in the kindling process are critical to the emergence of affective disorders, integrating this anatomical information with the appearance and disappearance of associated classical neurotransmitter and neuropeptide alterations may provide the key to unlocking the puzzle of both the positive and inverse relationship between seizures and affective disorders and their overall relationship to the temporal lobe and related structures.

CLINICAL IMPLICATIONS AND CONCLUSIONS

While we have emphasized that seizures, particularly those involving limbic structures, may provide a paradigm for understanding the relationship to the affective disorders, other paradigms may also be useful in elucidating possible relationships between limbic system function and dysfunction in the affective disorders. We have discussed elsewhere (Silberman *et al.*, 1985; Post *et al.*, 1991) that patients with affective disorders show a high incidence of psychosensory and psychomotor alterations typically observed in patients with complex partial seizures (CPS) of the temporal lobe and limbic system. The specificity of these signs and symptoms as a reference to temporal lobe pathology remains to be demonstrated. Nevertheless, to the extent that these psychosensory symptoms do mark temporal lobe dysfunction, they raise the question of whether such symptoms might also be used to delineate response to psychotropic medication in the recurrent affective disorders.

There is increasing recognition that a large segment of patients with bipolar affective disorders are not responsive to treatment with lithium carbonate, and require use of the anticonvulsants carbamazepine or valproate, either alone or adjunctively with lithium (Post *et al.*, 1990). There are currently no well validated clinical or biological markers to predict which patient may respond to which therapeutic modality, although there is some evidence of differential response between carbamazepine and lithium, with poorer lithium responders being those with more fulminant onset mania, more dysphoric mania, more rapid cycling, and a negative family history of affective illness in first-degree relatives. While we have not observed that the presence of psychosensory symptoms predicts successful acute antidepressant or antimanic treatment with carbamazepine (in fact more psychosensory symptoms appear to be associated with better responses to lithium carbonate in our initial studies of Silberman *et al.*, 1985), more recent data of Hayes and Goldsmith (1991) suggest that bipolar patients who require treatment with anticonvulsants do show a greater history of self-reported psychosensory symptoms.

Thus, it is hoped that clinical indices, or electrophysiological or regional brain imaging studies, might identify a cohort of affectively ill patients with limbic system dysfunction who are more amenable to treatment with agents such as carbamazepine and valproate, known to stabilize paroxysmal neuronal activity in limbic areas of brain (Albright and Burnham, 1980), in contrast with lithium, which is ineffective in this regard (Post *et al.*, 1984d; Weiss *et al.*, unpublished observation, 1991). Having raised this proposition, we would emphatically highlight the caveat that response to anticonvulsants such as carbamazepine and valproate in the affective disorders cannot be used to infer that a seizure disorder, even a covert one, underlies the pathophysiology of this illness. We have argued elsewhere that the time-frame of acute anticonvulsant response to these agents is very different from their longer-term requirements for psychotropic efficacy, and different biochemical or physiological effects of these agents in different time courses may be involved in their anticonvulsant versus psychotropic efficacy (Post, 1988; Post *et al.*, 1990, 1992). Nonetheless, there may be common elements in the ability of these agents to dampen paroxysmal neural activity associated with seizure disorders and dysrhythmic activity in temporal lobe and limbic areas of the brain (not associated with a seizure), that are important to their common therapeutic efficacy in both seizures and affective disorders. Similarly, the major motor seizures of electroconvulsive therapy appear to exert not only anticonvulsant effects in some patients and seizure models (Post *et al.*, 1984b), but also are themselves highly effective in the treatment of primary affective disorder. In this fashion, it might be conceptualized how both seizures themselves (via their associated induction of compensatory endogenous anticonvulsant mechanisms) and anticonvulsant drugs may both be effective in the treatment of the affective disorders.

We are hopeful that an evocative procedure using intravenous infusions of procaine may be helpful in further dissecting the role of temporal lobe dysfunction and affective disorders. We have previously found that intravenous procaine administration appears to produce selective increases in fast EEG activity over temporal lobe structures in association with secretion of ACTH, cortisol, and prolactin (but not growth hormone), dose-related psychosensory symptoms, and diverse effects on mood, ranging from euphoria to dysphoria (Kellner *et al.*, 1987).

It is noteworthy that patients with affective disorders may be more prone to euphoric responses than either those patients with borderline personality disorder or normal volunteer subgroups (Kling *et al.*, unpublished observations). Recent studies of regional blood flow using O-15 PET methodology also suggest that (concomitant with emotional changes) procaine may yield increases in blood flow in anterior temporal structures, providing further validation both of procaine as a probe of limbic system and anterior temporal lobe structures (Kellner *et al.*, 1987) and of the relationship of these structures to emotional processes. This may provide the groundwork for a series of studies not only to assess diagnostic group differences in response to procaine's effects on mood, behaviour, cerebral blood flow, EEG, and endocrine responsivity, but also potentially to identify patients who are or are not responsive to anticonvulsant modalities in the treatment of their affective disorder.

A final perspective may be of interest in considering how temporal lobe and limbic structures could play a role in the affective disorders. We have illustrated how an acute ictal event comes to evoke a brief induction of the proto-oncogene *c-fos*, which then leads to longer-lasting alterations in neuropeptide function. This paradigm might then be relevant in considering how acute events such as psychosocial stressors may trigger longer-lasting biochemical processes that could be associated with the development of primary affective disorders. Nakajima *et al.* (1989a,b) and others (Bullitt, 1989; Draisci and Iadarola, 1989) have demonstrated that stressors can induce *c-fos* in some of the same areas of brain activated by amygdala kindling. Specifically, the stress of the ear clips placed as the control procedure for animals not receiving electroconvulsive seizures is sufficient to produce notable increases in *c-fos* in pyriform cortex and hippocampus of mice (Nakajima *et al.*, 1989a). Others have demonstrated stress-induced *c-fos* in other areas of brain such as paraventricular and supraoptic nuclei with 24 h water deprivation (Sagar *et al.*, 1988).

Since it has long been recognized that critical psychosocial stressors may play an idiopathogenic role in the triggering of affective disorders (for reviews, see Post *et al.*, 1986b; Post, 1992), the same questions regarding the spatio-temporal consequences of *c-fos* and other proto-oncogene induction that were raised for acute ictal events become pertinent to the consequences induced by psychosocial stressors. This provides a mechanism for conceptualizing how acute psychosocial events may lead to longer lasting neurotransmitter and neuropeptide events in the brain associated with the affective disorders (Post, 1992). It is noteworthy that the pyriform cortex and dentate gyrus of the hippocampus (the two entry points into the critical early stages of amygdala kindling) are similarly implicated in the regional expression of *c-fos* induction following some types of stressors (Nakajima *et al.*, 1989a,b) and following injection of CRH (Clark *et al.*, 1991b). Is this a potential for conceptualizing how psychosocial stressors, like behavioural sensitization to the psychomotor stimulants, could progressively produce increases in activity upon subsequent reactivation, as postulated elsewhere (Post *et al.*, 1984c, 1987b; Post, 1990b)? While it is apparent that psychosocial stressors are intimately involved in the precipitation of initial episodes of major affective disorder, with successive recurrences, identifiable psychosocial stressors are less apparent (Post, 1992). Eventually, with enough repetitions of affective episodes, manias and depressions begin to occur autonomously. Could this represent the transition, akin to the transition to spontaneity in amygdala kindling, where the requisite for triggering by exogenous stimulation, which was apparent earlier in the evolution of the process, is no longer needed?

In this fashion, it is hoped that some of the analogies and lessons drawn from the data on amygdala kindling may be pertinent to conceptualizing the evolution of affective disorders, how initial acute events can lead to longer-lasting vulnerabilities to affective disorders, and how processes which were initially triggered can occur spontaneously. Perhaps in this fashion one can now reformulate questions and empirical tests, not of whether the temporal lobes and limbic structures are involved in affective disorders, but what are the specific time courses, anatomical areas, and mechanisms involved?

REFERENCES

Ackermann, R.F., Engel Jr, J. and Phelps, M.E. (1986). Identification of seizure-mediating brain structures with the deoxyglucose method: studies of human epilepsy with positron emission tomography, and animal seizure models with contact autoradiography. *Adv. Neurol.*, **44**, 921–934.

Adamec, R.E. (1990). Does kindling model anything clinically relevant? *Biol. Psychiatry*, **27**, 249–279.

Adamec, R.E. and Stark-Adamec, C. (1983). Limbic kindling and animal behavior-implications for human psychopathology associated with complex partial seizures. *Biol. Psychiatry*, **18**, 269–293.

Albright, P.S. and Burnham, W.M. (1980). Development of a new pharmacological seizure model: effects of anticonvulsants on cortical- and amygdala-kindled seizures in the rat. *Epilepsia*, **21**, 681–689.

Altshuler, L. (1991). Depression and epilepsy. In: Theodore, W.H. and Devinsky, O. (Eds), *Epilepsy and Behavior*, Wiley-Liss, Inc., New York, pp. 47–65.

Banki, C.M., Bissette, G., Arato, M. and Nemeroff, C.B. (1988). Elevation of immunoreactive CSF TRH in depressed patients. *Am. J. Psychiatry*, **145**, 1526–1531.

Bawden, H.N. and Racine, R.J. (1979). Effects of bilateral kindling or bilateral subthreshold stimulation of the amygdala or septum on muricide, ranacide, intraspecific aggression and passive avoidance in the rat. *Physiol. Behav.*, **22**, 115–123.

Baxter Jr, L.R., Phelps, M.E., Mazziotta, J.C., Schwartz, J.M., Gerner, R.H., Selin, C.E. and Sumida, R.M. (1985). Cerebral metabolic rates for glucose in mood disorders. Studies with positron emission tomography and fluorodeoxyglucose F 18. *Arch. Gen. Psychiatry*, **42**, 441–447.

Baxter Jr, L.R., Schwartz, J.M., Phelps, M.E., Mazziotta, J.C., Guze, B.H., Selin, C.E., Gerner, R.H. and Sumida, R.M. (1989). Reduction of prefrontal cortex glucose metabolism common to three types of depression. *Arch. Gen. Psychiatry*, **46**, 243–250.

Belenkov, N.Y.U. and Shalkovskaya, L.N. (1980). Role of dominant motivation in manifestation of the effects of electrical stimulation of the hypothalamus and limbic region. *Neurosci. Behav. Physiol.*, **10**, 112–117.

Brent, D.A., Crumrine, P.K., Varma, R., Brown, R.V. and Allan, M.J. (1990). Phenobarbital treatment and major depressive disorder in children with epilepsy: a naturalistic follow-up. *Pediatrics*, **85**, 1086–1091.

Bromfield, E.B., Altshuler, L., Leiderman, D.B., Balish, M., Ketter, T.A., Devinsky, O., Post, R.M. and Theodore, W.H. (1992). Cerebral metabolism and depression in patients with complex partial seizures. *Arch. Neurol.*, submitted.

Buchsbaum, M.S., Delisi, L.E., Holcomb, H.H., Cappelletti, J., King, A.C., Johnson, J., Hazlett, E., Dowling-Zimmerman, S., Post, R.M., Morihisa, J., Carpenter, W., Cohen, R., Pickar, D., Weinberger, D.R., Margolin, R. and Kessler, R.M. (1984). Anteroposterior gradients in cerebral glucose use in schizophrenia and affective disorders. *Arch. Gen. Psychiatry*, **41**, 1159–1166.

Buchsbaum, M.S., Wu, J., Delisi, L.E., Holcomb, H., Kessler, R., Johnson, J., King, A.C., Hazlett, E., Langston, K. and Post, R.M. (1986). Frontal cortex and basal ganglia metabolic rates assessed by positron emission tomography with [18F]2-deoxyglucose in affective illness. *J. Affective Disord.*, **10**, 137–152.

Bullitt, E. (1989). Induction of c-fos-like protein within the lumbar spinal cord and thalamus of the rat following peripheral stimulation. *Brain Res.*, **493**, 391–397.

Carroll, B.J., Feinberg, M., Greden, J.F., Haskett, R.F., James, N.M., Steiner, M. and Tarika, J. (1980). Diagnosis of endogenous depression. Comparison of clinical, research and neuroendocrine criteria. *J. Affective Disord.*, **2**, 177–194.

Clark, M., Post, R.M., Weiss, S.R.B., Cain, C.J. and Nakajima, T. (1991a). Regional expression of c-fos mRNA in rat brain during the evolution of amygdala kindled seizures. *Mol. Brain Res.*, **11**, 55–64.

Clark, M., Weiss, S.R.B. and Post, R.M. (1991b). Expression of c-fos mRNA in rat brain after intracerebroventricular administration of corticotropin-releasing hormone. *Neurosci. Lett.*, **132**, 235–238.

Dongier, S. (1960). Statistical study of clinical and electroencephalographic manifestations of 536 psychotic episodes occurring in 516 epileptics between clinical seizures. *Epilepsia*, **1**, 117–142.

Douglas, R.M., Dragunow, M. and Robertson, H.A. (1988). High-frequency discharge of dentate granule cells, but not long-term potentiation, induces c-fos protein. *Mol. Brain Res.*, **464**, 259–262.

Dragunow, M. and Robertson, H.A. (1987). Kindling stimulation induces c-fos protein(s) in granule cells of the rat dentate gyrus. *Nature*, **329**, 441–442.

Dragunow, M., Currie, R.W., Faull, R.L., Robertson, H.A. and Jansen, K. (1989). Immediate-early genes, kindling and long-term potentiation. *Neurosci. Biobehav. Rev.*, **13**, 301–313.

Draisci, G. and Iadarola, M.J. (1989). Temporal analysis of increases in c-fos, preprodynorphin and preproenkephalin mRNAs in rat spinal cord. *Mol. Brain Res.*, **6**, 31–37.

Edeh, J. and Toone, B. (1987). Relationship between interictal psychopathology and the type of epilepsy. Results of a survey in general practice. *Br. J. Psychiatry*, **151**, 95–101.

Ehlers, C.L., Henriksen, S.J., Wang, M., Rivier, J., Vale, W. and Bloom, F.E. (1983).

Corticotropin releasing factor produces increases in brain excitability and convulsive seizures in rats. *Brain Res.*, **278**, 332–336.
Engel Jr, J., Kuhl, D.E. and Phelps, M.E. (1982). Patterns of human local cerebral glucose metabolism during epileptic seizures. *Science*, **218**, 64–66.
Ervin, F.R., Mark, V.H. and Stevens, J. (1969). Behavioral and affective responses to brain stimulation in man. *Proc. Annu. Mtg. Am. Psychopathol. Assoc.*, **58**, 54–65.
Fink, M. (1984). Theories of the antidepressant efficacy of convulsive therapy (ECT). In: Post, R.M. and Ballenger, J.C. (Eds), *Neurobiology of Mood Disorders*, Williams & Wilkins, Baltimore, pp. 721–730.
Flor-Henry, P. (1969). Psychosis and temporal lobe epilepsy: a controlled investigation. *Epilepsia*, **10**, 363–395.
Flynn, J.P., Foote, W. and Edwards, S. (1970). Neural mechanisms involved in a cat's attack on a rat. In: Whalen, R.E., Thompson, R.F., Verzeano, M. and Weinberger, N.M. (Eds), *The Neural Control of Behavior*, Academic Press, New York, pp. 210–240.
Gloor, P., Olivier, A., Quesney, L.F., Andermann, F. and Horowitz, S. (1982). The role of the limbic system in experiential phenomena of temporal lobe epilepsy. *Ann. Neurol.*, **12**, 129–144.
Goddard, G.V., McIntyre, D.C. and Leech, G.K. (1969). A permanent change in brain function resulting from daily electrical stimulation. *Exp. Neurol.*, **25**, 295–330.
Gold, P.W., Chrousos, G., Kellner, C., Post, R.M., Roy, A., Avgerinos, P., Schulte, H., Oldfield, E. and Loriaux, D.L. (1984). Psychiatric implications of basic and clinical studies with corticotropin-releasing factor. *Am. J. Psychiatry*, **141**, 619–627.
Halgren, E. (1981). The amygdala contribution to emotion and memory: current studies in humans. In: Ben-Ari, Y. (Ed.), *The Amygdaloid Complex*, Elsevier/North-Holland Biomedical Press, Amsterdam, pp. 395–408.
Halgren, E., Walter, R.D., Cherlow, D.G. and Crandall, P.H. (1978). Mental phenomena evoked by electrical stimulation of the human hippocampal formation and amygdala. *Brain*, **101**, 83–117.
Hayes, S.G. and Goldsmith, B.K. (1991). Psychosensory symptomatology in anticonvulsant-responsive psychiatric illness. *Ann. Clin. Psychiatry*, **3**, 27–35.
Higuchi, T., Kato, N. and Noguchi, T. (1985). Kindling and somatostatin. In: Wada, J.A. (Ed.), *Kindling III*, Raven Press, New York, pp. 349–360.
Holsboer, F. (1989). Psychiatric implications of altered limbic-hypothalamic-pituitary-adrenocortical activity. *Eur. Arch. Psychiatry Neurol. Sci.*, **238**, 302–322.
Kalin, N.H. (1986). ACTH in plasma and CSF in the rhesus monkey. *Biol. Psychiatry*, **21**, 124–140.
Kato, N., Higuchi, T. and Friesen, H.G. (1983). Changes of immunoreactive somatostatin and beta-endorphin content in rat brain after amygdala kindling. *Life Sci.*, **32**, 2415–2422.
Kellner, C.H., Post, R.M., Putnam, F., Cowdry, R.W., Gardner, D., Kling, M.A., Minichiello, M.D., Trettau, J.R. and Coppola, R. (1987). Intravenous procaine as a probe of limbic system activity in psychiatric patients and normal controls. *Biol. Psychiatry*, **22**, 1107–1126.
Kopa, J., Szabo, I. and Grastyan, E. (1968). A dual behavioral effect from stimulating the same thalamic point with identical stimulus parameter in different conditional reflex situations. In: Gellhorn, E. (Ed.), *Biological Foundations of Emotion*, Scott, Foresman & Co., Glenview, Illinois, pp. 107–127.
Kristensen, O. and Sindrup, E.H. (1978). Psychomotor epilepsy and psychosis. *Acta Neurol. Scand.*, **57**, 370–379.
Kubek, M.J., Meyerhoff, J.L., Hill, T.G., Norton, J.A. and Sattin, A. (1984). Effects

of subconvulsive and repeated electroconvulsive shock on thyrotropin-releasing hormone in the rat brain. *Life Sci.*, **36**, 315–320.

Kubek, M.J., Fuson, K.S., Aydelotte, M.R. and Knoblach, S.M. (1990). Kindling increases neuronal production of thyrotropin-releasing hormone mRNA in seizure foci as determined by in situ hybridization histochemistry. *Epilepsia*, **31**, 633.

Landolt, A. (1958). Serial EEG investigations during psychotic episodes in epileptic patients and during schizophrenic attacks. In: de Haas, L. (Ed.), *Lectures on Epilepsy*, Elsevier, Amsterdam.

MacLean, P.D. (1990). *The Triune Brain in Evolution: Role in Paleocerebral Functions*, Plenum Press, New York.

Mayberg, H.S., Starkstein, S.E., Sadzot, B., Preziosi, T., Andrezejewski, P.L., Dannals, R.F., Wagner Jr, H.N. and Robinson, R.G. (1990a). Selective hypometabolism in the inferior frontal lobe in depressed patients with Parkinson's disease. *Ann. Neurol.*, **28**, 57–64.

Mayberg, H.S., Starkstein, S.E., Peyser, C.E., Folstein, S.E., Dannals, R.F., Folstein, M.F. and Wagner Jr, H.N. (1990b). Cerebral glucose utilization in Huntington's Disease: inferior frontal hypometabolism identifies patients with major depression. *Soc. Neurosci. Abstr.*, **16**, 139.

Meyerhoff, J.L., Bates, V.E. and Kubek, M.J. (1990). Elevated TRH levels in pyriform cortex after partial and fully generalized kindled seizures. *Brain Res.*, **525**, 144–148.

Milstein, V., Small, J.G., Klapper, M.H., Small, I.F., Miller, M.J. and Kellams, J.J. (1987). Uni- versus bi-lateral ECT in the treatment of mania. *Convulsive Ther.*, **3**, 1–9.

Mizrahi, E.M., Kellaway, P., Grossman, R.G., Rutecki, P.A., Armstrong, D., Rettig, G. and Loewen, S. (1990). Anterior temporal lobectomy and medically refractory temporal lobe epilepsy of childhood. *Epilepsia*, **31**, 302–312.

Morgan, J.I. and Curran, T. (1988). Calcium as a modulator of the immediate-early gene cascade in neurons. *Cell Calcium*, **9**, 303–311.

Morgan, J.I. and Curran, T. (1989). Stimulus-transcription coupling in neurons: role of cellular immediate-early genes. *Trends Neurosci.*, **12**, 459–462.

Mukherjee, S., Sackeim, H.A. and Lee, C. (1988). Unilateral ECT in the treatment of manic episodes. *Convulsive Ther.*, **4**, 74–80.

Nakajima, T., Daval, J.L., Gleiter, C.H., Deckert, J., Post, R.M. and Marangos, P.J. (1989a). C-fos mRNA expression following electrical-induced seizure and acute nociceptive stress in mouse brain. *Epilepsy Res.*, **4**, 156–159.

Nakajima, T., Post, R.M., Weiss, S.R.B., Pert, A. and Ketter, T. (1989b). Perspectives on the mechanism of action of electroconvulsive therapy: anticonvulsant, dopaminergic, and c-fos oncogene effects. *Convulsive Ther.*, **5**, 274–295.

Nemeroff, C.B., Widerlöv, E. and Bissette, G. (1984). Elevated concentrations of CSF corticotropin-releasing factor-like immunoreactivity in depressed patients. *Science*, **226**, 1342–1344.

O'Connell, R.A., Van Heertum, R.L., Billick, S.B., Holt, A.R., Gonzalez, A., Notardonato, H., Luck, D. and King, L.N. (1989). Single photon emission computed tomography with [123I] IMP in the differential diagnosis of psychiatric disorders. *J. Neuropsychiatry*, **1**, 145–153.

Pakalnis, A., Drake, M.E., John, K. and Kellum, J.B. (1987). Forced normalization: acute psychosis after seizure control in seven patients. *Arch. Neurol.*, **44**, 289–292.

Penfield, W. and Perot, P. (1963). The brain's record of auditory and visual experience: a final summary and discussion. *Brain*, **86**, 595–696.

Pinel, J.P.J. (1981). Kindling-induced experimental epilepsy in rats: cortical stimulation. *Exp. Neurol.*, **72**, 559–569.

Pinel, J.P.J. and Rovner, L.I. (1978). Experimental epileptogenesis: kindling-induced epilepsy in rats. *Exp. Neurol.*, **58**, 190–202.

Pinel, J.P.J., Treit, D. and Rovner, L.I. (1977). Temporal lobe aggression in rats. *Science*, **197**, 1088–1089.

Porrino, L.J., Esposito, R.U., Seeger, T.F., Crane, A.M., Pert, A. and Sokoloff, L. (1984). Metabolic mapping of the brain during rewarding self-stimulation. *Science*, **224**, 306–309.

Post, R.M. (1986). Does limbic system dysfunction play a role in affective illness. In: Doane, B.K. and Livingston, K.E. (Eds), *The Limbic System: Functional Organization and Clinical Disorders*, Raven Press, New York, pp. 229–249.

Post, R.M. (1988). Time course of clinical effects of carbamazepine: implications for mechanisms of action. *J. Clin. Psychiatry*, **49**, 35–46.

Post, R.M. (1990a). Alternatives to lithium for bipolar affective illness. In: Tasman, A., Goldfinger, S.M. and Kaufmann, C.A. (Eds), *Review of Psychiatry, Vol. 9*, American Psychiatric Press, Inc., Washington, D.C., pp. 170–202.

Post, R.M. (1990b). Sensitization and kindling perspectives for the course of affective illness: toward a new treatment with the anticonvulsant carbamazepine. *Pharmacopsychiatry*, **23**, 3–17.

Post, R.M. (1992). The transduction of psychosocial stress into the neurobiology of recurrent affective disorder. *Am. J. Psychiatry*, in press.

Post, R.M., Kennedy, C., Shinohara, M., Squillace, K., Miyaoka, M., Suda, S., Ingvar, D.H. and Sokoloff, L. (1984a). Metabolic and behavioral consequences of lidocaine-kindled seizures. *Brain Res.*, **324**, 295–303.

Post, R.M., Putnam, F.W., Contel, N.R. and Goldman, B. (1984b). Electroconvulsive seizures inhibit amygdala kindling: implications for mechanisms of action in affective illness. *Epilepsia*, **25**, 234–239.

Post, R.M., Rubinow, D.R. and Ballenger, J.C. (1984c). Conditioning, sensitization, and kindling: implications for the course of affective illness. In: Post, R.M. and Ballenger, J.C. (Eds), *Neurobiology of Mood Disorders*, Williams & Wilkins, Baltimore, pp. 432–466.

Post, R.M., Weiss, S.R.B. and Pert, A. (1984d). Differential effects of carbamazepine and lithium on sensitzation and kindling. *Prog. Neuropsychopharmacol. Biol. Psychiatry*, **8**, 425–434.

Post, R.M., Rubinow, D.R. and Gold, P.W. (1986a). Neuropeptides in manic-depressive illness. In: Nemeroff, C.B. (Ed.), *Neuropeptides in Psychiatric and Neurological Disease*, Johns Hopkins University Press, Baltimore, pp. 76–115.

Post, R.M., Uhde, T.W., Joffe, R.T. and Bierer, L. (1986b). Psychiatric manifestations and implications of seizure disorders. In: Extein, I. and Gold, M. (Eds), *Medical Mimics of Psychiatric Disorders*, American Psychiatric Association Press, Washington, D.C., pp. 35–91.

Post, R.M., Delisi, L.E., Holcomb, H.H., Uhde, T.W., Cohen, R. and Buchsbaum, M.S. (1987a). Glucose utilization in the temporal cortex of affectively ill patients: positron emission tomography. *Biol. Psychiatry*, **22**, 545–553.

Post, R.M., Weiss, S.R.B. and Pert, A. (1987b). The role of context in conditioning and behavioral sensitization to cocaine. *Psychopharmacol Bull.*, **23**, 425–429.

Post, R.M., Weiss, S.R.B., Nakajima, T., Clark, M. and Pert, A. (1990). Mechanism-based approaches to anticonvulsant therapy. In: Meldrum, B.S. and Williams, M. (Eds), *Current and Future Trends in Anticonvulsant Anxiety and Stroke Therapy*, Wiley-Liss, Inc., New York, pp. 45–90.

Post, R.M., Altshuler, L.L., Ketter, T. A., Denicoff, K. and Weiss, S.R.B. (1991). Antiepileptic drugs in affective illness: clinical and theoretical implications. In: Smith, D.B., Treiman, D.M. and Trimble, M.R. (Eds), *Advances in Neurology, Vol. 55, Neurobehavioral Problems in Epilepsy*, Raven Press, New York, pp. 239–277.

Post, R.M., Weiss, S.R.B. and Chuang, D.-M. (1992). Mechanisms of action of anticonvulsants in affective disorders: comparisons with lithium. *J. Clin. Psychopharmacol.*, **12**, 235–355.

Racine, R. (1978). Kindling: the first decade. *Neurosurgery*, **3**, 234–252.

Ring, H. and Trimble, M.R. (1992). Depression in epilepsy. In: Robinson, R.G. and Starkstein, S.E. (Eds), *Depression in Neurological Disease,* Johns Hopkins Press, Baltimore.

Risch, S.C., Lewine, R.J., Jewart, R.D., Kalin, N.H., Stipetic, M., Risby, E.D., Eccard, M.B., Caudle, J., Pollard, W.E. and Brummer, M. (1990). The relationship between structural brain imaging, limbic HPA activity and CSF CRF and catecholamine metabolites in affective disorders and schizophrenia. *Clin. Neuropharmacol.*, **13**, 601–602.

Robertson, M.M. and Trimble, M.R. (1983). Depressive illness in patients with epilepsy. *Epilepsia*, **24**, S109–S116.

Rosen, J.B., Cain, C.J., Weiss, S.R.B. and Post, R.M. (1992). Alterations in mRNA of enkephalin, dynorphin and thyrotropin releasing hormone during amygdala kindling: An in situ hybridization study. *Mol. Brain Res.,* in press.

Rubinow, D.R., Gold, P.W., Post, R.M., Ballenger, J.C. and Cowdry, R.W. (1984a). Somatostatin in patients with affective illness and normal volunteers. In: Post, R.M. and Ballenger, J.C. (Eds), *Neurobiology of Mood Disorders*, Williams & Wilkins, Baltimore, pp. 369–387.

Rubinow, D.R., Post, R.M., Gold, P.W., Ballenger, J.C. and Wolff, E.A. (1984b). The relationship between cortisol and clinical phenomenology of affective illness. In: Post, R.M. and Ballenger, J.C. (Eds), *Neurobiology of Mood Disorders*, Williams & Wilkins, Baltimore, pp. 271–289.

Rubinow, D.R., Davis, C.L. and Post, R.M. (1991). Somatostatin. In: Nemeroff, C. (Ed.), *Neuropeptides in Psychiatry*, APA Press, Washington DC, pp. 31–49.

Sagar, S.M., Sharp, F.R. and Curran, T. (1988). Expression of c-fos protein in brain: metabolic mapping at the cellular level. *Science*, **240**, 1328–1331.

Satinoff, E. (1978). Neural organization and evolution of thermal regulation in mammals. *Science*, **201**, 16–22.

Sato, M., Morimoto, K. and Wada, J.A. (1984). Antiepileptic effects of thyrotropin-releasing hormone and its new derivative, DN-1417, examined in feline amygdaloid kindling preparation. *Epilepsia*, **25**, 537–544.

Sato, M., Racine, R.J. and McIntyre, D.C. (1990). Kindling: basic mechanisms and clinical validity. *Electroencephalogr. Clin. Neurophysiol.*, **76**, 459–472.

Schwartz, J.A., Speed, N.M., Mountz, J.M., Gross, M.D., Modell, J.G. and Kuhl, D.E. (1990). ^{99m}Tc-hexamethylpropyleneamine oxime single photon emission CT in poststroke depression. *Am. J. Psychiatry*, **147**, 242–244.

Schwartz, J.M., Baxter, L.R., Mazziotta, J.C., Gerner, R.H. and Phelps, M.E. (1987). The differential diagnosis of depression: relevance of positron emission tomography studies of cerebral glucose metabolism to the bipolar-unipolar dichotomy. *J. Am. Med. Assoc.*, **258**, 1368–1374.

Shin, C., McNamara, J.O., Morgan, J.I., Curran, T. and Cohen, D.R. (1990). Induction of c-fos mRNA expression by afterdischarge in the hippocampus of naive and kindled rats. *J. Neurochem.*, **55**, 1050–1055.

Shinoda, H., Nadi, N.S. and Schwartz, J.P. (1991). Alterations in somatostatin and proenkephalin mRNA in response to a single amygdaloid stimulation versus kindling. *Mol. Brain Res.*, **11**: 221–226.

Silberman, E.K., Post, R.M., Nurnberger, J., Theodore, W. and Boulenger, J.-P. (1985). Transient sensory, cognitive, and affective phenomena in affective illness: a comparison with complex partial epilepsy. *Br. J. Psychiatry*, **146**, 81–89.

Slater, E., Beard, A.W. and Glithero, E. (1963). The schizophrenia-like psychosis of epilepsy. *Br. J. Psychiatry*, **109**, 95–150.

Smith, M., Weiss, S.R.B., Abedin, T., Post, R.M. and Gold, P. (1991). Effects of amygdala-kindling and electroconvulsive seizures on the expression of corticotropin releasing hormone (CRH) mRNA in the rat brain. *Mol. Cell. Neurosci.*, **2**, 104–116.

Stevens, J.R., Mark, V.H., Ervin, F., Pacheco, P. and Suematsu, K. (1969). Deep temporal stimulation in man. *Arch. Neurol.*, **21**, 157–169.

Theodore, W.H., Fishbein, D., Deitz, M. and Baldwin, P. (1987). Complex partial seizures: cerebellar metabolism. *Epilepsia*, **28**, 319–323.

Valenstein, E.S., Cox, V.C. and Kakolewski, J.W. (1970). Reexamination of the role of the hypothalamus in motivation. *Psychol. Rev.*, **77**, 16–31.

von Meduna, L.J. (1935). Die Knvulsionstherapie der Schizophrenie. *Psychiatr. Neurol. Wochenschr.*, **37**, 317–319.

Wada, J.A. and Sato, M. (1974). Generalized convulsive seizures induced by daily electrical stimulation of the amygdala in cats. *Neurology*, **24**, 565–574.

Wada, J.A., Sato, M., Wake, A., Green, J.R. and Troupin, A.S. (1976). Prophylactic effects of phenytoin, phenobarbital, and carbamazepine examined in kindled cat preparations. *Arch. Neurol.*, **33**, 426–434.

Weiss, S.R.B., Post, R.M., Gold, P.W., Chrousos, G., Sullivan, T.L., Walker, D. and Pert, A. (1986). CRF-induced seizures and behavior: interaction with amygdala kindling. *Brain Res.*, **372**, 345–351.

Wolf, P. (1991). Acute behavioral symptomatology at disappearance of epileptiform EEG abnormality: paradoxical or 'forced' normalization. In: Smith, D.B., Treiman, D.M. and Trimble, M.R. (Eds), *Advances in Neurology, Vol. 55, Neurobehavioral Problems in Epilepsy*, Raven Press, New York, pp. 127–142.

The Temporal Lobes and the Limbic System
Edited by M.R. Trimble and T.G. Bolwig

18

Brain and Consciousness

J.R. SMYTHIES
Department of Neuropsychiatry, Institute of Neurology, The National Hospital, Queen Square, London, UK

INTRODUCTION

The study of the brain–mind relationship has traditionally been done by philosophers, but with hardly any progress since Plato and Aristotle. Recently, however, it has seemed possible that the problem can be tackled by science. In this chapter I will suggest that the real brain–mind problem arises because we have two quite different ways of obtaining information about reality. One is ordinary seeing, or perception, in which we gain information about the brain and its workings. The other is introspection, as carried out by psychologists, in which case we observe our own sensations and can catalogue and classify their properties. An exact analogy is given by television. In TV we can either examine the images on the TV screen as they really are—a series of coloured parallel lines: or we can accept the TV picture as giving us a view of what is going on in the TV studio. Charlesworth (1979) has argued that television is a good model for how perception works, as first suggested by Grey Walter (1950). The TV image is in direct causal relation to the events it portrays and its images 'carry their own significance', i.e. are not coded. In the TV system the information is coded in the TV camera, is then transmitted and processed, and finally is decoded by the raster (or scanning) mechanism in the TV set. The brain–mind problem is not about how to locate *functions* such as memory or intelligence in the brain, there is little problem about that; it is about how to locate *phenomena*, i.e. our sensations.

Perception

We now know a good deal about how the brain works in visual perception. This is mediated by Hubel and Weisel analysers, parallel distributed processing in nerve nets, Freeman's neuronal cell assemblies co-ordinated by the 40 Hz (gamma) rhythm, Meyrand's central pattern generators and so on—a vastly complex pattern of *coded* information in the nerve nets of the brain.

Introspection

In introspection psychology we also have a vast body of data on the nature and properties of phenomenal consciousness; in the case of visual perception the properties and behaviour of the *visual field*—the array of our sensations that we experience in consciousness (see the comprehensive review by Vernon, 1962). The properties of the *basic* visual field are revealed by the Ganzfeld experiments. In this the stimulus is a uniform and featureless field of light. This is experienced as a misty two-dimensional film situated in front of the observer 'O'. A similar 'basic' field may be experienced in the pitch dark. Contrary to 'common sense', in the pitch dark we do not see just 'nothing'. On the contrary, 'As Locke well knew, and as Lord Brain has reminded us. . .' (Wright, 1981), darkness is a positive state which we experience and observe as a black field. This basic visual field is roughly circular in shape (certainly not square or triangular) and is coloured *black*, or in the Ganzfeld situation, *white*. We know this because in the Ganzfeld situation in about one third of the subjects quite a new phenomenon develops which is a complete disappearance of the entire faculty of vision, which they find very frightening. They will say they have gone blind and can no longer see even blackness. In this case they really do see nothing as they do not see at all. This 'field' or 'screen' is the terminal of the representative mechanism of visual perception on which are projected, when our eyes are open, the coloured and spatial sensations of our normal visual experience that *represent* external events, just as the pictures on the TV screen represent events in the TV studio. Thus we can say that the fundamental properties of our sensations are extension in space, colour, and movement.

THE BRAIN–MIND PROBLEM

The brain–mind problem may now be stated: (i) how can we relate the (coded) spatio-temporal pattern of events in the nerve nets in the visual areas of the cortex to the (quite different) spatio-temporal pattern of events in the visual field, and (ii) how does the visual brain, as a piece of communication mechanism, mechanically construct these images in the visual field, which is also a part of (the end stage of) this communication mechanism?

The most fashionable theory of the mind–brain relationship at present is some form of the Identity Theory, in which mental events are supposed to be *identical* to certain brain events. But, once we have grasped the intrinsic spatio-temporal nature of consciousness, we must come to realise that this theory is quite untenable: for two reasons: (a) the brain patterns are incongruous with the patterns in the visual field; and two spatio-temporal patterns must be *congruous* in order to be identical—a square, for example, cannot be identical with a circle, nor a sphere with a doughnut. This is a fact of basic geometry; (b) the events in the brain are a *coded* version of external events, whereas the corresponding events in the visual field are *uncoded*, and it is axiomatic that *x* and a coded version of *x* cannot be *identical.* Russell Brain (1960) was the first to draw attention to this problem, 'Somehow this coding of spatial information in a spatio-temporal pattern of frequencies [in the sensory cortex] is decoded into a static representation of a spatial pattern. How this is done goes to the heart of the brain–mind relationship'. Sherrington (1940) put it thus, 'It is a far cry from an electrical reaction in the brain to suddenly seeing the world around us, with all its colours, its distances and chiaroscuro'.

Problem (i) has recently surfaced in neuroscience in the form of the 'binding' problem discussed by Churchland (1986), Anderson and Palca (1988), and others quoted by these authors. The problem arises in the following manner. The visual pathways in the cortex have now been mapped in fair detail (Zeki and Schipp, 1988) and it appears that the three visual functions of colour, shape and motion are processed in three different mechanisms that remain anatomically separate, except for cross-links, for as far up the visual mechanism as they have been traced, i.e. to cortical visual areas V5 and V6. It is certain that, in the phenomenal object, the colour, the shape and the movement are located in one and the same spatial location. The correlated neuronal events in the brain are located in three different places. How, then, can they be identical? Churchland (1986) puts the problem thus: 'A fundamental puzzle concerning visual perception arises from the fact that cells in different areas of the cortex appear to be specialized to respond to different dimensions of the physical stimulus. . .In other words, perceptual features seem arranged by topic and dispersed hither and thither around the visual cortex. Our perceptions, by contrast, show no such disunity. One sees a unified composite, such as a running black dog or a falling yellow ball. We seem to be driven to the inference that there must be neuronal means for conjoining distinct properties—yellow colour and roundness—such that what is seen is seen as a yellow ball'. Anderson and Palca (1988) say, 'But if sensory pathways operate in parallel, how do they ever get back together to form the integrated image of the visual field that we see with the mind's eye? Hubel acknowledges that we "don't have the slightest idea. In fact we sometimes wonder if it is necessary to suppose that they get together at all.

Could they not be parallel and independent and not have any final pathway?"'.

This also becomes a problem in mathematics, i.e. in topology which is the mathematics dealing with fundamental spatial relations between spatial entities. Further light is thrown on the binding problem by the fact that this construction of the unitary perceptual object (Churchland's 'unified composite perception') can break down in the case of certain brain lesions to produce the phenomenon of 'space' or 'film' colours. In this the colour spreads out of the phenomenal object into the surrounding phenomenal space. Clearly the mechanism that normally keeps the colour *in* the object has gone wrong. Furthermore shape and movement can become dissociated in two ways—apparent movement (such as the phi phenomenon in which two adjacent blinking lights are seen as one light hopping from side to side), and a phenomenon seen under the influence of hallucinogenic drugs in which, for example, a lighted cigarette whirled rapidly round at arm's length in a circle is seen as a dozen or so stationary glowing balls strung out in a circle along the path of the cigarette. Under these drugs many types of these interchanges between shape and movement may be seen.

Freeman (1990), working particularly with olfaction, has discovered what the highest neural mechanisms concerned in perception are like. This concerns the role of neuronal cell assemblies (NCAs) and chaos in brain function. He reports that 'perception depends on the simultaneous, co-operative activity of millions of neurons spread throughout expanses of the cortex. . .every neuron in the [olfactory] bulb participates in generating each olfactory perception'. This information is carried by 40 Hz electrical rhythms that Freeman calls γ waves. The wave form does not carry information but the *amplitude pattern* across the entire olfactory cortex does. This pattern of γ wave activity is generated by a unique nerve cell assembly (NCA) that functions according to the principles of mathematical chaos. Gray *et al.* (1989) have provided evidence that a similar system may operate in the visual cortex.

Thus the problem reduces to discovering the relationship between one set of events, A, arranged with the introspectively observed properties of the phenomenological object in consciousness (e.g. in the case of the round yellow bouncing ball, experienced as spatially integrated, the yellow colour is *inside* the round shape and both *move* together) with a second set of neuronal events, B, arranged as three different sets of NCAs each spatially separated from the others, one for colour, one for shape and one for movement. The NCAs *code* the information in B that is presented *pictorially* in A. In all known information processing mechanisms this needs a raster to effect this transformation. Thus the question may be raised: what performs this function in the brain?

The so-called mind–brain problem, or brain–consciousness problem, has thus left the confines of philosophical debate, where it was for 2000 years, and may now be tackled by scientific and particularly mathematical means; and the relevant branches of mathematics are geometry and topology, as the great French logician Jean Nicod (1969) foresaw long ago.

But before we can tackle this we must first get four sources of today's confused thought about this problem out of the way. These are (i) the different meanings of 'consciousness'; (ii) the false philosophical theory of perception known as Direct or Naive Realism; (iii) the general confusion over the body-image; and (iv) Descartes' mistaken criterion of extension in space for distinguishing between mind and brain. The following sections will deal with these in turn.

Consciousness

The word 'conscious' or 'consciousness' has at least three quite separate meanings:

1. The medical/behavioural sense as in when we say 'The patient has now regained consciousness'.
2. The cognitive or attentive sense as in when we say 'She was conscious of an eerie feeling in the room'.
3. The phenomenological sense we employ when we define consciousness as the total of what we can introspect, i.e. our sensory fields, plus our images, thoughts and emotions as we experience these directly.

Much of the present confusion in the area of brain-consciousness relations arises because we tend to confuse these usages. The sense in which I will be using 'consciousness' in this paper is sense 3—the phenomenal one.

Perception

There are currently two theories of perception—Naive or Direct Realism (or DR) and Indirect Realism or the Representative Theory (RT). Direct realism is supported by a number of philosophers. As Richard Gregory says in his magnum opus *Mind in Science*: '[Direct] realism is popular among philosophers as it seems to give certainty to perception, and so to give an undoubted basis for empirical knowledge. This is not to be expected of perception regarded as *representations*, which is how we regard perception in this book'. RT is supported by some philosophers and by all scientists who deal with perception. DR espouses the naive common sense view that in perception—especially vision—we are in direct contact with the physical object. That is, the extended coloured patch that we experience directly is held actually to *be* the physical object, or at least the surface of the physical object. RT in contrast holds that these extended coloured patches that we experience directly—called 'sensations' by scientists and clinicians, and names like 'sense-data', 'sensa', and 'qualia' by philosophers—are not *direct* views of external objects but are *representations* of them constructed in some way by the representative mechanisms of perception.

The point is far too complex and involved to cover here but I will just sum up the verdict of most vision scientists which is that RT is undoubtedly correct and that DR is just another example of what Churchland (1986) has called 'folk psychology'.

Body-image

The third source of confusion at the heart of this matter is the present widespread confusion between the body-image and the physical organism ('body'). The term 'body-image' is widely used in neurology, but this use tends to muddle two quite different concepts, as first pointed out in 1953 (Smythies, 1953). If we simply describe the nature of our experience, we will describe our sensations in consciousness, including our somatic sensations making up the somatic sensory field. In addition to this we have a system of *beliefs* about our own bodies, e.g. that I have 10 fingers, blue eyes and a tendency to stoutness. Since the term 'body-image' is often used indiscriminately in the neurological literature to describe both the somatic sensory field and the body concept, nothing but confusion often results. And in this confusion we lose sight of the important fact that the somatic sensory field is not identical with the physical body, which of course 'common sense' thinks it is.

Paul Schilder concludes his book *The Image and Appearance of the Human Body* with these words '. . .the empirical method leads immediately to a deep insight that even our own body is beyond our immediate reach, that even our own body justifies Prospero's words "We are such stuff as dreams are made of, and our little life is rounded with a sleep"'. One of the founders of Gestalt psychology, Wolfgang Köhler (1947), put it thus: 'My body [somatic sensory field] is the outcome of certain processes in my physical organism, processes which start in the eyes, muscles, skin and so forth, exactly as the chair before me [visual sensation] is the final product of other processes in the same organism. If the chair is seen "before me", the "me" of this phrase means my body as an experience, of course, not my body as an organism in the physical world'.

Yet it is still undeniably true, some 50 years after those words were written, that most neuroscientists and neurologists, no matter how much they may support RT in theory, nevertheless lapse into the DR mode of thinking at all other times. For 'common sense' has an enormously deep-seated uncritical assumption that we experience our physical bodies directly; that is that the mass of somatic sensations always present in some form or other in consciousness, simply *is* the physical body. Yet Schilder, Köhler and the whole physiological account of perception assure us categorically that this is not so, and that it is really just another example of unreliable, indeed false, folk psychology. In terms of contemporary science, the somatic sensory field can only be identical with certain patterns of neuronal activity in the parietal lobes of the brain; just as the visual field—our visual sensations—can only be identical, not with the external objects they *represent*, but with certain neuronal activity in the higher visual centres of the brain. We can highlight this problem by asking, 'Where in the world of my direct experience is located my physical brain?'. Most people would instinctively locate it in the head of the experienced body, that is the head of phenomenological body image. But, of course, this is quite wrong, as the head of the somatic sensory field is itself *in* the brain. So how can the brain be in the 'head' when the 'head' is in the brain?

This essential point has been very effectively illustrated by Jonathon Harrison in his account of Ludwig, the brain-in-a-vat. Harrison (1985) recounts a tale of the far distant future when the skills of neurosurgery and the techniques of neurocybernetics are developed to a degree unimaginable today. Ludwig was born with a hideously deformed body but a magnificently developed brain. Dr Smythson, the leading neuroscientist and neurosurgeon of the day, removed Ludwig's brain from its shattered body and placed it in a life support system, in which, not only was the brain transfused with blood, but the cut ends of the cranial nerves and spinal cord were linked up to neurocybernetic machines of enormous complexity. The motor nerves were also connected to the machine. In this way, by appropriate stimulation via the neurocybernetic stimulators, Ludwig could be given brain stimulations, and thus 'life' experiences, exactly like we get. Dr Smythson programmed his neurostimulators in such a way as to give Ludwig all the experiences of a normal life, including that of having a perfectly normal body. All the brain stimulations we get from our sense organs, Ludwig got from his neurostimulators. As far as Ludwig was concerned, his life experience was just like ours and he had no way of knowing that he was just a brain-in-a-vat. Ludwig had a body image (somatic sensory field) just like we do and a similar body concept (the details of which, of course, depended on how Dr Smythson had programmed his computers running Ludwig's neurostimulators).

So if I ask myself, 'Where, relative to the spatial system in which my spatially extended visual and somatic sensations are extended, is the physical body itself?'. The answer is all around and very much larger—for the whole extent of consciousness is itself identical with a small volume in the brain not in the whole body (physical organism) itself. This is enough to make the stoutest mind boggle.

Descartes' extension in space

The fourth area of confusion that I would like to consider relates to Descartes' claim that extension in space provides *the* criterion for distinguishing between the mental and the physical. Descartes divided the world into *res extensa*, the physical world of extended physical objects; and *res cogitans*, unextended thinking spirits. This theory rests, however, on an entirely erroneous basis. For, once we come to realise that RT is true and DR is false, we must realise that our visual and somatic sensations are certainly mental entities, that is they are located at the *inner terminal* of the representative mechanisms of perception, and that they are equally certainly extended in space—in this case internal private phenomenal space and not external public physical space. Other contents of consciousness, such as thoughts and auditory and olfactory sensations and images, lack extension in space (although they may have location). That is to say a thought as experienced does not have geometrical properties (such as a left side and a boundary curve) that visual sensations have. Thus consciousness is much more complicated an entity than Descartes supposed. His criterion of extension in space represents as much a division *within* consciousness itself as it does between certain aspects of consciousness and external physical objects. This has the very important consequence that, when we come to relate consciousness and its contents to brain events, we must think primarily in terms of relating two *spatial* entities rather than trying to think up possible relations between an extended brain and unextended thinking spirits. Thus the problem becomes one in formal geometry and topology.

CONCLUSIONS

So to return to the mind–brain problem, if we reject the Identity Theory, what does this leave us with? Cartesian dualism fails to pass the very first test, since it describes the mind as unextended in space, a thinking spirit, whereas, as we have seen, spatial extension is a primary property of phenomenal consciousness. I believe that, if we stay within the confines of contemporary physics, there is only one even remotely possible current theory of mind–brain relation and that is Niels Bohr's complementarity theory. In a famous speech in 1932 he suggested that the mind/brain relation might be similar to the particle/wave complementarity of the electron in quantum mechanics. Here one entity, the electron, can have particle-like properties under one mode of observation, and another, rather different set of wave-like properties under another mode of observation. Thus one entity, the mind/brain, could present one set of properties when observed by a neurosurgeon and a different set of properties when observed by itself. Complementarity is a different logical relation to identity. This might solve the binding problem, but I am not sure that it solves Brain's problem, i.e. can such complementarity solve the problem of the missing raster system in the brain?

Recently two eminent physicists, Roger Penrose (1989) and Andrei Linde (1990) have warned us against taking it for granted that physics is now complete and so we can safely base our theories of consciousness on contemporary physics. In fact, Penrose predicts a new revolution in physics on a par with relativity and quantum theory, and that this theory may give us a better basis to explain the nature of consciousness and its relation to the brain. Linde suggests that consciousness may have a reality value in the world on a par with matter and space–time. We now know that consciousness has its own spatio-temporal structure (that described by introspection psychologists, see especially French (1987)). Space used to be thought of as merely an 'unreal' container for 'real' matter. Now, Linde says, we know that space can exist in its own right independent of matter, and can have detectable manifestations in the form of gravitational waves. In a similar vein consciousness is today widely viewed as a mere by-product of matter. But Linde suggests that consciousness may have its own 'degrees of freedom', that is it may exist in its own right independent of physical space–time and matter. In this new physical theory, space–time, matter and consciousness become co-equal partners in a single over-riding reality.

REFERENCES

Anderson, A. and Palca, J. (1988). Who knows how the brain works? *Nature*, **335**, 489–491.

Brain, W.R. (1960). Space and sense-data. *Br. J. Philos. Sci.*, **11**, 177–191.

Charlesworth, M. (1979). Sense-impressions: a new model. *Mind*, **88**, 24–44.

Churchland, P.S. (1986). *Neurophilosophy. Toward a Unified Science of the Mind–Brain.* MIT Press, Cambridge.

Freeman, W.J. (1990). The physiology of perception. *Sci. Am.*, **264**, 78–89.

French, R. (1987). The geometry of visual space. *Nous*, **21**, 115–137.

Gray, C.M., Konig, P., Engel, A.K. and Singer, W. (1989). Oscillatory responses in the cat visual cortex exhibit inter-columnar synchronization which reflect global stimulus properties. *Nature*, **338**, 334.

Gregory, R. (1984). *Mind in Science*, Penguin, Harmondsworth.

Grey, Walter, W. (1950). Features in the electrophysiology of mental mechanisms. In: Richter, D. (Ed.), *Perspectives in Neuropsychiatry*, H.K. Lewis, London, p. 77.

Harrison, J. (1985). *The Philsopher's Nightmare,* Nottingham University Press.

Köhler, W. (1947). *Gestalt Psychology*, New American Library, New York, p. 22.

Linde, A. (1990). *Particle Physics and Inflationary Cosmology*, Harwood, Chur.

Nicod, J. (1969). *The Foundations of Geometry and Induction*, Routledge & Kegan Paul, London.

Penrose, R. (1989). *The Emperor's New Mind*, Oxford University Press, Oxford.

Schilder, P. (1950). *The Image and Appearance of the Human Body*, International Universities Press, New York.

Sherrington, C. (1940). *Man on His Nature*, Cambridge University Press, Cambridge.

Smythies, J.R. (1953). The image and appearance of the human body. *Brain*, **76**, 132–145.

Smythies, J.R. (1992). *The Walls of Plato's Cave*, in press.
Vernon, M.D. (1962). *A Further Study of Visual Perception*, Cambridge University Press, Cambridge.
Wright, E. (1981). Yet more on epistemic seeing. *Mind*, **90**, 585–591.
Zeki, S. and Schipp, S. (1988). The functional logic of cortical connections. *Nature*, **335**, 311–317.

Index

Affective disorders
  bipolar, anticonvulsants in 256–257
  carbamazepine/valproate mode of action 93–95, 256–257
  complex partial seizures and, *see* Complex partial seizures (CPS)
  electroconvulsive therapy action 257
  frontal lobe hypometabolism 253
  GABA-hypothesis 93
  in diencephalic tumours 196
  in temporal lobe tumours 192
  mechanism of development,
    neuropeptide induction 255–256
    stressors and *c-fos* induction 258–259
  psychosensory and psychomotor alterations 256
  temporal lobe and 247–265
    clinical implications 256–259
    complexity of interactions 247–249, 250
    peptide changes in kindling, implications 253–256
    procaine infusion study 257–258
    progressive spread of kindling, implications 251–153
    see also Complex partial seizures (CPS)
  temporal lobe surgery and 250
Affective responses, temporal lobe stimulation 252–253
Affective symptoms, partial seizures 119–120, 249–250
Afferent fibres
  contact number with pyramidal cells 25
  impulse frequency 24
  single, activation methods 20, 21
After-discharge (AD) 74
  in kindling 74, 252
Aggression 247, 248
Akinetic mutism 189, 196
Alcohol, abuse, 'kindling' due to 75
'Alien' tissue lesions, schizophrenia-like pschoses and 193, 223, 226, 228, 230
Alzheimer's disease 200
2-Amino-5-phosphonovalerate (APV) 16, 17, 28
Ammon's horn 39
  see also Hippocampal formation
Ammon's horn sclerosis (AHS) 224, 226
  functional considerations 230–232
Ammon's horn sclerosis (AHS) (*cont.*)
  gangliogliomas and 226–230
  see also Hippocampal sclerosis; Mesial temporal sclerosis
Amnesia
  aetiology 200–201
  anterograde 201, 205, 205–207
    limbic-diencephalic circuits role 205, 207
    tests 205, 207
  automatisms, associated with 11
  basal forebrain 200
  in cerebrovascular disease of limbic system 191
  classification 200–201
  diencephalic 200, 201
    pattern of memory deficits 202
  ictal, psychosis in temporal lobe epilepsy 160
  organic 200
  post-traumatic 204
  rate of forgetting 203, 204
  retrograde 203, 204
    anterograde relationship 205–207
    frontal cortex and anterior temporal cortex 206, 207
    mechanism 206–207
    tests 205, 206, 208
  temporal lobe 200
    diencephalic amnesia comparison 203–204
    pattern of memory deficits 203
    rate of forgetting, controversy 203–204
  third ventricle tumours 195
  transient 200
  transient global, *see* Transient global amnesia (TGA)
  see also Memory
Amnesic syndrome 200
  aetiology 200
  neuropsychological studies 201–204
AMPA receptors 17
  blocker (CNQX) 16
  GluR subunits 18
    flip and *flop* expression 19
  as hetero-oligomer 20
  long-term potentiation (LTP) expression 28
  molecular studies 18–20
Amygdala 249
  in affective behaviour 249

Amygdala (*cont.*)
kindling, *see* Kindling phenomeon
lesions, seizures due to 189
self-preservation role 8
stimulation,
kindling and 72
sensations due to 122
Amygdala division, of limbic system 8, 9
Amygdalahippocampectomy, selective (AHE) 169
comparison with anterior temporal lobe resections 171
emotional decisions before/after 174–176
epileptological outcome 181–182
hypometabolism before/after 180–181
learning and memory after 170–174
preoperative risk assessment 173
pre-/postoperative antiepileptic drug modifications 182–183
Amygdala kindling, *see* Kindling phenomenon
'Amygdalo-hippocampal epilepsy' 155
Amytal test 173
Anosmia 189, 195
Anterior temporal gyrus of Heschl 122
Anterograde amnesia, *see* Amnesia
Anterograde Memory Quotient (AMQ) 205
Anticonvulsant activity, of TRH 254, 255
Antiepileptic drugs
mechanism of action 91–99
pre-/postoperative modifications in 182–183
psychosis risk factor in temporal lobe epilepsy 161–162
see also Carbamazepine; Valproate
Antipsychotic effect, dopamine receptors mediating 52
Antisocial behaviour 121
Anxiety, PET studies in 109
APV (2-Amino-5-phosphonovalerate) 16, 17, 28
Archicortex 8
'Architectural follies' 231, 233
in schizophrenia 218
Aspartate 17
release during seizures 65
Astrocytes, glial fibrillary acidic protein in 82
Astrocytic lesions 229, 230
Auditory seizures 117
Aura symptoms 160
Autobiographical memory 205, 206, 208
Automatisms 11, 120–121, 121
amnesia associated with 11
in frontal lobe seizures 124
Autonomic symptoms, of partial seizures 118
Awareness 115

Basal forebrain amnesia 200
Basal ganglia circuits
input and output 47
involving dorsal striatum 47, 48–49
involving ventral striatum 48, 50–51
organization 46–47
see also Striatum
Bear–Fedio Inventory (BFI) 141, 143, 144
Behaviour
after temporal lobe resection, *see* Temporal lobe resections

Behaviour (*cont.*)
changes in kindling 74–75, 247
lidocaine-induced 247, 248
disturbances, in temporal lobe epilepsy, *see* Personality disorders; Temporal lobe epilepsy
postictal, endogenous opioids role 109
reptilian and mammalian, evolutionary aspects 7–8
Beliefs 272
feelings, free-floating affective feelings 12
'Binding problem', in brain–mind relationship 269–270
Birth injury/difficulties
schizophrenia development 219
schizophrenia-like psychoses and 226
Body-image 272–273
Brain
areas involved in schizophrenia 216–218
damage,
lateralized, emotional/psychological effects 179, 180
psychosis risk factor in epilepsy 162
development,
disturbances in schizophrenia 218–219, 232, 233
in schizophrenia-like psychoses 231, 232
lesions,
'binding' problem and 270
complex partial seizures and 116
oedema 190
self-stimulation 248
structure, in schizophrenia 215–216
volumes in schizophrenia 215–216
Danish studies 240–241
fixed brain tissue, limitations 241
unbiased estimation 239–246
weight, in schizophrenia 215
Brain–consciousness problem 270, 271
body-image 272–273
consciousness meanings 271
Descartes' extension in space 273–274
perception, representations 271, 272
perception theories 271–272
Brain–mind relationship 267–276
'binding problem' 269–270
complementarity theory 274–275
Identity Theory, rejection 269, 274
physical theories 274–275
problem statement 268, 270

CA1 region, *see* Hippocampal formation
Calbindin 66
Calcium
buffering variations, hippocampal vulnerability to neuronal loss 66
in long-term potentiation (LTP) induction 28
Carbachol, kindling due to 75
Carbamazepine
in bipolar affective disorders 93–95, 256–257
effects of, summary 92
kindling phenomenon, effect on 94
modes of action 91, 92
in affective disorders 93–95, 256–257
antiepileptic 95–96

Carbamazepine (*cont.*)
modes of action (*cont.*)
dopamine turnover 94, 97
GABA turnover reduced 93, 97
glutamate release reduced 95
K^+ channels role 95, 97
Na^+ channels role 93, 97
NMDA receptors 96
Cavalieri principle 239, 241, 242
Cerebral angiography 104
Cerebral blood flow
PET studies 108, 191
procaine infusion studies 258
psychopathology in absence of epilepsy 194
SPECT study 109–110, 191, 194
Cerebral metabolism, *see* Glucose metabolism; Hypometabolism
Cerebrovascular disease 189–197
limbic system 190–191
symptomatology 191–192
symptomatology 190, 191–192
c-fos induction
in kindling mechanisms 77, 251, 258
stressors inducing 258
Chaos, in brain function 270
Cholinergic blockade 201, 203
Cingulate cortex 8
Cingulate gyrus 9
lesions, symptoms 195
role in emotional expression 10
CNQX, as AMPA receptor blocker 16
Coactivation, in long-term potentiation induction 27
Cocaine, kindling due to 75
Cognitive disturbances, in partial seizures 118–119
Comparator, hippocampal formation as 38, 53–54, 184
Complementarity theory 274–275
Complex partial seizures (CPS) 4, 115
affective symptomatology relationship 119–120, 249–250, 254–255
case histories 119, 120
inverse relationship 250
lag in onset 250, 255
neuropeptide induction role in 255
possible mechanisms 254–255
temporal lobe stimulation 252–253
assumptions related to 116
brain lesions and 116, 122
corticotropin releasing hormone (CRH) induction 255
epidemiology 125–126
frontal lobe 125
hypermetabolism region 108
incidence 125
interictal hypometabolism 106, 107, 108, 253
frontal lobe hypometabolism with 253
psychopathology 169
psychosis risk factor 162
site of seizure onset 116, 122
spatio-temporal evolution of biological changes 254, 255, 256
temporal lobe 122, 122–125, 125
anatomical–clinical correlations 122–125
see also Temporal lobe epilepsy
temporal lobe stimulation role 252–253
Complex partial seizures (CPS) (*cont.*)
in temporal lobe tumours 193
transient global amnesia attack 204
see also Partial seizures
Complex partial status 193
Computed tomography (CT) 102, 105, 191
in schizophrenia 214, 215
brain volumes 239
Conditioning 201
Confabulation 207
Congenital structural abnormalities 231
Consciousness 268
definition and meanings 115, 271
existence independent of matter/space–time 275
extension in space 274
impairment 115
seizure relationship 152
in partial motor seizures 116
in relation to brain–consciousness problem 271
Cooperativity 27
Corpus striatum, *see* Striatum
Cortical dysplasia lesions 228
Cortico-striato-pallido-thalamic-cortical circuit 46, 47, 48
Corticotropin releasing factor (CRF) 254, 255
transient inductions after seizures 255
Corticotropin releasing hormone (CRH) 247, 254, 255
increased mRNA in kindling 254
increased secretion in depression 255
Cortisol 254
CPP [(3-(+)-2-carboxypiperazin-4-yl)propyl-1-phosphonate], protection against hippocampal damage 65
Crying, relevance to emotion and limbic system 10–11

Decision-making ability, amygdalahippocampectomy (AHE) effect 174–176
Dementia 215
in temporal lobe tumours 192
Dendrites, spines on 24, 25
increase and shape changes 30
Dense core vesicles 231
Dentate-CA3 system, diffuse 38–39, 41–43
Dentate gyrus
in amygdala kindling 252
c-fos induction by stressors 258
granule cells 38, 40, 42, 130
ganglioglioma origin 231
loss in mesial temporal sclerosis 130, 131
neurogenesis 231
inhibition increased in, after kindling 76
input from entorhinal cortex 38, 40, 41
diffuse 41, 42
mossy fibre projections to CA3 38–39, 41, 42
perforant pathway 38
2-Deoxyglucose 77
Depolarization, post-synaptic
in long-term potentiation induction 27–28
minimal number of synapses 23–24
see also Excitatory post-synaptic potential (EPSP); Hippocampal synapses; Synapses

Depression
after complex partial seizures, reason for lag 255
corticotropin releasing hormone (CRH) hypersecretion 255
frontal lobe hypometabolism and 253
hypothalamic-pituitary-adrenal axis activation in 254
thyrotropin releasing hormone (TRH) hypersecretion 255
Depth electrode recordings, seizures and psychopathology 144
Descartes' extension in space 273–274
Developmental anomalies, *see* Brain, development
Diaschisis 190
Diencephalic amnesia, *see* Amnesia
Diencephalon
lesions, symptoms 195–196
tumours 195–196
Digital subtraction angiography 104
Direct Realism (DR) 271, 272
Dissector principle 242–243
Domoate poisoning 61
limbic system pathology 61, 63–64
Dopamine
depletion, kindling increased 78
effect on ventral striatum 52–53
increased activity in mania 94
role in striatum 49
turnover, carbamazepine/valproate depressant effect on 94, 97
Dopamine receptors
antagonist, effect on seizures 52
antipsychotic and extrapyramidal effects 52
D_1 and D_2 49–50, 52
effect on striatal output channels 49–50
Dopaminergic system 47–48, 49–50, 51
of hippocampal formation 51
manipulations, effect on epilepsy 51, 52
mesolimbic, hippocampal-striatal pathway as output to 51–53
ventral striatum influencing pathways 51
DSM IIIR classification 151
Dysmnesic symptoms 118

Electrical stimulus, kindling 72–75, 247
Electroconvulsive therapy 250, 257
Electroencephalogram (EEG)
basal, in psychomotor epilepsy 5
in kindling 72, 73
pre-/postoperative changes after amygdalahippocampectomy 183
psychosis in temporal lobe epilepsy 160, 179
temporal lobe epilepsy classification 152
Emotion
changes, in temporal lobe tumours 192
crying and laughter 10–11
expression,
hypothalamic role 4
limbic system role 4, 5, 7
Emotional preferences, amygdalahippocampectomy (AHE) effect on 174–176
Encephalitis 194, 200
Endogenous opioids 109
Entorhinal cortex 39
hippocampal connections with, *see* Entorhinal–hippocampal network
inputs to 40
lateral area,
fibres to distal CA1 44
fibres terminating in dentate gyrus 41
lateral-to-medial connectivity 40, 41, 44
layers II and III 40, 44
longitudinal fibres and input integration 40
medial area,
fibres to proximal CA1 44
fibres terminating in dentate gyrus 41
perforant pathway, *see* Perforant pathway
role in hippocampal comparator action 53, 184
subiculum projection to 45–46
Entorhinal–hippocampal network 37, 38–45
diffuse dentate-CA3 system 41–43
mossy fibre projections 41, 42
perforant pathway 41
Schaffer collaterals to CA1 43
transition to selective system 43
organization 38–40
as part of memory system 45–46, 53
pathway differentiation at entorhinal cortex level 40
pathway differentiation at perforant pathway level 40–41
reverberatory circuits 46, 53
selective CA1-subiculum system 44–45
Environmental factors
behavioural response to electrical stimulation 248
in schizophrenia-like psychoses 226
Epilepsia partialis continua 117
Epilepsy
behavioural changes without seizures 137, 146, 194
personality disorders and, *see* Personality disorders
see also Psychosis; Temporal lobe epilepsy
Epileptic equivalent 138
Epileptic insanity 138, 149
Epileptic personality 139
see also Personality disorders
Epileptiform after-discharge 74, 252
Epileptiform events, spontaneous, in kindling 74, 76
Euphoria 192, 258
Evolution
limbic system 7
mammalian forebrain 1, 2, 7
Excitatory neurotransmission, carbamazepine reducing 95
Excitatory post-synaptic currents (EPSC) 15–16, 21
facilitated responses 22
Excitatory post-synaptic potential (EPSP) 15
amplitude, spine number effect 25
in long-term potentiation 26
single-fibre 23
slow component 16, 17
time course 15–16
Excitotoxins 61–69
antagonists, in protection from limbic pathology 65–66
release during seizures 65

Excitotoxins (*cont.*)
  role in limbic system pathology 61–69
    antagonists protecting 65–66
    cytopathology 62
    domoate 61, 63–64
    focal hippocampal injection effects 64–65
    glutamate/aspartate release 65
  see also Glutamate; Kainate
Experimental models, status epilepticus 62–63
Extrapyramidal effects, via dopamine receptors in dorsal striatum 52
Eysenck Personality Inventory (EPI) 142

Facilitation 22, 26
Falret, J. 137–138
Family support 183, 184
Fascia dentata, granule cells, *see* Dentate gyrus
Febrile convulsions 226
Fluorodeoxyglucose (FDG) 77, 105, 180, 253
'Forced normalization' 179, 232
Forebrain, evolution 1, 2
Fos protein 77, 251
Fossils 7
Free-floating feelings 5, 12
Frequency potentiation 26
Frontal cortex, in retrograde memory 206–207
Frontal lobe
  dysfunction, limbic-diencephalic pathology with and amnesia 206
  hypometabolism 253
Frontal lobe seizures 124
  symptoms 124

GABA
  in kindling 78
  turnover, carbamazepine reducing 93, 97
  valproate interaction 94, 95, 97
GABAergic pathways, basal ganglia circuits involving dorsal striatum 49
GABA-hypothesis, of affective disorders 93
Gangliogliomas 226, 226–230
  Ammon's horn sclerosis comparison 226–230
  congenital structural abnormalities associated 231
  functional considerations 230–232
  location 227, 228
  morphology 230
  schizophrenia-like psychoses and 226, 226–230
Ganzfeld experiments 268
Gastaut–Geschwind syndrome 137–148, 179
  concept development 137–139
  see also Personality disorders
Gelastic seizures 120
Glial fibrillary acidic protein (GFAP)
  in astrocytes 82
  increased in kindled rats 81, 82, 85
    time course 82–85
Glial marker proteins, in kindling 80–85
Glial reaction 62, 218
Glioma, cell loss in 62, 63
Globus pallidus, striatal projections to 49
Glucose metabolism
  enhanced in kindling 77
  PET studies 106–108
  in self-stimulation of brain 248

Glucose metabolism (*cont.*)
  see also Hypometabolism; Positron emission tomography (PET)
Glutamate 61
  at excitatory hippocampal synapses 16–17
  hippocampal damage due to 63
  receptors 16–17, 17–20
    AMPA-receptor, *see* AMPA receptors
    L-AP4 receptor 17
    metabotropic receptor 17, 19, 20, 30
    molecular studies 18–20
    NMDA receptor, *see* NMDA receptors
  release,
    carbamazepine reducing 95
    during seizures 65
    in long-term potentiation 26
Graft, noradrenaline-rich, in kindling 79, 80
Grand mal epilepsy, psychosis risk 159
Granule cells, *see* Dentate gyrus
Grey matter, in schizophrenia 215–216, 216
'Growth ring hypothesis' 8
Gustatory sensations 123

Hallucinations, structured 120
Hamartomas 231
  cell loss in 62, 63
Head injury 204, 226
Hemisphere dominance 176, 220, 225
Heterotopia 62, 132
Hierarchical control in CNS 248
Hippocampal connections, organization 37–60
  entorhinal network, *see* Entorhinal–hippocampal network
  functional relevance 45–53
    as motor pathway 46–51
    as output to mesolimbic dopaminergic system 51–53
    as part of memory system 45–46, 53, 206
  schematic illustration 54
  selection between output channels 38, 39, 44–45, 54
Hippocampal formation 37, 39
  in affective behaviour 249
  Ammon's horn, *see* CA1, CA3 (*below*)
  Ammon's horn sclerosis, *see* Ammon's horn sclerosis
  antiepileptics mechanism 91–99
    see also Carbamazepine; Valproate
  CA1 39, 149
    cell loss 62, 129
    cell loss and psychosis associated 149–150
    input from CA3 39, 43
    input from layer III of entorhinal cortex 44
    lesions and memory impairment 206
    projections to subiculum 39, 44–45
    spines on dendrites 24, 25, 30
  CA3 39
    kainate action on 64
    mossy fibre projection from dentate gyrus 38–39, 41, 42
  dopaminergic system of 51, 52
  fields H_1, H_2, H_3 and neuron loss 130, 131, 133
  focal injection of excitotoxins 64–65

Hippocampal formation (*cont.*)
  functional role 184–185
    as cognitive map 184
    as comparator 38, 53–54, 184
    dorsal and ventral hippocampus 40, 249
    as inhibitor 184
    in kindling mechanism 76–77
    in memory, *see* Memory
    models 37–38, 53–55
    RAM (random access memory) 185
    as register or locomotion planner 185
  inputs to 5, 6, 38–45
  inputs to ventral striatum 46, 48, 50, 54
  lesions 189, 206
  neurone loss 62, 129–131, 133
    aetiology 132–133
  noradrenaline-rich graft, effect on kindling 79, 80
  pathology,
    in status epilepticus 62–63
    in transient global ischaemia 63
    see also Limbic system, pathology; Temporal lobe epilepsy
  regions 39
  in schizophrenia 216, 220
  seizure threshold 124
  Sommer sector, *see* Hippocampal formation, CA1
  stimulation, sensations due to 122
  see also Dentate gyrus; Subiculum
Hippocampal 'gliosis' 191
Hippocampal kindling, *see* Kindling phenomenon
Hippocampal sclerosis 63, 91, 106
  neuron loss in 133, 134
  see also Ammon's horn sclerosis, Mesial temporal sclerosis
Hippocampal-striatal pathway 46–47
  as motor pathway 46–51
  as output to mesolimbic dopaminergic system 51–53
  see also Striatum
Hippocampal synapses, excitatory 15–35
  activity-dependent changes 26–30
    long-term potentiation, *see* Long-term potentiation (LTP)
    short-lasting changes 26
  EPSP and EPSC 15–16
  equipotentiality of 24
  facilitation 26
  interaction between synapses 22–26
    afferent impulse frequency 24
    location/distribution in dendritic tree 24–26
    minimal number for cell discharge 22–24
  location and shape of dendritic spines 24, 25, 30
  long-term potentiation, *see* Long-term potentiation
  properties of single synapse 20–22
    methods of study 20–21
    transmitter quanta 22
  transmitters 16–17
    receptor studies 17–20
    see also Glutamate
  variability in 22
  see also Excitatory post-synaptic potential (EPSP)
Huntington's chorea 244, 253
6-Hydroxydopamine (6-OHDA) 78
Hypergraphia 144, 145
Hypermetabolism 108
  in complex partial seizures 108
Hypersomnia 195
Hypoglycaemia 63
Hypometabolism, interictal 106–108
  in complex partial seizures 106, 107, 108, 253
  frontal lobe 253
  opioids contributing to 109
  pre-/post amygdalahippocampectomy (AHE) 180–181
  in temporal lobe epilepsy 106–108
Hypothalamic lesions 195
Hypothalamus, role in emotion expression 4
Hypoxia, perinatal 63
  neurone loss due to 132, 133

Ibotenate 64
Identity Theory 269, 274
Illusions 120
Imaging, *in vivo* 101–114, 191
  functional 105–110
    positron emission tomography 105–109
    SPECT 105, 109–110
  structural 101–105
    MRI 102–104
    roentgenographic 102, 104–105
  see also individual techniques
Indirect Realism or Representative Theory (RT) 271, 272
Insanity, postepileptic 138, 149, 150
In situ hybridization 19, 251
Insula 122
Intellectual impairment 192
'Interictal behaviour syndrome of TLE' 179
Intracranial pressure, raised 190
Introspection 267, 268
In vivo imaging, *see* Imaging
Ischaemic lesions 190, 191
  see also Cerebrovascular disease

Jacksonian seizure 116

Kainate 61
  action on CA3 neurons 64
  agonists 64
  receptor 18
  status epilepticus induced by 75
Kindling phenomenon 71–90, 178
  afterdischarges (ADs) 74, 252
  aggression enhanced 247
  anatomical substrates 72, 74, 85
  behavioural changes/responses 74–75, 247
  carbamazepine and valproate action in 94
  clinical relevance 71
  CRH and TRH mRNA induction 254
  electrical stimulus 72–75, 247
  electrographic measures 72–74, 77
  hyperdopaminergic function induced 94
  mechanisms (studies) 76–85
    amygdala role 76–77
    c-fos induction 77, 251

Kindling phenomenon (*cont.*)
mechanisms (studies) (*cont.*)
inhibitory/excitatory interactions 76, 77
inhibitory systems relevant 78
LTP similarity 76
metabolic labelling 77
neurochemical (NMDA receptors) 77–78
neuronal degeneration association 85
neuronal and glial marker proteins 80–85
neurophysiological 76–77, 252
noradrenaline and 78–80
pathways activated 74, 252
peptide changes 78, 253–256
synaptic remodelling role 80
unilateral then bilateral 252
working hypothesis 85
as memory model 76
partial 77, 81
pharmacological 75–76, 247
progressive involvement of neural structures 74, 251–253
synpatic potentiation hypothesis 76
Kojevnikow's syndrome 117
Korsakoff syndrome 200, 201, 203

Language disturbances 192
L-AP4 receptor 17
Laughter, relevance to emotion and limbic system 10–11
Learning 201
in temporal lobe epilepsy, pre-/postoperative 170–174
Left handedness 225
Leucotomy 241
Lidocaine-induced seizures 75, 247
behavioural disturbances after 247, 248
Limbic cortex 1
features 8
see also Limbic system
Limbic-diencephalic circuits, in anterograde memory 205, 207
Limbic dyscontrol syndrome 178
'Limbic epilepsy' 4, 152, 155
see also Temporal lobe epilepsy
Limbic lobe 1, 3
olfactory functions 3
'Limbic loop', ventral striatum involvement 48, 50–51
Limbic system 1–14, 189
cerebrovascular disease, *see* Cerebrovascular disease
definition 1, 7, 189
development of concept 3–7
emotion expression 4, 5, 7
crying and laughter 10–11
evolution 7
heterogeneity in 249
impact on affective behaviour 249
inputs from intero- and exteroceptive systems 5, 6, 11
lesions 189
outside temporal lobe, symptomatology 194–196
personality disorders with 139, 193–194
Limbic system (*cont.*)
lesions (*cont.*)
symptoms 189, 191–194, 194–196
see also Temporal lobe limbic system
memory of ongoing experience and 11
pathology,
in domoate poisoning 63–64
due to excitotoxins, *see* Excitotoxins
in mesial temporal sclerosis 62
NMDA antagonists blocking 65–66
in status epilepticus 62–63
seizures 11
anatomical–clinical correlations 123
see also Complex partial seizures (CPS)
subdivisions 8–11
amygdala division 8
septal division 8
thalamocingulate division 9, 10
temporal lobe, *see* Temporal lobe limbic system
tumours, *see* Temporal lobe limbic system; Tumours, intracranial
Lithium 256
Lobectomy 232
see also Temporal lobe resections
Localization-related epileptic syndromes 115–127, 134
frontal lobe seizures 125
temporal lobe seizures 122–125
see also Partial seizures
Locus coeruleus, graft 79
Long-term potentiation (LTP) 26–30
criteria for 26–27
expression mechanisms 28–30
metabotropic glutamate receptor in 30
post-synaptic 29–30
presynaptic 28–29
receptor unmasking 29
induction 27–28
coactivation 27
cooperativity 27
kindling mechanism similar 76
in memory and learning 206
morphological correlates 30–31
protein kinases modulatory effects 20

Magnetic resonance imaging (MRI) 102–104, 191
normal brain 104
PET scans superimposition 104, 105, 108
risks 102
in schizophrenia 215
T1 images, hippocampal anatomy 102
T2 images, 'unidentified bright objects' (UBOs) 102
Mammalian forebrain, evolution 1, 2, 7
Mania 94
Mediodorsal thalamic nucleus, total neuronal number 243
Memory 199–212
anterograde 201, 205, 207
tests 205, 207
assessment 207–208
autobiographical 205, 206, 208
classification and concepts 201, 202

Memory (*cont.*)
  deficits, hypometabolism correlation (PET study) 109
  hippocampal-entorhinal projection role 45–46, 53, 206
  hippocampus role 172–173, 206, 207
    possible mechanisms of impairment effect 184, 206
  impaired consolidation 184
  impaired retrieval 184
  interference phenomena 184
  kindling as model 76
  models 76, 201
  of ongoing experience 11
  primary (short-term) 201
  remediation 208–209
  retrograde 201, 207
    tests 205, 206, 208
  secondary (long-term) 201
    explicit/semantic/implicit types 201, 207
  in temporal lobe epilepsy, pre-/postoperative 170–174
  tests 205, 206, 207, 208
    auditory nonverbal material 172
  see also Amnesia
Mental symptoms, in intracranial tumours 189, 190
Mesencephalon
  lesions, symptoms 195–196
  ventral, ventral striatal projections 51
Mesial temporal lobe, *see* Temporal lobe
Mesial temporal sclerosis 62, 63
  aetiology 129–136
  definitions 129–132
  pathology 62, 130–131
    aetiology of changes 132–133
  psychosis relationship 223
  see also Ammon's horn sclerosis, Hippocampal sclerosis
Mesocortex 8
Metabolic effects
  self-stimulation of brain 248
  see also Glucose metabolism; Hypometabolism
Metabotropic receptor 17, 19
  in long-term potentiation (LTP) 30
  molecular studies 20
N-Methyl-D-aspartate, *see* NMDA receptors
Microdysgenesis 132
Migraine 204
Minnesota Multiphasic Personality Inventory (MMPI) 139, 140, 141, 146, 160
Morel, B.A. 137–138
Mossy fibre connections 38–39, 41, 42
  reorganization, in temporal lobe epilepsy 132
Mossy fibre reactive synaptogenesis 133
Motor pathway, hippocampal-striatal pathway 46–51
mRNA
  AMPA receptor 20
  c-fos 251
  corticotropin releasing hormone (CRH) 254
  thyrotropin releasing hormone (TRH) 254

Nadig's test 171–172
Naive or Direct Realism (DR) 271, 272
Nasopharyngeal electrode 5
Neocortex 11, 122, 206
Neopallium 8
Neurobehavioural analysis 7–8
Neurodegenerative conditions 218
Neuron(s)
  degeneration, kindling association 85
  loss,
    aetiology in mesial temporal sclerosis 132–133
    clinical manifestations correlation 134
    in field H_1 130, 131, 133
    in mesial temporal sclerosis 62, 129–131, 132–133
    repeated brief seizures causing 63
    in schizophrenia 216, 243
    seizure-related 133
  quantification 130, 131, 241–243
  total number in schizophrenic brains 241–243, 244
Neuronal cell assemblies (NCAs) 270
Neuronal marker proteins, in kindling 80–85
Neurone specific enolase (NSE) 81
Neurotransmitters
  at excitatory hippocampal synapses 16–17
  in long-term potentiation (LTP) 28
  quanta, release 22
  see also Glutamate
NMDA receptors 17, 24
  abnormalities, in diencephalic amnesia 202
  activation, kindling induction 78
  agonists, focal intrahipppocampal injection 64
  antagonists 16, 17, 63
    kindling retarded by 78
    limbic system pathology blocked 65–66
    long-term potentiation blocked 28
  carbamazepine blocking 96
Noradrenaline, kindling and 78–80
  depletion, kindling increased 78
  graft to hippocampus, kindling retarded 79, 80
Nucleus accumbens, total neuronal number 243
Nucleus basalis 201

Obsessive compulsive behaviour 109
Olfactory bulb and tract
  kindling 72
  lesions 195
Olfactory cortex 3
Olfactory perception 270
Olfactory sensations 118, 123
Oligodendrocytic lesions 229, 230
Opercular syndrome 123–124
Opiate receptor studies 108–109
Opioids, endogenous 109
Oxygen metabolism, PET studies 108

Pallidum (globus pallidus), striatal projections to 49
Panic disorder 109
Panoramic vision 118
'Papez circuit' 4, 5, 10
Parahippocampal gyrus 39
  projections to 221
  removal 170
  in schizophrenia 216, 217, 220
Paralysis 117
Paranoid symptoms, in temporal lobe epilepsy 144, 159

Partial seizures 116–122, 134
anatomical–clinical correlations 122–125
with autonomic symptoms 118
with motor signs 116–117
with psychic symptoms 118–122
somatosensory 117–118
see also Complex partial seizures (CPS); Simple partial seizures
Perception 267, 268
olfactory 270
theories 271–272
Indirect Realism or Representative Theory (RT) 271, 272
Naive or Direct Realism (DR) 271, 272
visual, *see* Visual perception
Perforant pathway 38, 40–41
differential distribution of 43
layer II projections, to diffuse dentate-CA3 system 41
layer III projections, to CA1/subiculum 44
Periamygdaloid area, stimulation, sensations due to 122
Personality, premorbid 222
Personality disorders, epilepsy and 137, 138, 140, 193
clinical studies 144–145
concept development 137–139
limbic system lesions and 139, 193
personality features 141, 143, 146
rating scale studies 139–144, 146
bilateral/unilateral lesions 141, 176
MMPI 139, 140, 141, 146
non-MMPI 142–144
seizure type number 141
Personality disorders, in temporal lobe tumours 193–194
Petit mal
absences 108
insanity with 150
status 193–194
Pharmacological agents
in memory remediation 209
see also Antiepileptic drugs
Pharmacological stimulus, in kindling 75–76, 247
Phenomenal consciousness 268
Phenytoin, psychosis risk factor in temporal lobe epilepsy 161–162
Pilocarpine model 52
Pneumoencephalography (PEG) 104, 240
Positron emission tomography (PET) 105–109, 191
in complex partial seizures 253
hypometabolism 106–108, 253
MRI with 104, 105, 108
opiate receptor studies 108–109
pre-/post amygdalahippocampectomy (AHE) 180–181
tracers 105, 106
Post-epileptic insanity 138, 149, 150
Postepileptic stupidity 150
Posterior neocortical structures 122
Posterior temporal cortex 122
Posterior temporal neocortical syndrome 124–125
type I and II seizures 124
Postoperative psychosis 180
Post-traumatic amnesia (PTA) 204
Potassium channel, in carbamazepine mode of action 95, 97
Procaine 257–258
Proisocortex 8
Protein F1 28
Protein kinase 20
Protein kinase C (PKC), in long-term potentiation 28, 30
Proto-oncogenes 77, 251, 258
Psychical seizures 169, 179
Psychic equivalents 138
Psychic symptoms 118–122
Psychomotor epilepsy 4, 155
seizure classification 123–124
see also Complex partial seizures (CPS); Temporal lobe epilepsy
Psychomotor status 193
Psychopathology, in absence of epilepsy 137, 146, 194
Psychosensory symptoms 256
response to anticonvulsants in bipolar affective disorders 256–257
Psychoses 149, 155, 213–238
functional 215
neuropathology 213–238
organic 215, 218
see also Schizophrenia
Psychosis, and epilepsy 155–159, 220–222
affective features 250
forms of epilepsy and 158–159
frequency 158
generalized epilepsies and 158, 159
grand mal epilepsy 159
risk 156–157
explanations for 157
overestimation of rate (clinical) 156, 157, 159
underestimation of rate (epidemiological) 157
risk factors 160–163
unrelated to temporal lobe epilepsy 162–163
see also Psychosis, and temporal lobe epilepsy
Psychosis, and temporal lobe epilepsy 149–167, 179–180, 193, 194, 220–222
classification of epilepsy 152, 155
classification of psychoses 151–152, 152, 153–155, 179
alternative 155
ictal 153, 194
interictal 154, 194
parictal 154
postictal 153
controlled studies on relationship 158, 159
epidemiological studies 155–158
historical aspects 149–151
pathology 149–150, 161
psychoses in generalized epilepsy comparison 159
risk factors 160–161
directly linked 160–161
interlinked 161–162
severity of epilepsy 162
unrelated to TLE 162–163
schizophrenia relationship 150, 151, 157, 163, 193, 194
see also Schizophrenia-like psychoses

Psychosocial stressors 258–259
Pyriform cortex
  in amygdala kindling 72, 74, 252
  c-fos induction by stressors 258

Quisqualate 17, 64

Reading dominance 176, 178
Rehabilitation, memory, techniques 209
Religiosity 145
Representations 271, 272
Representative Theory (RT) 271, 272
Reptiles, neurobehavioural studies 7–8
Responsiveness 115
Retrograde Memory Quotient (RMQ) 205
Retrosplenial cortex 54, 55
Rhinencephalon 1, 3, 189
  see also Limbic system
Roentgenographic studies 104–105

Schaffer collaterals 39, 43
Schizophrenia
  as birth injury, evidence against 219
  brain volume estimation, *see* Brain, volumes
  definition/symptoms 157, 159
  as developmental disorder 219–220, 232, 233
  as neurodegenerative process, evidence against 218, 219
  neuropathology 213–220
    brain areas involved 216–218
    brain structure 215–216
    causes of changes 218
    cytoarchitecture 218, 219
    disturbed brain development 218–219
    left hemisphere 220, 225
    temporal horn enlargement 225
    total neurone number 241–243, 244
    unbiased estimation of brain volumes, *see* Brain
  prevalence and costs 213
  prevalence in epilepsy 157–158
  psychosis in epilepsy, relationship 150, 151, 157, 163, 193, 220–222
  schizophrenia-like psychoses relevance to 232–233
  vulnerability as emergent phenomenon 233
Schizophrenia-like psychoses, of epilepsy 157, 179, 194, 220–232
  age of onset 222
  basic parameters 224–225
    laterality and sex 224–225
  environmental factors 226
  functional considerations 230–232
  pathology 222–223, 226
    'alien' tissue lesions 193, 223, 226, 228, 230
    see also Gangliogliomas
  relevance to schizophrenia 232–233
  temporal lobe epilepsy 220–232
    incidence 224
  see also Psychoses, and temporal lobe epilepsy
Schneiderian first rank symptoms 157, 159, 225
  temporal lobe epilepsy parameters and 223–224
Seizures
  dopaminergic system manipulation, effect 51–53

Seizures (*cont.*)
  glutamate and aspartate release 65
  repeated brief, cell loss due to 63
  see also Complex partial seizures (CPS); Partial seizures; Simple partial seizures
Self-stimulation of brain, metabolic effects 248
Sensations 267, 268, 271
Sensory-limbic hyperconnection 178
Separation 10
Separation cry 9, 10
Septal division, of limbic system 8
Signs/symptoms of partial seizures, *see* Partial seizures
Simple partial seizures 115
  hypermetabolism 108
Simple partial status epilepticus 117
Single photon emission computer tomography (SPECT) 105, 109–110, 191, 194
  advantages 105
  hyper- and hypoperfusion zones 110
  tracers 110
Sleep disorders 195
Sodium channels, carbamazepine reduction of GABA turnover 93, 95, 97
Sodium valproate, *see* Valproate
Somatic sensations 272, 273, 274
Somatosensory seizures 117–118
Somatostatin 254, 255
Sommer's sector, *see* Hippocampal formation, CA1
Sommer, W. 149–150
Somnolence 195
Space, extension in 273–274
Space–time 275
Squirrel monkey, brain 6
Status epilepticus 62–63
  experimental models 62–63
  kainic acid injections inducing 75
  limbic pathology 62
  psychosis risk factor 162
  simple partial 117
Stereology 239, 242, 244
Stimulants, abuse, 'kindling' due to 75
Stressors, *c-fos* induction 258
Striatonigral projections 49
Striatopallidal projections 49
Striatum
  circuits involving 47–51
  dopamine role 47–48, 49, 52
  dorsal,
    basal ganglia circuits involving 47, 48–49
    direct and indirect channels 49–50, 52
    dopamine receptors 49, 52
    output pathways 49
    role 54–55
  ventral,
    circuits ('limbic loop') 48, 50–51
    comparison with dorsal circuits 50, 54–55
    dopamine effect on 52–53
    functional differentiation 46, 54–55
    hippocampal inputs 46, 48, 50, 54
    influence on dopaminergic pathways 51
    role 54–55
    temporal lobe structures modulating 249

Subiculum
CA1 projections to 44–45
input from layer III of entorhinal cortex 44
projections to entorhinal cortex 45–46
projections to ventral striatum 46
as selective output structure 44–45, 184
Substantia nigra, striatal output pathways 49
Superior temporal convolution 122
Surgery
in temporal lobe epilepsy, psychosis risk factor 161
see also Temporal lobe resections
Synapses, excitatory, *see* Hippocampal synapses, excitatory
Synaptic density, in schizophrenia development 233
Synaptic potentiation hypothesis 76, 78

Tacrine 209
Temporal lobe 216
affective disorders and, *see* Affective disorders
'alien' tissue lesions 193, 223, 226, 228
morphology 230
amytal procedure, selective 173
anterior, lesions, and retrograde amnesia 206, 207
left, in schizophrenia 225
memory and, *see* Memory
mesial 216
ganglioglial lesions 227, 228, 230
hypofunction, PET studies 109
in schizophrenia 216, 220
in schizophrenia-like psychoses 222–223, 226, 227, 232
see also Hippocampal formation; Parahippocampal gyrus
stimulation,
affective responses 252–253
responses to 122–123
volume reduction in schizophrenia 216
Temporal lobe amnesia, *see* Amnesia
Temporal lobe epilepsy 4
aetiology 191
behavioural disturbances 138–139, 144, 146, 178
MMPI studies 139, 140, 141, 146
non-MMPI studies 142–144
pathology 149, 176, 178
see also Personality disorders
bilateral, learning and memory 170
classification 152, 155
of seizures 123–124
hippocampal neuron loss and 130, 131, 132
aetiology 132–133
laterality 223–224
see also left lateralization (*below*)
learning and memory in 170–174
left lateralization,
frontal lobe hypometabolism 253
functional implications 176
psychosis and 161, 178
schizophrenia-like psychoses and 225
paranoid symptoms 144, 159
pathology 130, 131, 132, 149, 191, 233
age of onset and 224
Temporal lobe epilepsy (*cont.*)
psychosis and, *see* Psychosis, and temporal lobe epilepsy
schizophrenia-like psychosis, *see* Schizophrenia-like psychoses
seizures,
anatomical–clinical correlations 122–125
epidemiology 125–126
frontal lobe involvement 124
signs of 134
types 123–124
severity, psychosis risk factor 162
sex distribution 223
surgery,
in psychosis development 161, 180
see also Temporal lobe resections
symptomatology, psychosis risk factor 160, 162
synonyms 4, 155, 156
in temporal lobe tumours 193
unilateral, model for functional implications of seizures 176
unilateral mesiobasal seizures, pre-/postoperative changes 176–178
see also Complex partial seizures (CPS)
Temporal lobe limbic system
cerebrovascular disease 191, 191–192
in vivo imaging, *see* Imaging
lesions 189, 190–191
symptomatology 191–194
seizures 123
tumours 189, 190–191, 192, 231
dominant side 192
epilepsy and 193–194
symptomatology 192, 193
see also Amygdala; Hippocampal formation
Temporal lobe resections 134
affective disorders after 250
anterior, neuropsychological outcome 171
behavioural consequences 169–188
emotional decisions 174–176
learning and memory 170–174
postoperative improvement 169
pre-/postoperative performance 170–178
unilateral mesiobasal seizures 176–178
best outcome, factors for 183–184
disseminated abnormality remaining 232
epileptological outcome 181–182, 232
granule cell loss 131
neurone loss 131–132, 133
positron emission tomography findings 180–181
postoperative psychosis 161, 180
pre-/postoperative antiepileptic drug modifications 182–183
pre-/postoperative scalp EEG changes 183
psychopathology, effect on 179–180
seizures after, reasons 232
see also Amygdalahippocampectomy (AHE)
Temporal polar syndrome 123
Temporobasal-limbic syndrome 123
Tetanic stimulation 24, 26, 27
Thalamocingulate division, of limbic system 9, 10
Thalamocortical system 49, 50
Third ventricle, tumours in region of 195

Thyrotropin releasing hormone (TRH) 78, 254
anticonvulsant activity 254, 255
hypersecretion in depression 255
mRNA 254
Todd's paralysis 117
Topology 270
Total neuron number, unbiased estimation 241–243, 244
Transcriptional regulation 251
Transient global amnesia (TGA) 191, 204–205
as complex partial seizures manifestation 204
incidence and duration 204
Transient global cerebral ischaemia 63, 65
Tumours, intracranial 189–197
diencephalon and mesencephalon 195–196
limbic system 190–191
outside temporal lobe 195–196
personality disorders and psychosis 193–194
symptomatology 192, 193
see also Temporal lobe limbic system
olfactory bulb and tract 195
in region of third ventricle 195
slow-growing 190, 191
symptomatology 190, 191–194
see also Gangliogliomas

Valenstein effect 248
Valproate
in bipolar affective disorders 93–95, 256–257
effects of, summary 92
kindling phenomenon, effect on 94
Valproate (*cont.*)
modes of action 91, 93
in affective disorders 93–95
antiepileptic 95–96
dopamine turnover 94
GABA interaction 94, 95, 97
Van Gogh, V. 139
Ventral pallidum, total neuronal number 243
Ventricle/brain ratio (VBR) 240
Ventricular enlargement, in schizophrenia 215, 218, 220, 239, 241
time-course 240
Vigabatrin 161–162
Viral infections 63
'Visceral brain' 5
Visual field 268
defects 196
Visual functions, processing mechanisms 269
Visual perception 268, 269
Visual seizures 117

Wada test 104, 173
Warrington Recognition Memory Scale 208
Wechsler Memory Scale - Revised 208
White matter, in schizophrenia 215–216, 216
Whole-cell patching technique 20
Wieser seizure types 123–124

X-ray computed tomography (XCT), *see* Computed tomography (CT)